PLANT BASED COOKB
BEGINNERS

THE COMPLETE PLANT BASED COOKBOOK FOR
BEGINNERS: MORE THAN 600 PLANT-BASED
HEALTHY RECIPES TO COOK QUICK, EASY
AND TASTY MEALS

Michael Taylor

Table of Contents

Introduction

Switching to a plant-based diet is one of the most important lifestyles changes you can make, but it doesn't come without challenges. For starters, there are diet changes you'll need to make and getting your family on board can be tough. Plus, there's the matter of cooking for yourself or learning how to cook with vegan alternatives.

If you're over 22, chances are that now or sometime in your near future you'll no longer be working full time and now need to figure out how to afford those pesky health insurance premiums as well as your rent and mortgage payments. With this in mind, there are ways you may contribute to the resolution of these problems.

It's not about going on a strict diet to lose weight or pay your bills. There is more to a plant-based diet than that. If you're looking for ways to improve your health and/or save money and help the planet, by all means go explore the world of plant-based eating but make sure it's an informed decision from beginning to end. There are a lot of myths out there in this respect, so it's important to know what they are before diving in head first.

We've put together resources, tips and advice for everyone interested to start a plant based diet or those who are already doing so.

A plant-based eating plan that allows you to eat foods that contain no animal products. That means zero dairy, eggs, honey or other animal byproducts including gelatin (e.g., gummy candy), honey processed beeswax and lard or other fats that are created by rendering dead animals in order to be made into palm oil and coconut oil (such as mayonnaise).

A plant-based diet that allows you to eat foods with ingredients from plants and animals. These foods include eggs, dairy products and honey. Some vegans who follow this approach are called 'Lacto-ovo vegetarians' or 'Lacto Vegetarians.' Those that only consume their food in its natural state are called 'Vegan.'

We all make changes in our life at some point. Some of them are more difficult than others, and the switch to a plant-based lifestyle is one of those that can be tough to accomplish. Maybe you're not sure how to start or where to find the information you need for your specific needs and interests. Maybe you're searching for a way to make the switch easier.

Or maybe you know exactly what you need but don't know how to find it, or how to educate people about the benefits of your choice.

Chapter 1. What The Vegetable Diet Is

It's a diet. I know, you're thinking "oh this sounds like it's going to be heavy on salads and light on everything else." Not at all! This diet does not prohibit any type of food, but it does encourage eating vegetables with every meal. The end goal of the diet is to eat more vegetables and less sugar and processed food. By eating more vegetables you'll actually lose weight without even trying!

There are a few problems with most diets. First, most of them say to eat less and exercise more, which doesn't really work, usually. In addition, most diet plans encourage using fake foods like diet pills or shakes, which aren't good for your body. The Vegetable Diet is a diet that will actually help you lose weight and not just make you hungry or nauseous! This is a true diet, it's not a fad based on some kind of food pyramid that won't work in the long run. The Vegetable Diet will work for you, even if you're not overweight. As long as you eat a healthy diet and follow the diet, you should lose weight.

The vegetable diet focuses on fruits and vegetables, which are good for your health. Vitamins and nutrients are abundant in fruits and vegetables, which help to maintain your body healthy and alert. Fruits are high in fiber while vegetables are low in calories. Most vegetables have a low glycemic index which means they can still be eaten even if you have diabetes or high blood sugar issues. Basically, the Vegetable Diet encourages eating foods that benefit your body while limiting foods that will only make you tired or sick.

The Vegetable Plan is only one part of a healthy lifestyle. Eating healthy isn't just about losing weight. It's about being able to get up in the morning and not feeling like you want to go back to bed! Eating healthier is about being able to stay healthy for the rest of your life. Eating healthy will make you feel better, look better and be able to live a full and happy life. So why not consider trying this diet?

How a Plant Based Diet Differs from Other Diet Plans

When it comes to a plant-based diet, a person can never run out of options. There are hundreds of ways to enjoy the same ingredients with a different taste and aroma. It is true that people who consume plant source diets usually struggle to find the right ingredients for their meals, which would provide balanced amounts of nutrients without the use of any animal-sourced products. In the markets full of processed products, it gets twice as more difficult to find organic plant-based food items.

People often get confused about the differences between being vegetarian and vegan. And when you introduce the idea of a plant-based diet, it completely boggles their mind! It is simply a matter of perspective and the context of the diet that changes their meaning. The plant-based diet is a wholesome concept that recommends every food item sourced from the plant, ranging from plant oils, grains, fruits, vegetables, flours, legumes, seeds, nuts, and plant-based milk. All types of animal-sourced products, whether meat or dairy, are not consumed on this diet. Some people follow this dietary approach for better health while others for environmental reasons. Whatever the reasons may be, the diet has shown remarkable positive effects on human health. And with the rising awareness of its benefits, the diet is recommended to all those who are suffering from obesity, cancer, or heart problems.

Why a Plant-Based Diet?

There are several incentives for choosing a plant-based diet, the first being the health benefits it guarantees. To convince yourself, first imagine all the nutrients that can be sourced from a plant-based diet that include unsaturated fats, high amounts of fiber and minerals, along with a balanced proportion of macronutrients. In light of this nutritional composition, let's discuss some of the known benefits of a plant-based diet.

Plant-based food is full of phytonutrients, special chemicals that are present only in plants and serve as the antioxidants and detoxifiers in the human body. When the entire diet consists of plant-based items, there is an increased intake of this phytonutrient, which helps the body resist cancer and other health-affecting agents.

Since the plant-based diet is free from all the saturated fats, it's great for serving the needs of people suffering from high cholesterol. The plant-based oils do not increase cholesterol but provide high-density lipoproteins—the good fats. It also controls obesity and actually helps to achieve weight loss. Similarly, the diet has also been proven to control the body mass index in perfect balance through its healthy contents. Following are the major diseases that can be prevented (or contained to some extent) by using a plant-based diet plan:

- High blood pressure
- Obesity
- Cancers
- Heart stroke
- High cholesterol levels
- Type II diabetes
- Diabetes

How to Plan a Diet

It's is not easy to make a change in any diet that you quickly embrace. The decision to take on a plant-based meal plan is based on wanting to live healthier lives. The change might be inevitable later on after many realizations of what we get when we eventually abandon what we prefer to consume. The previous chapters have narrowed down to health issues with many studies leading to a better life in adopting the latter meal plan, which is plant-sourced.

Changing from regular life diets to start incorporating plant-based foods will meet some resistance at first if not well understood. It is now through this that we have come up with different tips to follow to start a plant-based diet. These several tips can help us and make our understanding much more comfortable when dealing with plant-based foods. These tips also are used as guidelines that will help us not only today but even in the coming generations.

With that said, some people prefer a diet full of meat just because of its taste than understanding the health issues associated with its high consumption. These tips have been explained below in detail. The following chapters keenly highlight the need for easier comprehension. So that each one of us can be in a better position to indulge in eating the plant-based plant meals, after all, all of us need to begin from somewhere.

The first tip is all about setting rules and making sure that you are being initiated to new recipes of plant-based meals even twice a week. Regulations created by yourself will be quickly followed as compared to the ones formed and forced on you. In this plant-based diet, it is all about loving what you are doing. The created recipes will always be easy to follow, and once mastered, you will only be improving on them. One rule that can be created here is the setting of a day. This day is preserved mainly for one purpose, and that's making a plant-based meal. Make it to the family and get their ultimate reviews on what you have done. Ask them to comment on the tastes and the food in general. The result will help you a lot, especially in your next meal.

The next tip here is all about creating a constant tendency towards plant-based meals. Make a plan for cooking this food more often within a week. Don't wait for ages to pass since you are getting induced to starting your plant-based diet. Practice makes perfect, and within a short time, your skills, especially necessary skills, will improve. Your experience will be a notch higher, and this will be reflected in your habits. Making cooking of plant meals frequent is one of the most excellent tips in jump-starting your plant-based meal. Along the way, you will get adapted to it. You'll also realize that you've changed your approach to how you always think of other types of food, such as diets full of meat and junk foods.

It's vital to grab recipes from the shelves or drawers where they are kept and reading. The habit can occur without necessarily making or preparing these foods. At the same time, the pattern can improve your skills and give you several tips and morale to embark on preparation later on. Reading equips one with the required skills and creativity needed in an area of expertise. After having enough knowledge and comprehension, especially on these plant-based recipes, you can now embark on that kitchen work. Follow your recipes slowly by slowly and get used to it after some trials. The action will make it even easier. You will start enjoying it, and without knowing, you will be in an excellent position to begin migrating from your current diet to plant-based diets.

Most of us usually use vegetables in our daily diets without knowing their value. They may also use the plants in meal preparation without having a rare view of what they do in our food. Some use vegetables because others have been using while some will try to incorporate it just because it is there. It is just well for your understanding about this, but if you want to jump-start into this diet, then go for the vegetables that people regard as unusual.

The ones that you have never used ever since you were born. The ones you have never even seen. Visit different fruits vendors store and have these unusual collections. Ask questions if in case you do not understand. Pick them and try using them already to check on their flavors and tastes. Your ability to pick the right plant-based meal plan will help you to choose which to use and not to use. It is good to note that these unusual vegetables can be used to compensate for flavors gotten from meat-related dishes. This choosing of particular types of plants is a good tip to start your plant-based diet.

As a beginner in this diet, the best tip for starting a plant-based diet meal plan will be, to begin with, vegetables. Try as much as possible to eat vegetables. The act can be during lunch and dinner or rather a supper. Make sure that your plate is always full of plants of different categories. Different colors can help you choose the different types you want to get to learn. Vegetables too can also be eaten as snacks, especially when combined with hummus or salsa. You can also use guacamole too in this combination and rest assured you will love it.

People eat meat, and it has been part and parcel of their daily diet. As said earlier, many prefer meat due to its taste. They don't go for it because of its nutritional value. In many cases, we can look for ways to change our thinking about meat. If we can all agree to reduce the level of intake of meat, our lives would be better. The reason is appended to the health benefits of taking vegetables and not meat.

Then, the same can be replaced with the high intake of the plant-based meal, and then we shall rest assured that at long last our thinking about meat will have to change. For us to improve our diet, then we need to know the side effects of taking meat in large quantities. One of the most dangerous side effects is its ability to build up within the body tissues. Together with fatty oils, your body loses shape and obesity will encroach. Life-threatening problems start arising, and this will only land you into the hospital as you seek medication. In the long run, your life will be affected by the economic challenges appended to it. As you realize you have wasted many resources in dealing with a condition, you could have controlled from the beginning. The action might cause some depression and stress. It's good to note that you are not supposed to withdraw all meat at once. In this case, you can change your approach towards meal intake. Reducing the level of consumption will help us to indulge in plant-based cooking meals plan. You can also use this meat as just a side dish. That's like garnish. Avoid using meat as a centerpiece.

The types of fats and oils being used should be highly considered. Well-Chosen fats or oils will come from avocados, olive oil, some specific seeds and even nuts like groundnuts and so on. By doing this, you will be in a high position of being initiated to plant-based cooking.

As we all know, changing from one diet to another diet will be challenging. The case is specific, especially within a short period. What you need to do is to cook at least twice, thrice or even once within a week. Cook some plant-based food once or twice a week depending on how you might want. You will learn how to jump-start your initiation period. You'll also understand what it takes to grasp the basic knowledge of plant-based meal planning. In most cases, try to use more vegetables, beans, and even whole grains. Never use processed foodstuffs like processed and refined flour since this has got fewer nutrients and mostly lacks enough fiber needed within the body.

Another tip that will help you in starting a plant-based diet meal is by using whole grains during breakfast. Use it in high quantities since it will help you in adopting this kind of diet within a short period. It is not always easy to use all of these whole grains. The best way forward is to choose meals that can suit you and the rest of your family at first. Good examples will be highly recommended. These might include oats, barley, or even buckwheat. Here, you can add some flavors provided by different types of nuts and several seeds. Don't forget to include fresh fruits next to your reach.

Greens are some of the best vegetables preferable in the plant-based diet. They are also crucial in helping you to maintain a healthy diet. And going for them will help you jump start your long journey in embracing plant-based foods. Greens can be used at different levels and embracing it at the initial level is the best. Go for greens such as kales, spinach, collards and much more.

Use a good mode of cooking to preserve their nutritional value and also their tastes and flavors. Excellent cooking Directions of food can include the use of steam, grilling, or even frying for a short period. All the mentioned styles of cooking or somewhat preparation will help in maintaining the nutrients found in these greens. The body tissues readily require these nutrients for the proper functionality of the body organs.

Another way to get induced to a plant-based diet is by using diets that revolve or contains salad. You can make the salad greens from leafy greens like spinach, romaine and sometimes the red leafy greens are preferred. Different kinds of vegetables are added here. These vegetables are added together with beans, peas, or even fresh herbs.

The best thing with fruits is that fruits can be consumed at any time and in any way. They don't have any form of rigid procedure or protocol that needs to be followed as far as their consumption is concerned. Eating fruits every day as dessert will help you get adapted to it. This will create some sorts of habits within you and without realizing you will be fully indulged in a plant-based meal.

Fruits play different roles in our diet plans. By consuming them every day, we can quickly boost our immunity. The same meals will help us to forget to focus more on eating healthy for the rest of our lives. For example, some fruits will help you reduce the level of craving for sugary sweets, especially after having the main meal. Fruits such as watermelon and apples can help in keeping hydrated. Therefore, you will be able to get used to it. Within the long run, you will be adapted to plant-based diet meals. Another way that can also help you start your meal plan is by having curiosity or instead of being extra curious. Many studies have solid proof of interest as a tip in starting plant-based meal plans. Sometimes in life, you want to venture into something you never knew. You want to do something that you have not been doing, especially when it comes to cooking different meal plans.

Many times people have been obsessed with junk food and other meat-related foods. Trying something new is just out of curiosity and may take a reasonable period to understand fully. In the long run, you will develop skills that will eventually help you to do every work within the kitchen. As has been said earlier, changing from your healthy diet to a plant-based diet is not simple. However, after an extended period, you will be in an excellent position to embrace it. This comes about after your curiosity to do something new every day. You will get used to it over time.

Sometimes you can jump-start this plant meal as a result of love. Many people are trying something new. If you have that love for plant-related dishes, then you will be in an excellent position to embrace it after some time. The move will help you manage your eating habits.

Embracing plant-based diet meal plans will come in handy with the broader choice of the food sector to choose from. You will have an alternative source of food in addition to what you have been consuming over the last years. Having led by your love to eat plant-based meals or rather to change the diet will vastly help you to get used to it.

Within the long run, you will get familiarized and used to it. You will then start practicing it in your daily routines, thus reducing your urge on meat-related meals. For this one to work better, you must love eating too. The eventual result is just an aspect of life that will accelerate your objective in starting plant-based diet meal plans. Another tip is about pairing foods. You can use this tool to have more excellent knowledge of which types of plant-based foods can be matched and results in good taste. You can do this pairing by combining several flavors. The result should give you a strong feeling that works for you.

The same is appended to the fact that trial and error works. When you comprehend food pairing completely, rest assured that your cooking skills and love of it are moving to the next level. The later will even enable you to cook your plant-based meal without checking or following your recipes. You shall also experience timely results in time reduction and saves energy too. Sometimes you need also to compare notes on different books about plant-based recipes and pick only the best that can help you begin on this.

You can choose a paper having a Mediterranean diet and another one having vegetarian food recipes or you can also go for the Nordic diet. Compare the notes and pick the similarities. The actions will make you understand much more about plant-based food and how to adequately prepare them. These books done by different authors will also help you with some inspiration and ideas on different flavors.

Watching is also regarded as another tip, which will help you to start plant-based meal plans. Have those videos concerning cooking at your reach. Several stations are dealing with cooking. Spend much time watching them as you dearly take notes. Make a date with your television and watch those food networks that talk much about plant-based diets. Many studies have concluded that cooking videos are essential tools, especially in cooking. This is because, in your mind, you will be in a position to know how the food will look like even if you are not cooking. Using videos create some perfection in the kitchen. You'll have no stress or pressure here. It is all about watching and doing the required practice. Practicing now and then gives you that experience you need and will later help you to get embraced to the plant-based diet.

Chapter 2. Benefits Of Plant-Based Diet

Support Your Immune System

Plants have essential nutrients that cannot be obtained from other foods. The vitamins and minerals, phytochemicals, and antioxidants found in plants help keep your cells healthy and your body in balance so your immune system can function optimally. "Plants provide your body with the nutrients it needs to combat illnesses," explains Andrea Murray, MD Anderson's health education specialist. "Eating a plant-based diet improves your immune system's ability to fight viruses and microbes."

A healthy immune system is important in reducing the risk of cancer because it can recognize and attack cell mutations before they turn into disease.

Help Reduce Inflammation

Essential plant nutrients trigger inflammation in your body. The same little phytochemicals and antioxidants that boost your immune system also circulate in your body, neutralizing toxins from pollution, processed foods, bacteria, viruses, and more.

"The antioxidants in plants scavenge all of these so-called free radicals that can throw your body out of balance," says Murray. "To reduce inflammation, it's important to follow a plant-based diet and listen to your body's signals about how food is working for you."Prolonged inflammation can damage cells and tissues in your body and has been linked to cancer and other inflammatory diseases, such as arthritis. A plant-based diet can protect you by eliminating some of the triggers for these diseases.

Rich In Fiber

Fiber can be found in all unprocessed plant foods. It forms the structure of the plant. The more you eat, the more benefits you can get. A plant-based diet increases your gut's ability to absorb nutrients from meals that boost your immune system and reduce inflammation by making it healthier. Fiber aids in bowel control by lowering cholesterol and stabilizing blood sugar levels.Fiber is very important in reducing the risk of cancer. This is especially true for your risk of getting the third most common cancer—colon cancer.

Help Reduce the Risk of Other Diseases

The benefits of consuming mostly plants don't just mean reducing the risk of cancer. The plant-based diet has also been shown to reduce the risk of heart disease, stroke, diabetes, and certain mental illnesses.

Help Maintain a Healthy Weight

One of the most essential things you can do to reduce your cancer risk is to maintain a healthy weight. The only thing more important than keeping a healthy weight when it comes to cancer prevention is not smoking.

This is due to the fact that being overweight produces a hormonal imbalance as well as inflammation. Colon cancer, postmenopausal breast cancer, uterine, oesophageal, kidney, and pancreatic cancers are among the 12 malignancies that persons who are overweight or obese are more prone to get. When you eat mostly plants, you are eliminating many foods that lead to weight gain. Add in some exercise and you are on your way to losing weight.

Chapter 3. Guidelines On What to Eat for The Plant-Based Lifestyle

There are plenty of fruits and vegetables available all year round because they can be grown in various parts of the country when the season is ideal. While you will only be able to get locally grown fruits and veggies at the farmer's market when they are at their peak or in season, quite a few of them can be purchased from local grocery stores any time of the year.

Fruits

Fresh or frozen fruits are a main component of a plant-based diet. There are plenty of options but some provide a more powerful nutritional punch. When shopping for fruit go to your local farmer's market first. These will often yield the highest nutritional value. At the grocery store look for organic fruits as these should not be treated with harsh and dangerous chemicals. You want to have a variety of fruits on hand, but you also want to know which fruits are seasonal so you can be sure to have a nice mixture all year round. Below you will find a list of fruits you can typically find all year round, and also the best fruit to look for based on the season.

Easily found all year:

- Apples
- Bananas
- Lemon
- Papaya
- Coconut

Spring fruits

- Apricots
- Mango
- Strawberries
- Honeydew
- Pineapple

Summer fruits

- Blackberries
- Blueberries
- Raspberries
- Peaches
- Plums
- Nectarines
- Watermelon
- Cantaloupe

Fall fruits

- Grapes
- Guava
- Kiwis
- Cranberries
- Pears
- Pomegranate
- Figs
- Passion fruit

Winter fruits

- Grapefruit
- Navel oranges
- Passion fruit

Vegetables

Most vegetables you can find throughout the year, but some peak during different seasons. The season they are harvested in may have different flavors such as carrots. Carrots can be found all year round but you will find that they are sweetest in the colder, winter months. Just as with your fruits, you want to buy vegetables locally or at least organic at the grocery store. You'll find a list of vegetables that you may eat at any time of year, as well as when they're at their best. While there are many vegetables listed, this is not a full or complete list. Any and all vegetables should be included in the whole foods plant-based diet. Last but not least, many veggies that are at their height in one season are also numerous in the following season.

- Carrots
- Bell peppers (red, green, yellow, and orange)
- Kale
- Celery
- Cremini, shiitake, portobello and button mushrooms
- Onions
- Scallions
- Shallots
- Spinach
- Arugula
- Lettuce

Spring Veggies

- Leeks
- Radish
- Asparagus
- Rhubarb
- Green Beans

Summer veggies

- Cucumber
- Zucchini
- Green beans
- Eggplant
- Okra

Fall veggies

- Broccoli
- Fennel
- Pumpkin
- Butternut squash
- Swiss chard
- Brussels sprouts
- Acorn squash
- Yams
- Sweet Potatoes
- Corn

Winter veggies

- Bok Choy
- Broccoli rabe
- Cabbage
- Turnips

Whole Grains

The grains you include in your whole food plant-based diet should be 100% whole grains. When shopping for bread products and pasta, you can find a variety of whole-grain options. Whole-grain tends to be the most popular and easiest to find in grocery stores. Always check the labels before you buy, be sure it states 100% whole wheat or that the grain it is claiming to be is at the top of the ingredient list. Looking at the fiber content can also be a good indication, whole wheat, and whole-grain products should have at least three grams of fiber, if not more.

- Whole grain barley
- Millet
- Quinoa
- Steel cut oats
- Brown rice
- Bulgar

- Red rice
- Black rice
- Wild rice
- Buckwheat
- Sorghum
- Amaranth
- Corn

Healthy Fats

There are both healthy and bad fats, but many people shun the word "fat" when they hear it. Healthy fats form in a number of plant-based sources can provide you with high doses of vitamins, fiber, calcium, omega-3 fatty acids and more. Some of the most beneficial plant-based fats include:

- Avocado
- Nuts
- Seeds
- Banana

Legumes

Legumes refer to the wide selection of beans. While dried beans are ideal, canned beans can help cut back on cooking time and add convenience. When using canned beans, you want to look at the salt content and purchase those that have the least added salt. It is also important to rinse the canned beans to remove excess salt and impurities before cooking with them. Beans are a versatile ingredient and often used as a source of protein for plant-based diets. You will often find recipes that use beans as a substitute for meat products such as burgers, meatloaf, and meatballs. Legumes include:

- Black beans
- Black-eyed peas
- Kidney beans
- Navy beans
- Soybeans
- Chickpeas
- Lentils
- Lima beans
- Pinto beans
- Peas
- Green beans
- Adzuki beans

Seeds And Nuts

Nuts and seeds are healthy fats that can be added to a number of recipes for extra crunch and flavor. Many nuts and provide you with omega-3 fatty acids, fiber, and are a good source of fiber. Nuts are also highly versatile and can be made into nut butters and even be pureed to make cheese or cream sauces.

- Walnuts
- Almonds
- Pumpkin seeds
- Brazilian nuts
- Cashews
- Chia seeds
- Flax seeds

Plant-Based Milks

When it comes to dairy substitutes, there is quite a selection to choose from. When choosing a plant-based milk, ensure it is non-GMO or organic and unsweetened. Read the labels and avoid products that contain sugar such as cane sugar, carrageenan, and glyphosate. Plant-based milks are also just as easy to make at home. The process is fairly simple and just requires soaking, draining, blending, and straining. Some plant-based milk options include:

- Almond milk
- Cashew milk
- Soy milk
- Oat milk
- Coconut milk

Plant-Based Proteins

There are a number of ways you can get a significant amount of protein into your diet even when you eliminate or reduce the consumption of animal meat. These plant-based protein sources are some of the best alternatives for anyone switching to a plant-based diet.

- Tofu (silken, soft, and firm)
- Soybeans
- Lentils
- Tempeh
- Chickpeas
- Legumes

Spices And Herbs

Spices and herbs are a great way to add flavor and keep your plant-based meals interesting and unique. These can be found in the whole form and ground up for use, dried or fresh. Some spices and herbs to consider stocking up on include:

- Nutritional yeast
- Basil
- Tarragon
- Turmeric
- Rosemary
- Peppercorn
- Cumin
- Thyme
- Red pepper flake
- Oregano
- Paprika
- Bay leaf

Condiments

There are plenty of sauces and spreads you can include in or with your plant-based meals for a boost in flavor. As with any other products from the stores, check the labels and carefully read over the ingredients list. Some of the condiments on this list can include animal product ingredients like anchovy or casein.

- Amino acids
- Mustard (dijon, honey, and other varieties)
- Tahini
- Soy sauce
- Worcestershire sauce
- Vinegar (balsamic, apple cider, red wine)
- Salsa
- Relish

Though the whole foods plant-based diet is less strict about what foods you can't have, in the next chapter we will discuss a few key food groups you will want to eliminate. We will explore in depth the reasons why you should cut these foods out of your diet and how you can spot unhealthy ingredients, such as added sugars and artificial sweeteners on food labels.

Chapter 4. Types of Plant-Based Diet

plant-based diet can fit into different kinds of people's lifestyles and gives room for various types of eating patterns. From a working mum to a bodybuilder to a yogi, there will always be ways to follow a plant-based diet regardless of your tastes or lifestyle. Below is a list of the various types of a plant-based diet.

Junk Food Vegan Diet

Those on this kind of diet essentially don't eat eggs, meat, dairy, or any other form of animal product. They regularly consume highly-processed foods that are produced primarily in science labs.

Whole Foods Plant-Based Diet

The whole foods plant-based diet is basically concentrated around the consumption of whole foods (i.e., vegetables, whole starches, nuts, fruits, legumes, whole grains, etc.) while excluding processed foods. This diet is a health-conscious diet that features salads, buddha bowls, smoothies, and oat-pancakes that are decked in fruits.

High Carb Low Fat

Also known as HCLF, the concept behind the HCLF diet is based around carbs and the mindset that the body functions best when you get calories from mostly carbohydrates. This diet can be followed by consuming whole foods or more processed kinds of carbs like bread, pancakes, and pasta.

Whole Starch Low Fat

Also known as WSLF, it was inspired by two vegans who are YouTubers/Bloggers, Kristin and Alex, better known as Mrs. & Mr. Vegan. Staple foods within this diet are oats, beans, brown rice, vegetables, potatoes, and fruits. The WSLF diet mainly focuses on legumes, starchy vegetables, and whole grains. The basis of this diet is complex carbs, which can keep you full and satisfied.

Raw Diets

The raw diet is considered to be on a very high level when talking about plant-based diets. This diet can be high in fat and can be a subset of HCLF. When on this diet, you are expected to eat only raw foods, which include smoothies, noodles, cashew cheese, salads, and raw cheesecakes.

Raw Till 4

This diet is a hybrid of the HCLF and raw diets, as the name implies. Raw Till 4 literally implies that you consume only raw foods until 4 p.m. After 4 p.m., you are free to consume cooked foods.

Fruitarian

From the word "Fruit," we can denote that this type of diet is very similar to the raw diet. It has to do with the consumption of mostly raw fruit, along with little amounts of vegetables or leafy greens and minimal amounts of fat from nuts, seeds, and avocados.

Paleo

When on a paleo diet, there is a need for the consumption of low carbohydrates, high fat, and moderate protein. The paleo diet promotes the consumption of animal fats and proteins, but it doesn't support the consumption of dairy, refined sugar, grains, salt, oils, and legumes. However, fruits, seeds, vegetables, nuts, and roots can be consumed.

Difference between a Plant-Based Diet, Vegan, and Vegetarian Diet

When on a vegan diet, there is a need to abstain from the consumption of animal products. Vegans try to avoid all forms of cruelty and exploitation of animals for food, clothing, or for any other purpose. This doesn't necessarily mean that vegans consume lots of whole food meals; they can consume processed foods and snub their veggies too. Just like anyone else, they can consume (vegan-friendly) gummy candy, potato chips, and even cookies.

A plant-based diet, on the other hand, places more emphasis on consuming whole fruits and vegetables, eating lots of whole grains, and avoiding or minimizing the consumption of processed foods or animal products for health reasons. There are no definitions or strict guidelines for what makes up a plant-based diet other than placing emphasis on the consumption of fresh produce and eating a minimal quantity of processed foods.

Lastly, a vegetarian diet prohibits the consumption of fish, meat, or poultry. Most vegans decide to go with this diet plan because of cultural, ethical, or religious reasons. For example, an individual might develop concerns for animal welfare or a mindset that the killing of animals for eating is unnecessary.

Chapter 5. Basic for The Plant-Based Diet

Fruit, vegetables, beans, seeds and nuts are the staples of a plant-based diet. The following is a basic list of ingredients that will be used in this article.

-Green leafy vegetables: Kale, spinach, chard

-Olive oil: red wine vinegar (for cooking), nonstick spray

-Nuts and Seeds: Ground flax seed mixed with water (1 tbsp); Pumpkin seeds mixed with water (1/3 cup) soaked overnight in the refrigerator

-Beans: Cannellini beans or white kidney beans cooked in boiling water for ten minutes

-Vegetable stock cubes and vegan bouillon powder are also essential staples to have on hand.

-Fats: Animal-based fats, including butter and coconut oil, should be avoided. Instead, you can use olive oil, and only in moderation (e.g., twice a day)

-Tapioca: Tapioca pearls are found at Asian grocery stores; they are the most accessible and reliable way to obtain this ingredient. They do not go bad, so they can be stored for weeks or months.

-Soy milk option: Soy milk is an excellent alternative to milk and dairy. Most soy milks are fortified (contain vitamins B12 and D), which make them an ideal option for people with a vegan diet. If you have or plan on having digestive problems caused by milk whey, rice milk is a good alternative as it doesn't contain lactose.

-Shirataki noodles (lychee flavor): Whole Foods Market, Kim's Naturals, Amazon

- (optional: agar powder and/or xanthan gum to thicken recipes if needed)

-Coconut oil and vanilla extract for baking: I use unsweetened coconut milk to make pudding in place of cow's milk.

-Almond meal: Trader Joe's brand.

-Cacao powder: Cocoa powder or Dutch processed cocoa or baking chocolate can be used in place of cacao.

-Pure vanilla extract: pure vanilla extract is best for cooking and baking.

-Ketchup: Cholula's Mexican ketchup, I also recommend making your own

-Vanilla bean paste: vanilla bean paste is a common ingredient in many recipes for baked goods. It can be purchased at Whole Foods Market or online. It has a more intense flavor than vanilla extract and should be used sparingly, as the sweetness it imparts is much stronger than that of sugar or white sugar.

-Flax oil or flax seed oil: Flax oil is a pressed ground flax seed. It is used in the same way as olive oil and can be used for cooking and baking

-Ghee: Ghee is clarified butter. It has a higher smoke point than coconut oil, so it maintains its quality in high heat. It is also more stable than lesser grades of coconut oil, so it will last longer without turning rancid or becoming moldy. Ghee is sold in most Indian grocery stores and health food stores.

This list is an example of a diet that can be used as a guide, where if you have found something else you think should be listed, list it. It is by no means complete. As with any diet, you should consult with your doctor and a registered dietician.

Chapter 6. Vitamins and Minerals on a Plant-Based Diet

For human health, food is the basis of life. However, quality of life and longevity can only be achieved with proper and balanced nutrition. It is critical to regularly supply the body with a variety of nutrients, such as vitamins and minerals, in the right amounts and quantities.

For a plant-based diet to be good for your health, it must be balanced. In most cases, any negative consequences are not associated with the transition to the diet itself, but with the wrong combination of food and, as a result, an imbalance of substances necessary for health.

Besides sunshine, all other vitamins come from dietary sources. Your decision to start a plant-based diet means that you have to be more attentive to the balance of nutrients in your diet.

To sustain your long-term health by following a plant-based diet, be sure to supplement with sources of vitamin B12, vitamin D2, and sources of iron.

Vitamin B12

The risk of B12 deficiency is considerably higher for those on a plant-based diet because the main sources of B12 are mostly meat-based.

When the body lacks an adequate amount of vitamin B12, it can lead to nerve damage, shortness of breath, fatigue, cardiovascular issues, ineffective transportation of oxygen in the blood, and lots of other dangerous health symptoms. B12 is essential for a lot of bodily functions such as nerve function, metabolism, red blood cell production, and DNA formation.

Deficiency and its effects might take time to be obvious, so you should pay close attention to it. If you happen to notice any signs, it is advisable to seek your doctor's advice.

Plant-based foods are said to have a lesser amount of vitamin B12 than meat. However, the reality is that neither animals nor plants make B12. Vitamin B12 can be gotten from mostly animal foods. B12 is formed by bacteria that can be found in the gastrointestinal tract of animals. When the consumption of animal products takes place, B12 is ingested into the body as a bystander.

Based on some estimations, 10 percent of vegetarians and 50 percent of vegans lack vitamin B12.

Therefore, supplementing with B12 when following a plant-based diet is non-negotiable. This is because it's crucial in helping the body to function effectively, and an adequate amount cannot be achieved by consuming plants.

Iron

Iron is considered to be the most common nutritional deficiency irrespective of if you're on a plant-based or animal-derived diet.

The recommended volume for people who are over 50 is 8mg/day. For women below 50, 18mg/day is recommended to account for the loss of blood that they experience during their period, and pregnant women are advised to consume 27mg/day.

Good sources of plant-based iron include legumes, fortified cereals, spinach, and tofu. There is still a debate on the differences between non-heme (plant-based) and heme (animal-driven) iron. However, it is widely agreed that non-heme is less bioavailable, and therefore when on a plant-based diet, you should aim higher on your intake of iron. Iron deficiency can cause anemia; consequently, it's critical to try to avoid it.

Iodine

Iodine is a mineral that is recognized to be necessary for a healthy metabolism and thyroid. Iodine deficiency can lead to slow metabolism, fatigue, weight gain, and hypothyroidism, etc. It's best to consider sea vegetables when talking about iodine and a plant-based diet.

The list below shows the sources of iodine and a guide on how to achieve the recommended 150mcg daily (lactating and pregnant women have an increased recommended daily consumption, which is about 270mcg for women lactating and 220mcg for pregnant women).

- Dulse Flakes: half teaspoon of this will give you the recommended 150mcg/day.

- Plant Proof Tip: Add the dulse flakes to your pepper/salt showered with these minerals. Therefore, there will be a hint of iodine whenever you season your food.

- Nori: to get the recommended 150mcg/day, ingest 1.5 sheets of standard Nori daily.

- Potatoes

- Wakame

- Cranberries

- Iodine sea salt: it is recommended to try to add the above food groups before including iodized salt as a source of iodine.

It is important to know that iodine is not a mineral you should go overboard with because when you overeat it you may develop hyperthyroidism or an overactive thyroid, which can lead to weight loss, fatigue, and heart palpitations, etc.

Zinc

Zinc is an essential nutrient for you to watch out for. The recommended dose for men is 11mg and 8mg for women. Zinc helps the body to remain healthy, and therefore, you should consume lots of nuts, peas, and beans because they are the best natural sources.

Calcium

Calcium is an essential mineral that helps maintain healthy teeth and strong bones. It is also crucial for muscle contractions, blood clotting, and the healthy functioning of the nervous system. Getting the RDI of calcium can easily be achieved while on a plant-based or vegan diet. For adults, it is recommended that 1000–1300mg of calcium should be consumed daily, depending on gender and age (females and older people require more). The upper level is fixed at 2,500mg (1 year and older).

Below is a list of the top calcium-rich foods to help you decide on where to get your calcium from if you choose to follow a plant-based diet.

- Fortified plant milk (1 cup)—300–500mg
- Kidney beans (1/2 cup)—132mg
- Collards (1 cup)—270mg
- Oats (1 cup cooked)—84mg
- Hemp seeds (3 tbsp)—20mg

- Tahini (2 tbsp)—120mg
- Blackberries (1 cup)—42mg
- Mustard greens (1 cup)—160mg
- Kale (1 cup cooked)—94mg
- Raspberries (1 cup)—31 mg

Vitamin D

Also known as the "Sunshine Vitamin" as a result of its ability to be synthesized by the body through the action of sunlight. Vitamin D plays an essential role in increasing the absorption of calcium when required and promoting phosphorus absorption, which promotions a healthy bone mineral density. The vitamin also plays a very crucial role in the brain, heart, immune system, muscles, and thyroid. It also helps to regulate the production of insulin in the pancreas, which helps to fight against diabetes.

However, there are 2 primary forms of vitamin D, which are Vitamin D3 and Vitamin D2. Vitamin D2 is mostly artificially made by humans and combined with food substances via fortification. Vitamin D3, on the other hand, is synthesized from the sun into the human skin. It can also be found in few animal-based foods.

In the winter months or when the exposure to the sun is limited, it is best to acquire vitamin D from a supplement. This is said to be the most dependable and simple method of avoiding a deficit. Several studies indicate that 30–50mcg per day (100–200 IU per day) is effective for an average person to reduce the risk of dangerous diseases and develop a healthy vitamin D level.

However, the supplement dosage per serving can be expressed in IU (International unit) or mcg. 1 mcg of vitamin D3 is equivalent to 40IU, therefore if you are looking to get 50mcg of vitamin D daily, make use of a 2000IU vitamin D vegan supplement.

Omega-3 Fatty Acids

Omega-6 and omega-3 are known to be the primary source of polyunsaturated fatty acids (PUFAs). But omega 6s and omega 3s are the only fats that the body doesn't manufacture. Therefore, they have to be acquired from food in our diet.

The average Western diet consists of 20 times less omega 3s than omega 6s. This imbalanced ratio has very dangerous health consequences because a large consumption of omega 6s can lead to obesity, autoimmune diseases, cancer, and heart diseases. Basically, the omega 3/6 ratios protect the outer fatty layer of the cell in the body. The effect of omega-3 deficiency often manifests in dry, scaly skin, and this can cause dermatitis.

The recommended daily consumption is 1.1g for females and 1.6g for males. The majority try and get these fatty acids from seafood, and therefore you will have to start consuming flaxseed, chia seeds, soy products, and walnuts to keep up. There are many great supplements available if you find it difficult to fit these into your meal plans.

One way of getting a long-chain of the recommended intake of omega 3s is by consuming adequate plant-based foods that have ALA. The NHMRC Dietary Guidelines recommend the consumption of 400mg/day of DHA/EPA omega-3 for optimal health. However, it is advisable to target a total of 8,0000mg of ALA daily because the body transforms at least 5 percent of ALA into DHA/EPA.

Achieving the recommended dose is very possible, but it can be difficult to maintain daily.

•   1 tablespoon of Ground Flaxseed gives 1600mg of ALA.

•   1 tablespoon of Hemp Seeds provides 850mg of ALA.

•   1 tablespoon of Chia Seeds provides 2000mg of ALA.

Therefore, you would require the consumption of 5 tablespoons of ground flaxseeds or 4 tablespoons of chia seeds daily, to make sure that your body gets adequate omega 3s.

Chapter 7. How To Eliminate Bad Eating Habits

Cooking is all about preparing food that best suits you with the rest of the family. We all cook food for different reasons or rather goals. Some objectives are good, while others might sound vague, but all in all, we all cook with one primary purpose of improving our health. We all try our best to make different plans for doing our kitchen work. It also becomes vital to make sure that everything comes out in its perfect order with enough tastes and flavors. Sometimes we go for taste and forget that the nutrients content also matters a lot, especially when our health is considered.

Our health has been a significant factor in many situations. Therefore, that's why we prefer to deal with anything affecting it, by all means, using different ways. We are more inclined to health issues when types of food we are preparing have been put into significant consideration. These types of food referred to junk foods, and most of them have got a higher level of meat as a single ingredient. They are preferred due to their quick or natural mode of preparation.

In many cases, this occurs without knowing that some food such as meat, if not well cooked, will accelerate the thriving conditions of the internal worms. These warms include tapeworms that have severe complications with the internal body organs. These people have beliefs that the best restaurants within the world have been reserved for some high-class personality. This is just a belief since anyone with enough resources can visit those high-end restaurants. But these restaurants are served meat-related foods that have severe complications within the long run. Even though we are much aware of this, many argue that they lack time to prepare plant-based meals. That being creative enough to play with the plant-based recipes are time-consuming.

This has eventually affected the lives of many. Many have got health issues that hinder them from being productive in their capacity or even at work. These health issues include cancer-related complications, especially within the colon, breast, and even prostate cancer. Obesity has been another health issue over the years now. Many studies have been carried out on the possible ways to control these health issues, and many findings have narrowed down to plant-based cooking.

It is, therefore, possible for all of us to look for critical ways to understand plant-based food and how we can embark on it. Understanding plant-based cooking will even make you better and start making or preparing excellent plant-based meals, which are delicious and yummy. This knowledge will also help you in indulging in this kind of diet that you have never belonged to. Over some time, your cooking skills will improve, and having these basics; you will never require additional time or effort to prepare this food. You will be ultimately an experienced guru in the field of cooking plant-based meals without following even the recipes.

The plant-based cooking or preparation of food can be precisely defined as the type of cooking which involves or revolves around food prepared from plants. This implies that your diet will have more plant food as compared to other kinds of food. In other words, your food will be more of plant sources than meat and sometimes will even have no traces of meat at all — these diets composed of nuts, legumes, beans, whole grains and much more.

Apart from that, the nutrition recommendation also covers almost all types of vitamins. These meals have higher levels of fiber. They also contain other types of nutrients needed within the body. This type of cooking also offers enough minerals that are helpful in the optimal healthy life of a person, thus leading to a long lifespan. They also and also act as a preventive mechanism towards different diseases or infections. These diseases arise from heart complications and involve coronary thrombosis and other blood-related disorders such as blockage of blood vessels and much more. These types of food comprise of vegetables and fruits which have red, orange and yellow colors such as carrots, tomatoes, mangoes and much more. The same also includes green vegetables such as spinach, kales, romaine lettuce, broccoli, bok choy, among others. Traces of leeks, onions and even garlic can also be regarded as part and parcel of phytonutrient.

Plant-based cooking has more to offer in terms of disease curbing. As usual, this is compared to a vegetarian diet. The same meal plan is also compared to the Mediterranean diet even though the latter two have been found to support the health issues. This also leads us to an urge to understand these differences to be able to comprehensively understand what we shall be doing in the kitchen when preparing plant-based dishes.

The Mediterranean diet has its initial roots from plant-based sources and also incorporates other foods like fish, yogurt, poultry, and so on. Things such as meat and sweets are offered in fewer quantities even though not very often. This Mediterranean diet has been inclined to the positive side of our health. Studies have shown that the risk of getting heart diseases have reduced tremendously. There is a decreased level of metabolic syndrome with a good number of people showing a reduction in the level of health issues arising from this syndrome. Cases like cancers have also reduced.

This diet was found to be of help to people suffering from cancerous diseases such as colon, prostate, and even breast cancer. With this diet, if well offered, the frailty in older people will reduce too. This diet can also help to improve the functionality of your brain and physical body in general. However, this diet is slightly different from a vegetarian diet.

A vegetarian diet is gotten purely from plant-based meals. The same meal is also harvested from cooking meals with the plan in mind. Currently, only a few people are taking additional dietary supplements.

Vitamin B12 is one of these supplements. It's used to help their consumers in acquiring all the nutrients needed by their bodies. The vegetarian diets come in handy in different forms or rather types. It's now upon you to choose the best that fits you and the rest of your family. It is good to understand that your health issues should give you a direction when it comes to choosing the type of vegetarian food. There are different types which include a semi-vegetarian diet. This type consists of eggs, products of dairy, meat but not always, seafood, fish, and even poultry. A different kind of vegetarian diet is a pescatarian. It also includes eggs, it has fish in it, has seafood and some dairy products. However, this diet lacks meat or poultry. The last type though not often is called lactose vegetarian diet, which comprises using eggs and dairy foods only. This implies that this diet does not entertain anything to do with meat, fish, poultry, or even seafood.

Another related plant-based diet is the Nordic diet. This diet has some features similar to the Mediterranean cooking plan. It also has a high level of whole grains and berries. Other meals that you can look at include fatty fish such as salmon and so on. There are also vegetables, fruits, and even legumes. This diet also contains eggs and some dairy products with a high limitation of red meat and other processed foods. It does not involve sweets too.

The human race is funny when it comes to choosing between a diet comprising of meat in abundance supply and the one which has plant-based sources. It is now clear that many people eat meat not because of its nutritional value but because of its taste. They have forgotten that flavor and nutrition cannot go hand in hand. They are always going into different directions. The same implies that it will take some more time to instill this kind of information into the current generation. For them to digest it, they will still need much more time. And as a result of this, many will suffer from health-related diseases.

Many people argue that the actual plant-based cooking plan has no dairy and its products, that they have no meat at all or even oils and eggs. Many seem not to understand the difference that has been stipulated above concerning vegetarian diets, Mediterranean food, and even Nordic dishes. Others go ahead to hardening of the blood vessels such as arteries which later lead to heart disease.

Again there are a lot of talks that cover the consumption of eggs and meat. In the opinion of such individuals, the incorporation and their intake lead to the thriving of cancerous cell multiplication. It's now clear that many people have had a severe misconception about foods like oils. Surprisingly, to some point, they are not aware of the sources of these oils to be from plants like sunflower, avocados, canola, or even olives.

We are much obsessed with the word "plant" without taking much consideration, the word "plant-based." And, in this scenario, many argue that dairy products even if offered in fewer quantities, will still have various side effects on the body. This is true based on the knowledge that these fewer quantities are critical supplements in the building of muscles. Apart from that, the meals also lower blood pressure. This low quantity also helps in the reduction of tooth decay, reduces obesity, and also can help in the prevention of cancer.

Many people have argued that diet is perfect for your health. However, when it comes to discussing some of the issues affecting our bodies, the results have been overwhelming towards the plant-based meals. The idea is based on the fact that it can quickly help in curbing and controlling many diseases.

A group of scholars, however, argued that, even though plant-based meal plans are best for our diets, not all should be preferred. Their study found that the best plant-based meal plans are those who emphasized on ingredients that are fresh and whole. And due to this, they cautioned on the use of processed plant foods like fully refined maize flour, fully refined wheat flour and so on. As a result, they argued that when all these are observed, then the issue of health will be solved a notch higher. All these are meant to help us understand the plant-based cooking and their benefits. Understanding the plant-based diet plan can be a cumbersome task, especially when you have a family who hates fruits and vegetables. The only way to go about it is to show them the source of food.

It's also vital to discuss the side effects of the food on the body. Besides, it's essential to provide good reasons why the best options for cooking are embracing organic meals and natural cooking meals. Giving a clear view on why some foods are better than others will at least help them to understand the plant-based cooking. Also, having that passion and love boosts the morale of adopting plant-based sources of food.

The first benefit of understanding plant-based cooking is that it will help us in restoring our health and curbing of diseases. Many studies have proved beyond doubts that focusing on the plant-based cooking plan helps a lot in returning our healthy initial condition or rather situation. This involves the entire use of these meals in our daily diets. Diseases like cancer, especially cancer of the colon, prostate cancer, and even breast cancer, have been found to have a negative result with the plant-based foods. This implies that the cancerous cells are entirely affected by the presence of this food within the body system. As a result, their day to day thriving or growing is diminished and may even fail to show up. Due to this, the effect of cancer reduces, and those already diagnosed can also get healed.

Again, people who are mainly into this diet are not risky in cases or issues touching disease. Therefore they will never be prone to this disease. Following this diet will tremendously reduce heart-related conditions such as coronary thrombosis, arteriosclerosis, and so on. This leads to enough flow of blood within the blood vessels and with the required pressure. As a result, cases of heart attack will be nothing to worry about. We have other kinds of blood-related diseases such as elephantiasis which come as a result of poor blood circulation within the lower organs of the body, especially the limbs. Well, observation and considering this diet will help us to eliminate this.

Understanding of plant-based food or meal plans can also help us in improving our way of eating. The idea refers to eating habits. We are coming from a rigid society obsessed with much technology that doesn't allow us to concentrate on plant-based food. This over obsession, especially on fast food such as junks and the rest, has misled us to channel our way to poor eating habits.

With the help of this handbook, we can improve our eating habits. With that said, excellent plant-based meal plans have an accurate idea of what to eat and when to it. The same implies that the meal has specified breakfast, lunch as well as supper. At the same time, snacks and dinner have been organized categorically.

We are living in a world where taste seems to be better than nutrition. A good number of people eat junk foods, especially meat just because of how these food taste and not their value. This leads to a high level of build-up fats within the muscles and walls of the stomach. Unhealthy eating habits later result in obesity and other health-related diseases. By understanding the benefits of plant-based cooking, we get the chance to meet a world free from excess unhealthy meals such as junk food. The case also implies that the level of meat-related disease is reduced. Plant-based diets eliminate all these thus making us lead a good and a better life.

Our understanding of plant-based food or rather meal plans help us to decrease in weight. That's losing weight. Plant-based cooking relies mainly on foods that have their sources from plants. These types of foods include vegetables like kales, spinach, broccoli, and much more. This diet also contains fruits like mangoes, tomatoes, lettuce, and so forth. Cereals such as wheat, maize flour, oats, and much more are also part of this.

When plant-based cooking plans are fully understood and followed, health sectors within the society or a community improves. Lots of medications become a past tense thing. The people live a happy life. The immune system of everyone increases and falling sick diminishes. As a result, drugs become eliminated or somewhat reduced to a minimal level. The same instance will lead to a rise in the economy within the community since not much will be spent on medication. This is made possible by the help of a careful comprehension of plant-based cooking. An excellent plant-based diet also has fewer complications within the body as compared to the diets full of meat and other fatty foods. And due to this, there is no build-up of disease within the body tissues that will eventually require medications.

Knowledge of plant-based cooking if fully implemented can help us eradicate cruelty within the world, thus making the sustainability of the world to be more manageable. Chaos and cruelty always come as a result of sheer misunderstanding within different sectors. This is the same for even health sectors. Maintaining good health is the main objective of our daily lives, and without doing this, then the world will be full of chaos.

Imagine a world where the health sector is below standards. This implies that many people will be suffering from diseases such as heart attacks plus other blood related or heart-related diseases. This will eventually leave many industries with fewer people in terms of employees. Competent personnel within the ranks of the company will reduce, and obesity increases. All these will create cruelty and chaos that will be hard to eradicate. In a situation where the knowledge of this diet is well understood, then the correct implementation is followed, chances of cruelty become low. This makes the world to be easily manageable.

This type of diet always saves time. Also, its preparation is based on cooking using the purest forms of recipes. The result is you enjoying a healthy diet. Additional cooking and meal preparation plans don't involve complicated methods that take time to understand. All the skills required to make these recipes are easy to acquire. The duration of cooking is also less since they take the shortest time possible to get prepared. This leads to saving of your precious time that can be invested in other productive responsibility within the community or in an organization. Understanding the plant-based cooking diet will eventually allow us to be more productive in other areas since preparations of these foods require less time.

These types of food from plant-based sources require less fuel. A less or little amount of energy will often be used in their preparations. As a result, energy is saved. When this occurs, the high energy levels lead to a better economy. The world economies grow and thrive well. A good economy is characterized by good governance. Apart from that, the people comprising that economy will lead a better life. The result is usually courtesy of our well comprehensive nature towards our plant-based cooking.

Chapter 8. How To Start with A Plant-Based Diet

Studies suggest that the consumption of plant-based food is linked to sustainable weight management, minimal risk of heart disease, and a reduced risk of mortality. It's also associated with the treatment and prevention of high cholesterol and hypertension, and a lower risk of specific cancers.

Before you transition to a plant-based diet, note that launching a new diet entails boatloads of willpower, effort, and planning. Therefore, going cold turkey from day one is never a great idea.

You may simply shift to a plant-based diet by following these seven simple steps.

Start Slow

Select a few plant-based foods and start with them throughout the week. Begin with plant-based meals you enjoy eating, like oatmeal, jacket potatoes, pasta primavera, rice burrito, veggie stir-fry, three-bean chili, or lentil stew. However, you should then build on these foods. We as humans are known to be creatures of habit; therefore, we are likely to settle for less variety of dishes. Begin slowly and study this modern language of food with little or no pressure to be perfect.

Reduce Meat and the Consumption of Processed Food

Rather than going cold turkey from the start, begin by reducing the amount of animal-based and processed foods that you consume. It will help your body and mind to adapt to the new diet plan. Make fewer complex changes like including a large amount of fresh fruit or salad in your everyday meals. Next, avoid the consumption of dairy products and meat that you don't like so much anyway. After doing that, gradually work on trading animal-based ingredients for plant-based alternatives. For instance, if you like eating beef chili, replace meat with portobello mushrooms or dried bulgur. Or, if you love eating tacos, choose plant-based options, such as Quinoa Taco Meat and Mexican Spiced Cauliflower Tacos.

Settle for Plant-Based Breakfast

The next step is for you to commit yourself to eat a minimum of one plant-based meal a day. A healthy vegetarian breakfast is a great place to begin. Foods like muffins, waffles, toasts, parfaits, pancakes, and smoothie bowls are great to start with. After that, you should work on vegetarian zing your meals.

Watch Your Protein

The average protein that the body needs is about 1 gram for each kilogram of body weight and a lot of people consume more than enough. Of course, just because something is wonderful doesn't make it great if there are more of it. The excessive intake of protein is not only unnecessary, but it can also be dangerous to your health. You don't have to consume protein; what the body needs is for you to meet the requirements for the 9 essential amino acids that the body cannot synthesize by itself. Plant-based foods have amino acids in various quantities and contain enough protein to keep up with the requirements. It isn't possible to become deficient in protein as long as you are taking in adequate calories to maintain the body and are focusing on the consumption of whole foods and avoiding refined foods.

Know Your Food

You can drink Diet Coke and decide that you are a vegan. Knowing ways to ensure that your meal tastes delicious while still being wholesome and healthy is very important. A lot of commercial products, such as faux cheese and meat, are extremely processed and have the same ingredients that can be found in animal products, and this makes them very dangerous to health. These products are mostly packed with refined oils, salt, sugar, and flour. Thus, it is advisable to consume these kinds of foods only occasionally. It's better to settle for whole foods as much as possible. Educate yourself on nutrition and ways to make a variety of ingredients, or you can decide to pay a plant-based dietitian to guide you through the basics of transitioning to a plant-based diet.

Live on Healthy Foods

There are a variety of great products currently on the market, and it's easier to add foods that are plant-based to your diet. From dairy-free milk and kale chips to tofu and tempeh—there's always something available for every budget and palate. Therefore, leisurely explore the fresh produce and vegetarian aisles at your local stores and fill your cupboards with nutritious, plant-based products and store healthy snacks in accessible areas such as your bag, desk drawer, fridge, and kitchen counter.

Make Your Meals Exciting

Emphasize foods you love, which you can easily access. If you are not well skilled in the kitchen, then you go for more effortless recipes. For example, throw together frozen veggies and canned beans in a pan, include sauce, and cook to get a tasty pot of soup. Next, you should study new steps to make your simple recipes a lot more flavorful and fun.

Chapter 9. Improving Human Health and Environmental

A plant-based diet has various advantages, leading me to believe that it is not only a moral but also a long-term solution. Food choices ultimately depend on what people are willing to accept at an individual level. That is why I have been practicing a plant-based diet for over twenty years with complete joy and satisfaction. I do this because it just feels suitable for my body as well as my mind too.

Mind Benefits

1. Neuroprotection: A study found that a Plant-based diet helped protect the brain against inflammation, oxidative stress, and cell death in mice models for Alzheimer's disease

2. The foods found in a plant-based diet are generally easy to digest. Our body's digestive system doesn't have to work as hard to process these foods. This means our digestive system has more energy and can perform better overall, creating less waste that can harm us.

3. Plant-based diets have been linked to anti-aging effects on the brain.

4. Better mood: A plant-based diet has been shown to make people calmer, happier, and less stressed.

5. Better concentration: It's easier to pay attention and focus if you get enough protein from plants instead of meat.

6. Reduced risk of depression: A diet based on plants has been linked with lower rates of depression in multiple studies and there is evidence that suggests this is because it reduces the risk for anxiety disorders like panic attacks.

7. Better memory: A Plant-based diet is more effective at improving short-term memory than a meat-based diet.

8. Reduced stress: Studies show that plant-based diets can lower cortisol levels, the "stress hormone."

How You Will Feel Lighter, Cleaner, And Healthier Throughout The Day

Plant-based meals are widely recognized as some of the healthiest diet options, but there are several methods to achieve this. This plant-based diet cookbook for beginners will help you find a healthy and easy plant-based lifestyle with many delicious recipes. You'll feel lighter, cleaner, and healthier throughout the day.

A plant-based diet is effortless to follow. It is pretty simple. You can easily make changes to your diet daily, weekly, or monthly, which will help your motivation and allow you to try out new recipes without feeling overwhelmed by all the rules and regulations you have to follow.

A plant-based diet can also be easily followed by people with different aims depending on their personal health goals and nutritional needs. Eating healthy is easier than ever with the help of this book. You can also travel with your plant-based foods, so no matter where you are going or how long your trip is, you can be sure that your meals will be full of vitamins and nutrients with little to no prep time needed. Some foods are easily made into snacks for an on-the-go lifestyle. This is a fantastic approach to maximize your plant-based diet and the dishes in this book.

Eating vegan is easier than you think!

A plant-based diet may seem very difficult to follow; however, eating vegan is easier than you think when you get started and this book will help you find a way to maintain your new healthy eating habits.

The main thing to remember with plant-based foods is to focus on eating foods that you can grow yourself or find in the grocery store. Find recipe magazines, blogs and get ideas from friends. Once you start eating healthier and start experimenting on your own, you will find limitless options to continue with your new eating style and not get bored about it.

You won't feel like you're missing out on any of your favorite types of foods when you switch to a plant-based diet. You can also enjoy plant-based versions of all your favorite desserts. You won't have to give up the delicious foods you love. You just have to adjust them slightly to make them plant-based.

Plant-based meals can be very filling and are easier to digest than meals containing meat, which also helps with weight loss. Not only is plant-based eating lower in saturated fat, but it is also high in fiber, protein, and vitamins, all of which help with weight loss.

There are so many different recipes for plant-based meals that you will never get bored with them! This book gives you tons of healthy vegan meals for breakfast, lunch, dinner, snacks, and even dessert. You will feel lighter, cleaner, and healthier throughout the day with each of these delicious recipes.

More Environmentally Sustainable

Deforestation is exacerbated by the vast quantity of land required for livestock husbandry. This means the loss of habitat for wild animals, a decline in oxygen levels, and even an increase in greenhouse gases! Every hour, approximately 100 acres are bulldozed to make room for beef farming. To feed livestock, the U.S. uses more than half of its grain production (63 million tons) and 30% of its fossil fuels approximately. We could lower up to 75% of the current amount of land used for agriculture if all humans changed to a plant-based diet.

Water Consumption

No other activity consumes more fresh water in the U.S. than agricultural production, including food for direct human consumption and livestock feeding.

Gas Emission

In addition, animal agriculture is responsible for 18% of greenhouse gas emissions. It's no wonder that the United Nations has stated that "Livestock is one of the most significant contributors to today's most serious environmental problems."

Animal Cruelty

In addition, by relying on plants, animal pain can be avoided. Factory farming causes many animals to suffer immensely, including confinement indoors or enclosure in cages. They are exploited and denied a free life, only to become food for humans.

Water Contamination

Industrial farms also produce a large amount of waste that pollutes water sources and causes a reduction in biodiversity due to the loss of natural habitat.

Costs

Plant-based diets can be more affordable than ones based on animal products. This is because plant-based foods are also cheap and easy to produce.

The intelligent production of vegetables requires less effort in terms of machinery, water, and land than the production of animal products. A plant-based diet uses less water because plants do not need to be fed as much as animals. In addition, a plant-based diet uses less land than an omnivorous diet.

It takes much less space to grow just vegetables than it does to grow animals in a minimally decent space. I don't even want to consider intensive animal husbandry as an option for growing them. In addition, animals also need to be fed, so the space used to produce the food for them must also be taken into account.

Distribution

Moreover, due to their low cost, plant-based foods are widespread and available in almost all local markets. Consuming locally produced products also has a benefit related to the reduction of transportation energy consumption and pollution.

Feel In Harmony With Our Planet

You commit to living in harmony with the world when you consume a plant-based diet. Some people may choose to ignore the fact that human activities are the primary origin of our planet´s current struggles. Still, when you decide to change to a plant-based diet, you take responsibility for your actions and choose to be part of the solution for some of these big problems that the Earth is facing.

The plant-based diet has positive aspects also from an ethical point of view that are mostly similar to those of a vegan diet. Indeed, a plant-based diet does not exclude at all the option of eating animal products sometimes, but this is irrelevant if we think about what a daily diet based on meat entails, as discussed in the previous points.

But perhaps the most important decision you will make when plant-based dieting is choosing health over disease is choosing harmony with the rest of the world, and feeling good about yourself for making it happen.

Chapter 10. Cooking Equipment Used to Prepare Plant-Based Diet

You've probably already begun gathering some essential kitchen items and appliances to cook your own nutritious meals. Even with only these instruments, you can make beautiful and enjoyable foods.

Cutting Board

Cutting boards come in helpful when it comes to cutting and slicing your items before cooking. Wood or plastic may be used to make them. It's often a great idea to keep aromatic vegetables like garlic and onions on a separate chopping board so they don't contaminate the taste of other vegetables & fruits.

Sharp Knife

To invest in an excellent chef's knife is really a smart place to start since they will be your frequently used kitchen utensils. Because prices vary, you may select a sharp knife for cutting that fits your budget. Preparing ingredients with a decent knife is fast, simple, and considerably safer.

Large & Small Pot

To cook sauces, soups, cereals, curries, stews, and other meals may all benefit from having at minimum 1 small and 1 big pot. Large pots are ideal for cooking in bulk or for feeding a large household. It makes sense to have many pots since you may have to cook some grains as well as sauce or vegetables simultaneously.

Mixing Bowl

A mixing bowl made up of metal is ideal for making delicious baked items, stirring salads, and mixing pancake mixture. Metal bowls are less heavy than glass and take up less space. We suggest obtaining ones with lids so that they may be used as food storage boxes as well.

Non-Stick Frying Pans

When making vegan omelets or pancakes without oil, water-sautéing your veggies or dry-frying your tofu, a non-stick skillet, or a frying pan is an essential thing. We wouldn't recommend spending a lot of money on this since non-stick frying pans seldom survive more than just a few years. As a result, they are highly cost-friendly although useful kitchen addition. We utilize ours on a daily basis.

Whisk

When it comes to preparing pancake batter, blending up a sauce, or obtaining a light, fluffy mixture of cake, whisks are essential. Choose a balloon stainless steel design to avoid flavor transfer in acidic dishes.

Measuring Spoons & Cups

Get some purposeful measuring spoons and cups & stop working with guesses. They're essential if you really want to go with baking Directions and always obtain the greatest results. Measurement cups are also useful for determining how much quantity of water to add to the cooking oats or grains.

Baking Sheets

Friendly not only for baking bread or cookies, as well as for roasting potatoes and vegetables, also for making beanballs from home and burgers. Line it with parchment paper or place a silicone-baking mat on the top to minimize sticking.

Dinner Bowls

We like a delicious supper bowl brimming with spaghetti, noodles, or a lovely Buddha bowl dish. Bowls are actually more multipurpose than plates since they may be used to handle a variety of foods.

Peeler

A peeler, which comes in various designs and shapes, is necessary for peeling sweet potatoes, potatoes, carrots, & some other veggies. A peeler may also be used to prepare veggie spaghetti.

Spatula

Spatulas are particularly handy for flipping foods such as burgers, pancakes, and waffles and serving meals from casserole dishes or baking pans. Ours are often used to keep veggies from sticking together when sautéing.

Wooden Spoons

This vintage kitchenware is ideal for stirring gravies & sauces as they simmer and mix batter for cake and preparing oatmeal. The handle will not get hot when cooking, and it will not leave a mark on your ceramic pans and pots.

Food Processor

Food processors are better at breaking down and mixing items than blenders to purify them into a fine liquid form. For example, suppose you want to create homemade vegetarian burgers, brownies or energy balls using chickpeas or beans. In that case, a food processor may help you achieve the exact consistency you desire while mixing the flavors throughout. You can even use this appliance to prepare your homemade nut butter and flour at home from either oats or almonds for nutritious baked products.

Blender

High-powered blenders are a lifesaver when it comes to making healthful and fresh soups or smoothies that retain all of the fiber. For a smoother consistency, some brands may even be used to blend sauces, gravies, and dressings.

Tongs

When presenting challenging foods like spaghetti or noodles or scooping up hot products like vegan sausages, burgers, falafels, hot dumplings, or veggies, some firm tongs might come in very handy.

Cast-Iron-Skillet

A cast-iron skillet is a heavier-duty pan that maintains heat so well, making it ideal for frittatas, sautéed vegetables, cornbread, and even gooey desserts. It'll also survive for years, ensuring that you receive your money's payback. Furthermore, research has revealed that food cooked in a cast-iron pan has more iron, making it ideal for plant-eaters.

Wok

Woks are great pieces of equipment with a wide range of applications. You may use woks for curries, stir-fries, stews, stir-frying veggies, and even as a different frying pan. They are also reasonably priced and come in a variety of sizes.

Steamer Basket

Steaming potatoes, vegetables, and other items is an excellent technique to prepare them since nutrients are not wasted in the water as they are when they are boiled. As a consequence, the vegetables are firm yet tender, fast to cook, and flavorful.

Mandoline

A mandoline reduces the time it takes to slice, cut, chop and shred vegetables by almost half. So, if you dislike the preparation phase of cooking food, this one can be a good option. This instrument also allows you to obtain uniformly sized pieces, which benefits with processing times and makes your meal appear nice.

Grater

Most graters have a box-like shape and many sides, allowing them to be used for more than simply grating vegan cheese. They may also be used for shredding and slicing vegetables, as well as zesting out citrus fruits.

Silicone-Baking-Mats

Baking mats made up of silicone are an excellent low-waste substitute for parchment paper or tin foil. They may be used to roast veggies and potatoes and bake biscuits and cookies in an oven without using any oil when spread over a baking pan. They may simply be cleaned in warm water with soap also dried after each usage.

Food Containers

Having food storage containers on hand to keep any remains for another day is among the easiest ways to decrease waste in your kitchen. Glass, followed by metal, is the safest choice for keeping food and preserving its freshness. If you have the option, choose these. If you just have plastic containers, you may put them to good use first. If at all possible, make sure they're airtight.

Mason Jars

Mason jars are quite multifunctional, in addition to being extremely attractive. They're fantastic for preserving leftover sauces & dressings in your fridge, bringing a stacked salad to work for lunch, keeping prepared vegetables in water, freezing bulk cooked meals, and even bringing a self-made smoothie.

Food Wraps

These kitchen wares have been renowned in the zero waste sector for a time, not only as plant-based wraps but also as beeswax wraps. You may wash and then reuse these wraps made of organic cotton, coconut oil & soy wax to wrap your self-prepared meals again and again.

Nut-Milk-Bag

Are you concerned about the cost of plant-based replacements of milk, or do you wish to decrease your disposal? Nut-milk-bags lets you prepare your homemade milk by using any seed or nut, including cashews, almonds, macadamia nuts, rice, and sesame seeds. Of course, we used to prepare our homemade soy milk as well. This little cost-friendly piece of cotton is quite multipurpose and may have been used as a tea bag or to prep your homemade juice while using a blender, so this milk bag. Definitely one of our favorite little shenanigans.

Casserole Dish Or Baking Pan

Pasta bakes, stews, lasagnas, vegetable casseroles, and other set-and-forget dinners benefit greatly from casserole dishes & baking pans. They can also be used to make baked foods like oatmeal or risotto, which aren't your typical baked foods.

Slow Cooker Or Crock Pot

Make huge amounts of curries, spaghetti sauces, risottos, stews, or even oatmeal in a slow cooker or crock pot. Simply add your ingredients, spices, and liquids, then close the lid, and adjust the temperature to your requirement. The slow cooker performs all the job for you, whether you keep it while you are at work or on overnight, so you can arrive back to a great dinner with very little effort.

Tofu Press

A tofu press, which is made up of two parts, will strain all of the liquid from your tofu in mins without even using paper towels. As a consequence, you'll have delightfully firm tofu that's ready to absorb all of your fav sauces. Of course, if you do not want to spend the money on one, a dry towel and several weighty books will do.

Air Fryer

An air-fryer is such an amazing appliance whether you're looking for a healthy substitute for fries or want to prepare the tastiest crispy tofu. The air fryer enables you to cook a variety of your favorite recipes more healthily by using just a little or no oil. For example, a fryer may be used to prepare tacos, sushi, cauliflower wings, falafel, potato chips, roasted chickpeas, and sometimes even toast, in addition to potato wedges or fries. The possibilities are limitless.

Spiralizer

Spiralizing is an excellent method to get more vegetables into your own meals and into the meals of your kids as well. Spiralizers come in a variety of sizes and shapes, but they all accomplish the same stuff, they transform zucchini, sweet potatoes, carrots, as well as other vegetables into long, delicious spaghetti or noodles. Toss them into Thai meals, salads, or pasta sauces for a tasty alternative.

Knife Types For Cutting Plant-Based Diet

Granton Edge

The Granton edge appears as evenly distributed dimples around a centimeter through from the cutting edge. This knife was originally created for cutting meat, but then it has since been adopted by other knife kinds to allow air as well as water to release, making it simpler to cut both vegetables and fruit. These really are entertaining to practice with, but we've not discovered any big benefits.

Serrated

Serrated or scalloped knives are almost a must for tomatoes, bread, pineapple, or something with a considerably tougher outside than an inside. Tomatoes, in particular, may be effectively sliced with an extremely sharp, well-maintained flat blade. Among soft fruit, getting at least a serrated knife on hand is a smart idea.

Hollow Ground

These knives are useful for delicate jobs like peeling because the tip of the knife is worn down from the depth of the knife. However, they are fragile and should not be used for something hard, and they require more regular sharpening. The paring knife seems to be more versatile and may do the same duties as a chef's knife.

Paring Knife

Paring knives come in a variety of shapes and sizes. The first is a spike tip paring knife that is ideal for most fruits, tiny vegetables, or peeling by hand. The other is a stylet, sometimes known as a sheep's feet paring blade, which has a curved tip and a plain cutting edge and is useful for tiny jobs such as slicing garlic. Depending on your customary applications, this knife is less of a day-to-day knife than a regular paring knife. Finally, a bird's mouth paring blade, which curls in from the tip, can help you make your masterpieces if you have ever wanted to get into food artistry, transforming apples into the swan and melons into the flowers.

Straight & Curved Knives

Plain blades are choppers that work well with hard fruits and veggies like squash and sweet potatoes. For almost everything else, the curved or chef's knife is preferred. A sufficiently sturdy and sharp chef's knife, on the other hand, will operate very well on the hard veggies.

Cutting Techniques According to Food
Watermelon

A particular watermelon knife appears like a green and pink bread blade but doesn't have the hollow ground. A chef's blade or bread knife can readily cut through watermelon unless you eat it twice a day. The problem is that watermelons are bigger than the tools we use to cut them, resulting in uneven slices.

Leafy Greens

Serrated knives work well with leafy greens, particularly ones with tough stems such as Swiss chard or certain types of cut kale. Flat blades have a tendency to etch lines onto greens rather than slicing all completely through them.

Root Vegetables & Hard Squash

A sharp, sleek chef's knife is ideal for cutting tough vegetables. A sharpened knife will need to be hacked or pressed harder, and it is possibly deadly.

Onions

While cutting with a non-serrated knife is feasible, a serrated knife cuts through more readily and without slipping. Also, once you've become accustomed to cutting onions, they're really rather simple.

Soft Fruit

Use a serrated knife for anything soft, particularly with a harder hide like tomatoes, a keen paring blade, or a chef's knife for more accurate slices. Most people, particularly amateur cooks, prefer a serrated knife for tomatoes, figs, and other similar fruits. If you like non-serrated knives or don't have one, use a chef's knife for bigger fruits and vegetables and a paring blade for smaller ones, but this isn't a hard and fast rule.

Garlic

Garlic is easy to cut with almost any knife. A pairing blade or chef's knife can suffice, but a specialist knife such as a sheep's feet paring blade or similar flat-edged knife will make mincing simpler. Use a paring blade for complete slices, such as those seen in classic Chinese broccoli & garlic dishes.

Things To Keep In Your Mind While Cutting

The best sort of knife is determined by how a person cooks, cuts, as well as maintains their knives. Carbon steel blades are often pricey and regarded to be of good quality, although they do need some maintenance. If exposed to moisture, the carbon steel, as well as iron-carbon alloys, may rust. Nevertheless, these are popular among professional cooks because they can withstand a great deal of usage and damage, so they're a favorite for hard labor. Knives should be sharpened twice a year at home or more often when used regularly. Dull knives take more force to wield and are potentially hazardous in order to make prep work very difficult.

Ceramic blades are intended to hold their sharpness for far longer than that of the ordinary blade without honing. Still, they are hard to polish non-professionally whenever they run out or need a specific knife rock made of a harder substance than ceramic.

Stainless steel seems to be a widely used material for cookware since it's simple to clean and doesn't trust easily. In addition, stainless steel blades are easy to break and hone than carbon steel knives, although they are less costly, needless sharpening, and more suitable for the home cook.

Chapter 11.   Advice On Appliances and Accessories

A Good Kitchen Gadget is worth its weight in gold because it can often be the difference between a great dish and a dismal failure. Cooking is an art form and depending on the type of appliance you use; you will be able to create delicious dishes from scratch or make food that was not possible before with your existing kitchen tools. With these cooking appliances and accessories, it's likely that your recipes will turn out just as well as any chef's.

Choosing The Best Cookware

The cookware market has a variety of options to suit different needs, tastes, and budgets. Cookware sets are available in a large range of prices and the quality of the set depends on how much you spend on it. For example, if you want to invest in a high-end set of copper cookware, you can choose to purchase copper pots and pans that are made from flat discs of copper joined together at their edges with soldering. This sturdy form of cookware will last for many years, but the price for one pot or pan is about $300.

If you want to cook without spending a lot of money, you can check at several non-copper cookware sets made of aluminum or stainless steel, for example. This type of cookware is also durable and will last for many years. It's available at an average price of $100.

Copper Cookware Coils

Copper cookware coils are the best option when you want to get the finest quality cookware with the strength of a steel pot or pan. These coils are not made in one piece (like most other types of pots and pans). Instead, they are made from a series of flat pieces that are joined together by soldering to make pots and pans with a tight-fitting lid, which is great for hot food cooking. These coils can be disassembled and cleaned easily. These pots and pans are available at an average price of $300.

Stainless-steel Cookware

If you are looking for a high-quality non-copper cookware set, then stainless steel cookware is a good option. These products are usually made from high-grade, 18/10 stainless steel with a polished finish and rounded edges to reduce the chances of cuts and scratches, which make them more durable than other types of cookware. Online shopping is a good option if you want to buy stainless steel cookware at a reasonable cost because the prices for this sort of product are significantly lower than at department stores or supermarkets.

Cast-iron Cookware

For those of you who do not want to spend more than $100 for a good cookware set, then cast-iron cookware is a good option. These products are made of cast iron that is quite durable but has a lower thermal conductivity than regular steel, so food will take longer to cook in the cast iron pot than in a stainless-steel pot or pan. However, there are cases when it is better to use this type of cookware and other types of pots and pans at the same time to make sure that no food is left uncooked on the bottom of the pan. This type of cookware is available at an average price of $100.

Copper Cookware Sets

If you want to buy a good set of copper cookware, then you should pay attention to premium technology and quality materials for the pots and pans. You can choose from many different forms of copper cookware, such as copper pots and pans that are soldered in several pieces or coils made from one flat piece, but generally speaking a high-quality cookware set includes two pots and pans; a large pot that holds more food than the small pan; a thicker bottom metal (usually 2½ inches thick); an included lid; and a matching saucepan lid. You can purchase this type of cookware for about $500.

Aluminum Cookware

Aluminum is a good choice for those who want to buy cookware that is strong and durable but does not cost much money. These products are sold at an average price of $100 and can be used on all stovetop surfaces, which makes them perfect for anyone who wants a convenient cooking tool. When subjected to intense heat, these items have the disadvantage of not lasting very long. You should purchase these pots and pans if you want to save money but still want cooking products that are made from high-quality materials, such as heavy-gauge aluminum.

Cuisinart Rice Cooker

The most popular rice cookers are from Cuisinart and Zojirushi. They are much better than most other brands because they have a wider variety of settings. While some Cuisinart rice cookers have the ability to make sushi rice, the Zojirushi models have a more advanced textured-paddle system, which shreds ingredients for buttered steamed rice. These two brands also offer more delicate, slow cooking settings for cooking side dishes like oatmeal or soup. Also, the Cuisinart appliances are more durable than other brands and will last longer than others of their kind. However, you should not use either of these products to make porridge. Only Zojirushi offers a porridge cooker and never uses a heat element to cook food.

Waring Pro Rice Cooker

When it comes to rice cookers, Waring is the best brand because they are very durable. These products do not have any moving parts and are designed to stand up to the elements. They are ideal for making rice, oatmeal, and soups without burning your food. These appliances do not use heat settings or surfaces and have a nonstick interior that eliminates the need for constant washing of pots after each use. This type of appliance is available at an average price of $100.

Hamilton Beach Rice Cooker

The best thing about Hamilton Beach rice cookers is that they are easy to clean. They are also built from heat-resistant BPA-free plastic. If you want to add flavor to your rice, then you can use Hamilton Beach's "fuzzy logic" setting, which is one of the best features of these products. This feature uses a detector that determines the type of grain used and automatically adjusts cooking times and temperatures accordingly. The collapsible steaming basket, which allows you to steam veggies or meat on top of your rice while it cooks, is another great feature of this device. This type of appliance is available at an average price of $50.

Best Oil-less Fryer

Having a high-quality oil-less fryer is important if you want to save money and cook a lot of food. Most oil-less fryers do not have as many special features as regular oil canners, but they are more affordable and are easy to clean. They also require less maintenance because they do not require any oils to be added. On the other hand, some of these fryers are not designed for cooking vegetables and fish, but you can use them for that purpose too. The best oil-less fryer is available at an average price of $200.

Cuisinart Oil-less Fryer

The fact that it has six preset settings, 375 degrees F, 350 degrees F, 325 degrees F, 300 degrees F, 275 degrees F, and 225 degrees F, sets it apart from other oil-free fryers. This allows you to cook a wide range of foods without the need to read a temperature chart or do any adjustments. The Cuisinart oil-less fryer can also be used to cook chicken, fish and ground meat. This type of fryer is available at an average price of $200.

T-Fal Voila Sous Vide Immersion Circulator

A sous vide immersion circulator is a great way to prepare food. This product heats food at precise temperatures and circulates it through a system that creates an even temperature in each chamber. This allows you to cook food for long periods at low temperatures, which makes it tastier and prevents spoilage. This type of appliance is available at an average price of $350.

Anova Culinary Controller Sous Vide Recipes Kit

This product allows you to make barbecue, pasta, soup and more with your sous vide machine. This type of appliance is available at an average price of $200.

Best Juicer

There are many juicers on the market, and choosing one can be difficult. The best juicer is designed to reduce the time needed to juice produce so that you can make more juice at lower cost per unit. The best juicer has a high-quality warranty and comes with additional features, such as a digital screen, automatic spout, a special mesh filter and an easy-to-clean stainless-steel exterior. The Breville BJE510XL Juice Fountain Plus 850-Watt Juice Extractor is a fantastic choice if you're looking for a good juicer with attachments. It comes with an extra-large feeding chute, which allows you to juice large pieces of fruit without the need for a separate container. Another good product is the Breville JE98XL Juice Fountain Plus 850-Watt Juice Extractor, which comes with a machine that can be used to make various types of juice. You can use it to make orange or apple juice, or even banana and mango juices. This type of juicer is available at an average price of $120.

Ultraviolet Sterilizer

Instead of steam or ultra violet light, this type of heat source uses heat from the sun as its source of energy. The best ultraviolet sterilizer is easy to use and healthy because it allows you to keep food fresh for up to six months. It also comes with a digital display that allows you to monitor the temperature while cooking or baking. This type of product is available at an average price of $300.

Instant Pot 7-in-1 Multi-Use Programmable Pressure Cooker

The most popular pressure cookers are from Instant Pot, which is the best brand for this type of device. These products are designed with a steam release valve, which prevents food from burning on the bottom and eliminates the need for constant stirring. The Instant Pot is also the only brand that allows you to steam food while it cooks. This type of product is available at an average price of $180.

Best Blender

A blender is an essential kitchen appliance that can help you make a variety of different drinks and smoothies. Deciding on the best blender for your needs depends on how you intend to use it. If you decide to use it to make soups, smoothies or other food items, then a high-quality model will work best. If you are only planning on using it for drinks, then a high-quality blender will not be necessary. The best blender is available at an average price of $75.

Ninja Professional Blender, Black

This product has a lot of features that make it better than other blenders. For instance, it has a patented safety cover with a leak-proof seal that prevents splattering and leaking while processing the product slowly. It also has a large pitcher and come with two blades, which create less mixing time in the process. This type of blender is available at an average price of $90.

Vitamix Professional Series 750 Blender

The Vitamix Elite 750 has many features that make it one of the best blenders on the market. The high-powered motor is able to crush and pulverize even the hardest seeds and stems. This type of product is available at an average price of $600.

Best Food Processor

One of the best foods processors is a great way to make a variety of different meals quickly. It can also be a great way to cut down on costs by making your own meals at home. The best food processor comes with a large capacity and many useful features, such as a built-in knife sharpener that allows you to use this appliance for cutting meat, fish, vegetables and more. This type of product is available at an average price of $600.

Breville Sous Chef All in One Food Processor, 800-Watt

This product has an interesting design, which allows you to process food quickly and easily. It comes with a large bowl, which can be easily removed when processing large quantities of food. The stainless-steel jar is easy to clean and has a lid that locks in place so that the container is protected from leaks. This type of processor is available at an average price of $120.

KitchenAid 5-Speed Hand Blender with Attachment Kit, 3-Qt

A hand blender is good for making small amounts of food because it can be used in many different ways. It has a compact design and a fast motor that makes this type of appliance good for use in most kitchens. This product is available at an average price of $60.

Best Digital Kitchen Scale

A digital kitchen scale is a great way to ensure that your recipes are accurate so that you can make the food taste good. Many modern foods contain ingredients that cannot be measured by cups, such as molasses, honey or eggs. Using a high-quality kitchen scale is also a great way to make sure that you are not overpaying for your food by putting too much into the measuring cup and throwing out the rest because it falls off when you remove it from the container. This type of product is available at an average price of $50.

Sunbeam Digital Recipes Digital Kitchen Scale, Silver

This digital scale comes with a large display for easy reading in any lighting condition. It has a tare button, which lets you make sure that the container is empty before measuring. The unit also comes with a safety latch to prevent accidental misuse while processing your food. This type of product is available at an average price of $50.

Best Slow Cooker/Crockpot

A slow cooker is a great way to cook your food slowly so that it can be tender and flavorful without the need for constant stirring or heating on the stovetop. The best slow cooker is easy to use and allows you to cook a variety of different foods, including meat, vegetables and even desserts. The best slow cooker is available at an average price of $50.

Cuisinart Slow Cooker/Crock Pot

This type of product has many features that make it one of the most popular on the market today. It comes with a large digital display, which makes it easy to read while you are preparing your food. The cooking pot on this model is also dishwasher safe so that you can clean up easily. This type of product is available at an average price of $85.

Chapter 12.   Shopping List

Here are a few cupboard essentials you will need to start with:

Oils, Fats, And Spreads Substitutes

- Organic coconut oil
- Tahini
- Organic unsweetened applesauce
- Egg white substitute
- Coconut butter (or another nut butter)
- PAM vegan cooking spray

  Fruits, Berries, Vegetables, And Nuts

- Frozen mixed berries (or buy them individually or fresh)
- Fresh or frozen blueberries
- Fresh or frozen strawberries
- Fresh or frozen pomegranate seeds
- Chia seeds
- Sunflower seeds

- Flax seeds
- Pumpkin seeds
- Nuts (if you can eat them, must be raw and unsalted)
- Fresh fruit of your choice, such as peaches, plums, watermelon, kiwi, mangoes, oranges, lemons, and limes
- Mixed vegetables of your choices fresh or organically frozen
- Potatoes (yellow, purple, or red—avoid Russets for high sugar content)
- Sweet potatoes
- Tomatoes
- Cherry tomatoes
- White onions
- Red onions
- Spring onions
- Scallops

- Carrots
- Avocados
- Celery
- Mixed salad leaves
- Baby spinach
- Cabbage or Choi
- Aubergine/eggplant
- Coconut
- Jackfruit
- Fresh chilies
- Mushrooms
- Basil
- Thyme
- Dill
- Mint
- Rocket
- Garlic

- Milk/Dairy Substitutes
- Coconut milk, almond milk, hemp milk, rice milk, soy milk, and other plant-based "milks" Make sure it's non-sweetened and organic.
- Plant-based cream, non-sweetened and low fat
- Plant-based yogurt, non-sweetened and low fat

Meat Substitutes :

- Tofu
- Tempeh

- Mock meats (limit these, as they can be highly processed and high in sodium and sugars)

Other

- Coconut sugar
- Organic brown sugar
- Chickpeas (unsalted)
- Full mineral salt, like Himalayan Pink
- Ground black pepper
- Chili powder
- Turmeric powder
- Mixed herbs
- Italian seasoning
- Cajun spice
- Curry powder
- Cayenne pepper
- Ground cinnamon
- Ground ginger
- Garlic powder
- Organic low sodium vegetable broth
- Organic balsamic vinegar
- Organic white grape vinegar

Shopping On a Budget

The plant-based diet is a lot cheaper than when you are eating meat and other animal projects. But buying organic and looking for certain products can become costly when you are on a budget.

Buy your fresh products from fresh product markets, and don't go for big name brands that cost a fortune. There are lesser name brands that are just as good. Try buying from local farmers and smaller mom-and-pop-type stores.

When it comes to canned goods, condiments, sauces and frozen products, don't attempt to buy everything at once; instead, set a budget and buy some items two to three at a time. Make fresh produce your priority and those processed/packaged goods your second priority.

Chapter 13.   Planning Recipes For 28 Days

Day	Breakfast	Lunch	Snack	Dinner
1	Tofu & Mushroom Muffins	Garlic and Pepper Spiced Eggplant	Hydrated Apples	Summer Bell Peppers Mix
2	Quinoa Bread	Sesame with Bean Stir-Fry	Banana and Walnut Bread	Cabbage Skillet
3	Zucchini & Orange Bread	Ginger Garlic Spiced Chickpea Potato Curry	Choco-Peanut Mug Cake	Creamy Brussels Sprouts Mix
4	Coconut & Nuts Granola	Harvest Vegetable Sauté	Raspberry-Coco Desert	Zucchini-Rice Casserole
5	Chocolate Zucchini Bread	Provençal Summer Vegetables	Almond Cherry Bars	Vegetable Casserole
6	Corn Muffins	Stuffed Tomatoes with Bulgur	Coffee Flavored Doughnuts	Three-Bean Barley Chili
7	Quinoa Black Beans Breakfast Bowl	Eggplant Stuffed with Rice and Herbs	Simple Strawberry Cobbler	Peppery Black Beans
8	Corn Griddle Cakes with Tofu Mayonnaise	Yam and Carrot Casserole	Easy Pumpkin Pie	Walnut, Coconut, and Oat Granola
9	Savory Breakfast Salad	Zucchini Noodles with Tomatoes	Simple Cheesecake	Ritzy Fava Bean Ratatouille
10	Almond Plum Oats Overnight	Broccoli with Bell Pepper	Strawberry Donuts	Mashed White Beans, Potatoes, and Kale
11	High Protein Toast	Mushrooms with Bell Peppers	Apricot Blackberry Crumble	Spicy Chickpea Curry with Mango
12	Hummus Carrot Sandwich	Tomato Soup	Chocolate Coconut Cookies	Red Jerk Beans
13	Overnight Oats	Harvest Bowl	Shortbread Fingers	Easy Tahini Green Beans
14	Avocado Miso Chickpeas Toast	Cauliflower Fried Rice	Cinnamon Rolls	Red Beans with Cauliflower Rice

15	Banana Malt Bread	Curried Quinoa Salad	Fudge Brownies	Gold Chickpea Poppers
16	Banana Vegan Bread	Lettuce Wraps with Smoked Tofu	Vanilla Spiced Souffle	Black Beans and Avocado on Toast
17	Berry Compote Pancakes	Brussels Sprouts & Cranberries Salad	Chocolate Cup Cakes	Hummus Pizza with Tomatoes and Olives
18	Southwest Breakfast Bowl	Quinoa Avocado Salad	Air Baked Cheesecake	Sloppy Joe Sandwiches
19	Chia Seed Pudding	Roasted Sweet Potatoes	Air Roasted Nuts	Gnocchi With Sauce
20	Pumpkin Porridge	Greek Zoodle Bowl	Air Fried White Corn	Minestrone Soup
21	Quinoa Porridge	Vegetable Burritos	Fruit Cake	Tomato And Spaghetti Soup
22	Buckwheat Crepes	Twice-Baked Potatoes	Banana Walnut Bread	Asparagus Cream Soup
23	Chickpeas Spread Sourdough Toast	Creamy Mushroom Stroganoff	Cashew Chickpea Bars	Arugula Salad
24	Chickpeas with Harissa	Carrot Pesto Chili	Chocolate Avocado Pudding	Smoky Tofu and Bean Bowls
25	Quinoa and Rice Stuffed Peppers (Oven-Baked)	Spicy Chickpeas	Cranberry and Almond Muffins	Sloppy Black Bean Burgers
26	Eggplant Sandwich	Farro with Pistachios & Herbs	Chocolate Chip Cashew Bites	Super Three-Bean and Grains Bowl
27	Blueberry Muffins	Broccoli Soup	Banana Orange Nice Cream	Quick and Easy Veggie Pasta Soup
28	Banana Bread	Pumpkin Soup	Pineapple Coconut Macaroons	Homemade Garlic Black Bean Burgers

Chapter 14.   Planning Recipes For 28 Days for Athletes

Day	Breakfast	Lunch	Snack	Dinner
1	Pancakes	Tofu with Broccoli	Roasted Garlic Asparagus With Dijon Mustard	Almond Crackers
2	Granola	Tempeh with Bell Peppers	Tofu Zucchini Kabobs	Cauliflower Black Bean Rice
3	Overnight Oatmeal	Pasta with Asparagus	Chili Toasted Nuts	Skillet Quinoa
4	Pumpkin Pie Oatmeal	Tofu Lettuce Wraps	Chocolate Protein: Bites	Green Beans with Balsamic Sauce
5	Chocolate And Peanut Butter Quinoa	Tofu & Oat Burgers	Spicy Nuts and Seeds Snack Mix	Grain Dishes Cranberry and Walnut Brown Rice
6	Breakfast Scramble	Chickpea Lentil Burgers	Lentil Cakes	Curried Rice
7	Sweet Potato Breakfast Skillet	Lentil Falafel	Balsamic Green Beans Bowls	Cilantro and Avocado Lime Rice
8	Corn with Tofu	Stuffed Avocados	Kale Bowls	Fried Veggie Brown Rice
9	Cauliflower Oatmeal	Stuffed Bell Peppers	Green Bean Fries	Vegetable Stir-fry
10	Pumpkin Oatmeal	Stuffed Sweet Potatoes	Chili Walnuts	Sweet Coconut Pilaf
11	Berry Cobbler	Tangy Broccoli Salad	Seed and Apricot Bowls	Vegetable Quinoa Tots
12	Protein Bars	Summer Rolls with Peanut Sauce	Spiced Lentil Burgers	Easy Millet Nuggets
13	French Toast	Cheesy White Bean Cauliflower Soup	Filled Dough Pieces In Carrot Shape	Millet Fritters
14	Acai Bowl	Split Pea Soup	Banana Cream Stuffed Strawberries	Classic Garlicky Rice

15	Banana Almond Granola	Quinoa & Chickpea Tabbouleh	Tahini String Beans	Brown Rice with Vegetables and Tofu
16	Honeydew Smoothie	Cauliflower Caesar Salad with Chickpea Croutons	Black Beans Burger	Basic Amaranth Porridge
17	Chocolate Blueberry Smoothie	Vegetable Rose Potato	Mushroom Burger	Country Cornbread with Spinach
18	Chickpea Omelet	Rice Arugula Salad	Seitan Burgers	Rice Pudding with Currants
19	Sweet Polenta with Pears	Tomato Salad	Maple Roasted Squash	Chard Wraps with Millet
20	Tropi-Kale Breeze	Kale Apple Roasted Root Vegetable Salad	Carrot And Red Onion Sauté	Corn Kernel Black Bean Rice
21	Cinnamon Congee with Apricots and Dates	Rice Arugula Salad with Sesame Garlic Dressing	Avocado Tomato Bruschetta	Rice & Cuban Beans
22	Potato Medley	Garden Pasta Salad	Thai Snack Mix	Potato & Corn Chowder
23	Orange French Toast	Roasted Vegetables and Tofu Salad	Broccoli Poppers	Tomato Pesto Quinoa
24	Almond Butter Banana Overnight Oats	Roasted Lemon Asparagus Watercress Salad	Cauliflower Poppers	Oatmeal Cookies
25	Peach & Chia Seed Breakfast Parfait	Pumpkin and Brussels Sprouts Mix	Buffalo Cauliflower Bites	No-Bake Peanut Butter Oat Bars
26	Blueberry Pancakes	Almond and Tomato Salad	Veggie Nuggets	Peanut Butter Rice Crispy Treats
27	Apple Cinnamon Cut Oats	Best Avocado Zucchini Sushi	Fried Ravioli	Easy Chickpea Tacos
28	Ful Medammes Breakfast	Walnut Pesto Broiled Cauliflower	Tofu Bites	Instant & Yummy Steel Cut Oats

Chapter 15.   Breakfast

1. Hemp Breakfast Cookies

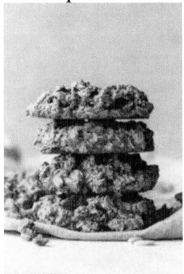

Preparation Time: 10 minutes
Cooking Time: 15 minutes
Servings: 6

Ingredients:

* 3 cups almond flour
* 1 cup dried dates, pitted
* ½ cup hemp seeds
* 1 cup almond milk

Directions:

1 - Mix almond milk with hemp seeds and dates in a bowl and leave for 1hour.
2 - Blend almond flour with the rest of the ingredients and milk mixture in a mixer until it makes a smooth dough.
3 - Preheat your oven to 350° F.
4 - Divide the dough into nine portions and shape each into a cookie.
5 - Place these cookies in a baking sheet lined with wax paper.
6 - Bake the cookies for 15 minutes in the oven and flip them once cooked halfway through.

Nutrition: Calories: 217; Fat: 25 g; Sodium: 132 mg; Carbs: 29 g; Fiber: 3.9 g; Sugar: 3 g; Proteins: 8.9 g.

2. Zucchini Oatmeal

Preparation Time: 15 minutes
Cooking Time: 4 minutes
Servings: 4

Ingredients:

* 2 cups rolled oats
* 6 tablespoons pea protein
* 2 teaspoons cinnamon
* 1 teaspoon nutmeg
* 2 ¼ cups almond milk
* 1 cup zucchini, grated
* ¼ cup maple syrup
* 1 teaspoon vanilla extract

Toppings:
* Banana
* Nuts
* Seeds
* Sugar-free chocolate chips
* 1 teaspoon coconut oil, melted

Directions:

1 - Cook oats with coconut oil in an Instant Pot for 2 minutes on Sauté mode.
2 - Stir in the rest of the ingredients, cover and seal its lid.
3 - Cook for 2 minutes on high pressure.
4 - When done, release all the pressure and remove the lid.
5 - Allow the oatmeal to cool and garnish with desired toppings.

Nutrition: Calories: 232; Fat: 12 g; Sodium: 202 mg; Carbs: 26 g; Fiber: 4 g; Sugar: 8 g; Proteins: 7.3 g.

3. Broccoli Oatmeal

Preparation Time: 15 minutes.
Cooking Time: 15 minutes.
Servings: 2

Ingredients:

* 1 cup broccoli
* ½ cup unsweetened almond milk
* ½ teaspoon cinnamon
* 1 tablespoon maple syrup

- ½ tablespoon peanut butter
- 1 strawberry, sliced

Directions:

1 - Mix milk with broccoli, maple syrup and cinnamon in a saucepan.
2 - Cook the rice mixture to a boil, then reduce the heat to low.
3 - Now cook the mixture for 10 minutes on a simmer.
4 - Allow the oatmeal to cool, then garnish it with a strawberry.

Nutrition: Calories: 234; Fat: 4.7 g; Sodium: 1 mg; Carbs: 18 g; Fiber: 7 g; Sugar: 3.3 g; Proteins: 6 g.

4. Peanut Butter Muffins

Preparation Time: 15 minutes
Cooking Time: 27 minutes
Servings: 6

Ingredients:

- ¾ cup oat flour
- ¼ cup coconut sugar
- 2 tablespoons pea protein powder
- 1 tablespoon baking powder
- 2 teaspoons baking soda
- 3 large bananas, mashed
- ½ cup peanut butter
- 2 tablespoons flaxseed
- ½ cup water
- ½ cup almond milk
- 1 teaspoon vanilla extract

Directions:

1 - Preheat the oven to 350 F and layer two muffin trays with cupcake liners.
2 - Soak flaxseed with ½ cup of water in a bowl for minutes.
3 - Mix mashed banana with milk, peanut butter and flaxseed mixture in a large bowl.
4 - Now, stir it with the rest of the muffin ingredients and mix well evenly.
5 - Divide the prepared batter into the muffin tray and bake for 27 minutes.

6 - Allow the muffins to cool and serve.

Nutrition: Calories: 297; Fat: 15 g; Sodium: 548 mg; Carbs: 35 g; Fiber: 4 g; Sugar: 1 g; Proteins: 9 g.

5. Veggie Quiche

Preparation Time: 20 minutes
Cooking Time: 1 hour
Servings: 4

Ingredients:

- 1 cup water
- Pinch of salt
- 1/3 cup bulgur wheat
- ¾ tablespoon light sesame oil
- 1½ cups fresh cremini mushrooms, sliced
- 2 cups fresh broccoli, chopped
- 1 yellow onion, chopped
- 16 ounces firm tofu, pressed and cubed
- ¾ tablespoon white miso
- 1¼ tablespoons tahini
- 1 tablespoon low-sodium soy sauce

Directions:

1 - Preheat oven to 350 °F.
2 - Lightly grease a pie dish.
3 - In a saucepan, add the water over medium heat and salt bring to a boil.
4 - Stir in the bulgur and again bring to a rolling boil.
5 - Now, lower the heat to low and simmer, covered for about 12-15 minutes or until all the liquid is absorbed.
6 - Remove from heat and set the saucepan aside to cool slightly.
7 - Now, place the cooked bulgur into the pie dish evenly and with your fingers, press into the bottom.
8 - Bake for approximately 12 minutes.
9 - Remove from the oven and set aside to cool slightly.
10 - Meanwhile, in a skillet, heat oil over medium heat.
11 - Add the mushrooms, broccoli and onion and cook for about 10 minutes, stirring occasionally.
12 - Remove from the heat and transfer into a large bowl to cool slightly.

13 - Meanwhile, in a food processor, add the remaining ingredients and pulse until smooth.

14 - Transfer the tofu mixture into the bowl with veggie mixture and mix until well combined.

15 - Place the veggie mixture over the baked crust evenly.

16 - Bake for approximately 30 minutes or until top becomes golden brown.

17 - Remove from the oven and set the pie dish aside for at least 10 minutes.

18 - With a sharp knife, cut into 4 equal-sized slices and serve.

Nutrition: Calories: 211 Fat: 10.4g Carbohydrates: 19.6g Dietary Fiber: 5.7g Sugar: 3.6g Protein: 14.4g

6. Carrot Muffins

Preparation Time: 15 minutes
Cooking Time: 18 minutes
Servings: 6

Ingredients:

- 1/3 cup water
- 2 tablespoons ground flaxseeds
- 2 cups all-purpose flour
- 1 cup plus 2 tablespoons rolled oats, divided
- ¾ cup brown sugar
- 2 teaspoons baking powder
- 2 teaspoons ground cinnamon
- ½ teaspoon ground ginger
- ½ teaspoon ground nutmeg
- Pinch of ground cloves
- ¼ teaspoon salt
- 1 cup unsweetened almond milk
- ½ cup coconut oil, melted
- 2 teaspoons pure vanilla extract
- 2 cups carrots, peeled and grated finely

Directions:

1 - Preheat your oven to 375 °F.

2 - Grease a standard sized 12 cups muffin pan.

3 - In a small bowl, add water and flaxseeds and mix well. Set aside.

4 - In a large mixing bowl, add flour, 1 cup of oats, brown sugar, baking powder, spice and salt and mix well.

5 - In another medium mixing bowl, add almond milk, oil and vanilla extract and beat until well combined.

6 - Add flaxseeds mixture and stir to combine well.

7 - Add oil mixture into the bowl with flour mixture and mix until well combined.

8 - Gently, fold in carrots.

9 - Transfer the mixture into prepared muffin cups evenly. Sprinkle with remaining oats evenly.

10 - Bake for approximately 15-18 minutes or until a wooden skewer inserted in the center comes out clean.

11 - Remove the muffin tin from oven and place onto a wire rack to cool for about 10 minutes.

12 - Carefully invert the muffins onto the wire rack to cool completely before serving.

Nutrition: Calories: 472 Fat: 20.9g Carbohydrates: 65,2g Dietary Fiber: 4.7g Sugar: 19.9g Protein: 7.1g

7. Tofu & Mushroom Muffins

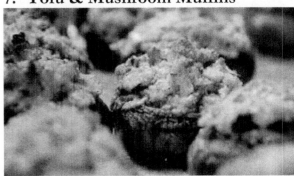

Preparation Time: 15 minutes
Cooking Time: 30 minutes
Servings: 6

Ingredients:

- 1 teaspoon olive oil
- 1½ cups fresh mushrooms, chopped
- 1 scallion, chopped
- 1 teaspoon garlic, minced
- 1 teaspoon fresh rosemary, minced
- Ground black pepper, as required

- 1 (12.3-ounce) package firm silken tofu, drained
- ¼ cup unsweetened almond milk
- 2 tablespoons nutritional yeast
- 1 tablespoon arrowroot starch
- ¼ teaspoon ground turmeric
- 1 teaspoon coconut oil, softened

Directions:

1 - Preheat your oven to 375 °F.
2 - Grease a 12 cups muffin tin.
3 - In a non-stick skillet, heat oil over medium heat and sauté scallion and garlic for about 1 minute.
4 - Add the mushrooms and sauté for 5-7 minutes.
5 - Stir in the rosemary and black pepper and remove from the heat.
6 - Set aside to cool slightly.
7 - In a food processor, add the tofu and remaining ingredients and pulse until smooth.
8 - Transfer the tofu mixture into a large bowl.
9 - Fold in the mushroom mixture.
10 - Pour the batter into prepared muffin cups evenly.
11 - Bake for 20-22 minutes or until a toothpick inserted in the center comes out clean.
12 - Remove the muffin tin from the oven and place onto a wire rack to cool for about 10 minutes.
13 - Carefully invert the muffins onto the wire rack and serve warm.

Nutrition: Calories: 184 Fat: 3.7g Carbohydrates: 6.8g Dietary Fiber: 1.8g Sugar: 1.9g Protein: 7.7g

8. Quinoa Bread

Preparation Time: 10 minutes
Cooking Time: 1½ hours
Servings: 12

Ingredients:

- 1¾ cups uncooked quinoa, soaked overnight and rinsed
- ¼ cup chia seeds, soaked in ½ cup of water overnight
- ½ teaspoon bicarbonate soda
- ¼ teaspoon Salt
- ¼ cup olive oil

- ½ cup water
- 1 tablespoon fresh lemon juice

Directions:

1 - Preheat your oven to 320 °F.
2 - Line a loaf pan with parchment paper.
3 - In a food processor, add all the ingredients and pulse for about 3 minutes.
4 - Pour the mixture into prepared loaf pan evenly.
5 - Bake for 1½ hours or until a toothpick inserted in the center comes out clean.
6 - Remove the loaf pan from the oven and place onto a wire rack to cool for about 10 minutes.
7 - Now, invert the bread onto the wire rack to cool completely before slicing.
8 - With a sharp knife, slice each bread loaf to the desired sized slices and serve.

Nutrition: Calories: 137 Fat: 6.5g Carbohydrates: 16.9g Dietary Fiber: 2.6g Sugar: 0g Protein: 4g

9. Zucchini & Orange Bread

Preparation Time: 15 minutes
Cooking Time: 1 hour 10 minutes
Servings: 16

Ingredients:

- 3 cups all-purpose flour
- 1 cup brown sugar
- 3 tablespoons flaxseeds
- ½ teaspoon arrowroot powder
- 1 teaspoon baking soda
- ½ teaspoon baking powder
- 2 teaspoons ground cinnamon
- 1 teaspoon salt
- ¾ cup canola oil
- 1 cup white sugar
- 1 cup unsweetened applesauce
- 2 teaspoons pure vanilla extract
- 2½ cups zucchini, shredded and squeezed
- 2 teaspoons fresh orange zest, grated finely

Directions:

1 - Preheat your oven to 325 °F.
2 - Grease and flour two (9x5-inch) bread pans.

3 - In a large mixing bowl, add flour, brown sugar, flaxseeds, arrowroot powder, baking soda, baking powder, cinnamon and salt and mix well.

4 - In another medium mixing bowl, add oil, white sugar, applesauce and vanilla extract and beat until well combined.

5 - Add oil mixture into the bowl with flour mixture and mix until well combined.

6 - Gently, fold in zucchini and orange zest.

7 - Divide the bread mixture into prepared bread pans evenly.

8 - Bake for approximately 70 minutes or until a toothpick inserted in the center comes out clean.

9 - Remove the bread pans from oven and place onto a wire rack to cool for about 10 minutes.

10 - Now, invert each bread onto the wire rack to cool completely before slicing.

11 - Cut each bread loaf into the desired sized slices and serve.

Nutrition: Calories: 276 Fat: 10.9g Carbohydrates: 42.5g Dietary Fiber: 1.5g Sugar: 23.3g Protein: 2.9g

10. Coconut & Nuts Granola

Preparation Time: 10 minutes
Cooking Time: 20 minutes
Servings: 12
Ingredients:
- 3 cups unsweetened coconut flakes
- 1 cup walnuts, chopped
- ½ cup flaxseeds
- 2/3 cup pumpkin seeds
- 2/3 cup sunflower seeds
- ¼ cup coconut oil, melted
- 1 teaspoon ground ginger
- 1 teaspoon ground cinnamon
- Pinch of salt

Directions:

1 - Preheat your oven to 350 °F.

2 - Lightly grease a large, rimmed baking sheet.

3 - In a bowl, add the coconut flakes, walnuts, flaxseeds, pumpkin seeds, sunflower seeds, coconut oil, spices, and salt and toss to coat well.

4 - Transfer the mixture onto the prepared baking sheet and spread in an even layer.

5 - Bake for approximately 20 minutes, stirring after every 3-4 minutes.

6 - Remove the baking sheet from the oven and let the granola cool completely before serving.

7 - Break the granola into desired sized chunks and serve with your favorite non-dairy milk.

Nutrition: Calories: 256 Fat: 23g Carbohydrates: 8.5g Dietary Fiber: 4.6g Sugar: 0.3g Protein: 4.8g

11. Chocolate Zucchini Bread

Preparation Time: 15 minutes
Cooking Time: 55 minutes
Servings: 6

Ingredients:

- 1 ¼ cup whole wheat flour
- ¾ cup coconut sugar
- ½ cup raw cacao powder
- 3 teaspoons baking powder
- 2 teaspoons baking soda
- 1 cup zucchini, shredded
- ½ cup almond milk
- 1/3 cup unsweetened applesauce
- 1/3 cup coconut oil, melted
- 2 teaspoons vanilla extract
- 2/3 cup sugar-free chocolate chip

Directions:

1 - Preheat your oven to 350 F and layer a 9-inch loaf pan with wax paper.

2 - Pat dries the shredded zucchini and keep it aside.

3 - Mix flour with baking soda, baking powder, cacao powder, coconut sugar and flour in a bowl.

4 - Stir it with vanilla, applesauce, milk, and peanut butter, then mix until smooth.

5 - Fold in sugar-free chocolate chips and zucchini shreds.

6 - Spread this batter in the prepared loaf pan.

7 - Bake this bread for 55 minutes in the oven.

8 - Allow the bread to cool, then slice.

Nutrition: Calories: 218; Fat: 22 g; Sodium: 350 mg; Carbs: 22 g; Fiber: 0.7 g; Sugar: 1 g; Proteins: 2.3 g.

12. Corn Muffins

Preparation Time: 15 minutes
Cooking Time: 20 minutes
Servings: 6

Ingredients:

- 1½ tablespoons ground flaxseed
- 1 cup almond milk
- ½ cup applesauce
- ½ cup pure maple syrup
- 1 cup corn meal
- 1 cup oat flour
- 1 teaspoon baking soda
- 1 teaspoon baking powder
- ½ teaspoon salt
- 1 cup corn kernels

Directions:

1 - Preheat your oven to 375° F.

2 - Mix almond milk with flaxseed in a large bowl, then leave it for 5 minutes.

3 - Stir it in maple syrup and apple sauce, then mix well.

4 - Add salt, baking powder, baking soda, oat flour and cornmeal, then mix until smooth.

5 - Add corn kernels and mix evenly.

6 - Divide the corn batter into 12 muffin cups and bake for 20 minutes in the oven.

7 - Allow the muffins to cool and serve.

Nutrition: Calories: 257; Fat: 12 g; Sodium: 48 mg; Carbs: 32 g; Fiber: 2 g; Sugar: 0 g; Proteins: 14 g.

13. Quinoa Black Beans Breakfast Bowl

Preparation Time: 15 minutes
Cooking Time: 25 minutes
Servings: 1

Ingredients:

- 1/4 cup brown quinoa, rinsed well
- Salt to taste
- 1 tablespoon plant-based yogurt
- ½ lime, juiced
- 1 tablespoon chopped fresh cilantro
- 1 (5 oz) can black beans, drained and rinsed
- 1 tablespoon tomato salsa
- ¼ small avocado, pitted, peeled, and sliced
- 1 radish, shredded

- 1/4 tablespoons pepitas (pumpkin seeds)

Directions:

1 - Cook the quinoa with 2 cups of slightly salted water in a medium pot over medium heat or until the liquid absorbs, 15 minutes.

2 - Spoon the quinoa into serving bowls and fluff with a fork.

3 - In a small bowl, mix the yogurt, lime juice, cilantro, and salt. Divide this mixture on the quinoa and top with beans, salsa, avocado, radishes, and pepitas.

4 - Serve immediately.

Nutrition: Calories: 131; Fats: 3.5 g; Carbs: 20 g; Proteins: 6.5 g.

14. Corn Griddle Cakes with Tofu Mayonnaise

Preparation Time: 15 minutes
Cooking Time: 35 minutes
Servings: 1

Ingredients:

- 1 tablespoon flax seed powder + 3 tablespoons water
- 1 cup water or as needed
- 1 cup yellow cornmeal
- 1 teaspoon salt
- 1 teaspoon baking powder
- 1 tablespoon olive oil for frying
- 1 cup tofu mayonnaise for serving

Directions:

1 - In a medium bowl, mix the flax seed powder with water and allow thickening for 5 minutes to form the flax egg.

2 - Mix in the water and then whisk in the cornmeal, salt, and baking powder until soup texture forms but not watery.

3 - Heat a quarter of the olive oil in a griddle pan and pour in a quarter of the batter. Cook until set and golden brown beneath, 3 minutes. Flip the cake and cook the other side until set and golden brown too.

4 - Plate the cake and make three more with the remaining oil and batter.

5 - Top the cakes with some tofu mayonnaise before serving.

Nutrition: Calories: 896; Fats: 50.7 g; Carbs: 91.6 g; Proteins: 17.3 g.

15. Savory Breakfast Salad

Preparation Time: 15 to 30 minutes
Cooking Time: 20 minutes
Servings: 1

Ingredients:

For the sweet potatoes:
- 2 smalls sweet potatoes
- 1 pinch salt and pepper
- 1 tablespoon coconut oil
  For the Dressing:
- 3 tablespoons lemon juice
- 1 pinch salt and pepper
- 1 tablespoon extra-virgin olive oil
For the Salad:
- 4 cups mixed greens
  For Serving:
- 4 tablespoons hummus
- 1 cup blueberries
- 1 medium ripe avocado
- Fresh chopped parsley
- 2 tablespoons hemp seeds

Directions:

1 - Take a large skillet and apply gentle heat.

2 - Add sweet potatoes, coat them with salt and pepper, and pour some oil. Cook till sweet potatoes turn brown.

3 - Take a bowl and mix lemon juice, salt, and pepper. Add salad, sweet potatoes, and the serving together. Mix well, dress and serve.

Nutrition: Calories: 523; Carbs: 57.6 g; Proteins: 7.5 g; Fats: 37.6 g.

16. Almond Plum Oats Overnight

Preparation Time: 15 to 30 minutes

Cooking Time: 10 minutes
Servings: 1

Ingredients:

- 60 g rolled oats:
- 3 plums, ripe and chopped
- 300 ml almond milk
- 1 tablespoon chia seeds:
- A pinch nutmeg
- A few drops of vanilla extract
- 1 tablespoon whole almonds, roughly chopped

Directions:

1 - Add oats, nutmeg, vanilla extract, almond milk, and chia seeds to a bowl and mix well.

2 - Add in cubed plums and cover and place in the fridge for one night. Mix the oats well the next morning and add into the serving bowl.

3 - Serve with your favorite toppings.

Nutrition: Calories: 248; Carbs: 24.7 g; Proteins: 9.5 g; Fats: 10.8 g.

17. High Protein Toast

Preparation Time: 30 minutes
Cooking Time: 15 minutes
Servings: 1

Ingredients:

- 1 white bean, drained and rinsed
- ½ cup cashew cream
- 1 ½ tablespoon miso paste
- 1 teaspoon toasted sesame oil
- 1 tablespoon sesame seeds
- 1 spring onion, finely sliced
- Lemon: 1 half for the juice and half wedged to serve
- 4 slices rye bread, toasted

Directions:

1 - In a bowl, add sesame oil, white beans, miso, cashew cream, and lemon juice and mash using a potato masher. Make a spread.

2 - Spread it on a toast and top with spring onions and sesame seeds. Serve with lemon wedges.
Nutrition: Calories: 332; Carbs: 44.5 g; Proteins: 14.5 g; Fats: 9.25 g.

18. Hummus Carrot Sandwich
Preparation Time: 30 minutes
Cooking Time: 25 minutes
Servings: 1

Ingredients:

- 1 cup can chickpeas, drain and rinsed
- 1 small tomato, sliced
- 1 cucumber, sliced
- 1 avocado, sliced
- 1 teaspoon cumin
- 1 cup carrot, diced
- 1 teaspoon maple syrup
- 3 tablespoons tahini
- 1 garlic clove
- 2 tablespoons lemon
- 2 tablespoons extra-virgin olive oil
- Salt as per your need
- 4 bread slices

Directions:

1 - Add carrot to the boiling hot water and boil for 15 minutes. Blend boiled carrots, maple syrup, cumin, chickpeas, tahini, olive oil, salt, and garlic together.
2 - Add in lemon juice and mix.
3 - Add to the serving bowl, and you can refrigerate for up to 5 days. In between two bread slices, spread hummus and place 2-3 slices of cucumber, avocado, and tomato and serve.

Nutrition: Calories: 490; Carbs: 53.15 g; Proteins: 14.1 g; Fats: 27 g.

19. Overnight Oats
Preparation Time: 30 minutes
Cooking Time: 15 minutes
Servings: 1

Ingredients:

- A pinch cinnamon
- 200 ml almond milk
- 120 g porridge oats
- 1 tablespoon maple syrup
- 1 tablespoon pumpkin seeds
- 1 tablespoon chia seeds

Directions:

1 - Add all the ingredients to the bowl and combine well. Cover the bowl and place it in the fridge overnight. Pour more milk in the morning.
2 - Serve with your favorite toppings.

Nutrition: Calories: 298; Carbs: 32.3 g; Proteins: 10.2 g; Fats: 12.7 g.

20. Avocado Miso Chickpeas Toast

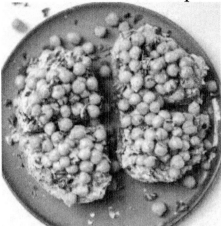

Preparation Time: 30 minutes
Cooking Time: 15 minutes
Servings: 1

Ingredients:

- 400 g chickpeas, drained and rinsed
- 1 medium avocado
- 1 teaspoon toasted sesame oil
- 1 ½ tablespoon white miso paste
- 1 tablespoon sesame seeds
- 1 spring onion, finely sliced
- 1 lemon, half for the juice and half wedged to serve
- 4 rye bread slices toasted

Directions:

1 - In a bowl, add sesame oil, chickpeas, miso, and lemon juice and mash using a potato masher.
2 - Roughly crush avocado in another bowl using a fork. Add the avocado to the chickpeas and make a spread. Spread it on a toast and top with spring onion and sesame seeds. Serve with lemon wedges.
Nutrition: Calories: 456; Carbs: 33.3 g; Proteins: 14.6 g; Fat: 26.6 g.

21. Banana Malt Bread

Preparation Time: 30 minutes
Cooking Time: 1 hour and 20 minutes
Servings: 1

Ingredients:

- 120 ml hot strong black tea
- 150 g malt extract + extra for brushing
- 2 bananas, ripe mashed
- 100 g sultanas
- 120 g pitted dates, chopped
- 250 g plain flour
- 50 g soft dark brown sugar
- 2 teaspoons baking powder

Directions:

1 - Preheat the oven to 140° C (284°F).
2 - Line the loaf tin with the baking paper.
3 - Brew tea and include sultanas and dates in it. Take a small pan and heat the malt extract, and gradually add sugar to it. Stir continuously and let it cook.
4 - In a bowl, add flour, salt, and baking powder, and now top with sugar extract, fruits, bananas, and tea.
5 - Mix the batter well and add to the loaf tin.
6 - Bake the mixture for one hour
7 - Brush the bread with extra malt extract and let it cool down before removing it from the tin.
8 - When done, wrap in a foil; it can be consumed for a week.

Nutrition: Calories: 194; Carbs: 43.3 g; Proteins: 3.4 g; Fat: 0.3 g.

22. Banana Vegan Bread

Preparation Time: 30 minutes
Cooking Time: 1 hour and 15 minutes
Servings: 1
Ingredients:

- 3 large bananas, overripe mashed
- 200 g all-purpose flour
- 50 ml unsweetened non-dairy milk
- ½ teaspoon white vinegar
- 10 g ground flaxseed
- ¼ teaspoon ground cinnamon
- 140 g granulated sugar
- ¼ teaspoon vanilla
- ¼ teaspoon baking powder
- ¼ teaspoon baking soda
- ¼ teaspoon salt
- 3 tablespoons canola oil
- ½ cup chopped walnuts

Directions:

1 - Preheat the oven to 350º F and line the loaf pan with parchment paper. Mash bananas using a fork.

2 - Take a large bowl, and add in mash bananas, canola oil, oat milk, sugar, vinegar, vanilla, and ground flax seed.

3 - Also, whisk in baking powder, cinnamon, flour, and salt. Add batter to the loaf pan and bake for 50 minutes. Remove from pan and let it sit for 10 minutes. Slice when completely cooled down.

Nutrition: Calories: 240; Carbs: 40.3 g; Proteins: 2.8 g; Fat: 8.2 g.

23. Berry Compote Pancakes

Preparation Time: 30 minutes
Cooking Time: 30 minutes
Servings: 1

Ingredients:

- 200 g mixed frozen berries
- 140 g plain flour
- 140 ml unsweetened almond milk
- 1 tablespoon icing sugar
- 1 tablespoon lemon juice
- 2 teaspoons baking powder
- A dash of vanilla extract
- A pinch salt
- 2 tablespoons caster sugar
- ½ tablespoon vegetable oil

Directions:

1 - Take a small pan and add berries, lemon juice, and icing sugar. Cook the mixture for 10 minutes to give it a saucy texture and set it aside. Take a bowl and add caster sugar, flour, baking powder, and salt. Mix well.

2 - Add in almond milk and vanilla and combine well to make a batter. Take a non-stick pan, and heat 2 teaspoons of oil in it, and spread it over the whole surface.

3 - Add ¼ cup of the batter to the pan and cook each side for 3-4 minutes. Serve with compote.

Nutrition: Calories: 463; Carbs: 92 g; Proteins: 9.4 g; Fat: 5.2 g.

24. Southwest Breakfast Bowl

Preparation Time: 30 minutes
Cooking Time: 15 minutes
Servings: 1

Ingredients:

- 1 cup mushrooms, sliced
- ½ cup chopped cilantro
- 1 teaspoon chili powder
- 1/2 red pepper, diced
- 1 cup zucchini, diced
- 1/2 cup green onion, chopped
- 1/2 cup onion
- 1 vegan sausage, sliced
- 1 teaspoon garlic powder
- 1 teaspoon paprika
- 1/2 teaspoons cumin
- Salt and pepper as per your taste
- Avocado for topping

Directions:

1 - Put everything in a bowl and apply medium heat until vegetables turn brown.

2 - Add some pepper and salt as you like and serve with your favorite toppings

Nutrition: Calories: 361; Carbs: 31.6 g; Proteins: 33.8 g; Fat: 12.2 g.

25. Chia Seed Pudding

Preparation Time: 10 minutes
Cooking Time: 0 minutes
Servings: 3

Ingredients:

- 2 cups unsweetened almond milk
- ½ cup chia seeds
- 1 tablespoon maple syrup
- 1 teaspoon vanilla extract

Directions:

1 - In a large bowl, add the almond milk, chia seeds, maple syrup, and vanilla extract and stir to combine well.

2 - Refrigerate for at least 3-4 hours, stirring occasionally.
3 - Serve with your favorite topping.

Nutrition: Calories: 125 Fat: 9g Carbohydrates: 14g Dietary Fiber: 7.3g Sugar: 4.2g Protein: 4.7g

26. Pumpkin Porridge
Preparation Time: 10 minutes
Cooking Time: 25 minutes
Servings: 4

Ingredients:
- 1 cup water
- Pinch of salt
- 1 cup almond flour
- 2 tablespoons maple syrup
- ½ cup sugar-free pumpkin puree
- ½ teaspoon ground cinnamon
- Pinch of ground nutmeg

Directions:

1 - In a saucepan, add the water and salt over medium-high heat and bring to a boil.
2 - Slowly, add the almond flour, stirring continuously.
3 - Lower the heat to medium and cook for about 15-20 minutes or until all the liquid is absorbed, stirring continuously.
4 - Add the remaining ingredients except the almonds and stir to combine well.
5 - Serve immediately.

Nutrition: Calories: 218 Fat: 15.1g Carbohydrates: 14.5g Dietary Fiber: 4.1g Sugar: 7g Protein: 0.4g

27. Quinoa Porridge
Preparation Time: 10 minutes
Cooking Time: 15 minutes
Servings: 4

Ingredients:

- 1 cup uncooked red quinoa, rinsed and drained
- 2 cups water
- ½ teaspoon vanilla extract
- ½ cup unsweetened coconut milk
- ¼ teaspoon fresh lemon peel, grated finely
- 10-12 drops liquid stevia
- 1 teaspoon ground cinnamon
- ½ teaspoon ground ginger
- ½ teaspoon ground nutmeg
- Pinch of ground cloves
- 4 tablespoons almonds, chopped

Directions:
1 - In a large saucepan, mix together the quinoa, water, and vanilla extract over medium heat and bring to a boil.
2 - Now, lower the heat to low and simmer, covered for about 15 minutes or until all the liquid is absorbed, stirring occasionally.
3 - In the saucepan with the quinoa, add the coconut milk, lemon peel, stevia, and spices and stir to combine.
4 - Immediately remove from the heat and fluff the quinoa with a fork.
5 - Serve warm with the topping of almonds.

Nutrition: Calories: 265 Fat: 12.8g Carbohydrates: 431.1g Dietary Fiber: 4.8g Sugar: 1.4g Protein: 8g

28. Buckwheat Crepes
Preparation Time: 30 minutes
Cooking Time: 25 minutes
Servings: 1

Ingredients:
- 1 cup raw buckwheat flour
- 1 and 3/4 cups light coconut milk
- 1/8 teaspoons ground cinnamon
- 3/4 tablespoons flaxseeds
- 1 tablespoon melted coconut oil
- A pinch of sea salt
- Any sweetener as per your taste

Directions:

1. Take a bowl and add flaxseed, coconut milk, salt, avocado, and cinnamon.
2. Mix them all well and fold in the flour.
3. Now take a nonstick pan and pour oil; provide medium heat.
4. Add a big spoon of the mixture.

5.   Cook till it appears bubbly, then flip side. Perform the task until all crepes are prepared. For enhancing the taste, add the sweetener of your liking.

Nutrition: Calories: 71; Carbs: 8 g; Proteins: 1 g; Fat: 3 g.

29. Chickpeas Spread Sourdough Toast

Preparation Time: 30 minutes
Cooking Time: 15 minutes
Servings: 1

Ingredients:

- 1 cup chickpeas, rinsed and drained
- 1 cup pumpkin puree
- ½ cup vegan yogurt
- Salt as per your need
- 2 slices sourdough, toasted

Directions:

1 - In a bowl, add chickpeas and pumpkin puree and mash using a potato masher. Add in salt and yogurt and mix.
2 - Spread it on a toast and serve.

Nutrition: Calories: 187; Carbs: 33.7 g; Proteins: 8.45 g; Fat: 2.5 g.

30. Chickpeas with Harissa

Preparation Time: 30 minutes
Cooking Time: 20 minutes
Servings: 1

Ingredients:

- 1 cup can chickpeas, rinse and drained well
- 1 small onion, diced
- 1 cup cucumber, diced
- 1 cup tomato, diced
- Salt as per your taste
- 2 tablespoons lemon juice
- 2 teaspoons harissa
- 1 tablespoon olive oil
- 2 tablespoons flat-leaf parsley, chopped

Directions:

1 - Add lemon juice, harissa, and olive oil in a bowl and whisk.
2 - Incorporate onion, cucumber, chickpeas, and salt.
3 - Add parsley from the top and serve.

Nutrition: Calories: 398; Carbs: 55.6 g; Proteins: 17.8 g; Fat: 11.8 g.

31. Quinoa and Rice Stuffed Peppers (Oven-Baked)

Preparation Time: 30 minutes
Cooking Time: 35 minutes
Servings: 1

Ingredients:

- 3/4 cup long-grain rice
- 2 bell peppers (any color)
- 1 tablespoon olive oil
- 1 onion diced
- 1 clove chopped garlic
- 1 can (11 oz) crushed tomatoes
- 1 teaspoon cumin
- 1 teaspoon coriander
- 2 tablespoon ground walnuts
- 1 cup cooked quinoa
- 1 tablespoon chopped parsley
- Salt and ground black pepper to taste

Directions:

1 - Preheat your oven to 200° C or 400° F.
2 - Boil rice and drain in a colander.
3 - Cut the top stem piece of the pepper off, remove the remaining pith and seeds, rinse peppers.
4 - Heat oil in a big frying pan, then sauté garlic and onion until soft.
5 - Add tomatoes, cumin, ground almonds, salt, pepper, and coriander; stir well and simmer for 2 minutes, stirring constantly.
6 - Remove from the heat and add the rice, quinoa, and parsley; stir well.
7 - Taste and adjust salt and pepper.
8 - Fill the peppers with a mixture, and place peppers cut side up in a baking dish; drizzle with little oil.
9 - Bake for 15 minutes.
10 - Serve warm.

Nutrition: Calories: 335; Fibers: 10 g; Carbs: 35 g; Proteins: 21 g; Fat: 14 g.

32. Eggplant Sandwich
Preparation Time: 30 minutes
Cooking Time: 30 minutes
Servings: 1

Ingredients:
- 1 eggplant, sliced
- 2 teaspoons parsley, dried
- Salt and black pepper to the taste
- 1/2 cup vegan breadcrumbs
- 1/2 teaspoons Italian seasoning
- 1/2 teaspoons garlic powder
- 1/2 teaspoons onion powder
- 2 tablespoons almond milk
- 4 vegan bread slices
- Cooking spray
- 1/2 cup avocado mayo
- 3/4 cup tomato sauce
- A handful basil, chopped

Directions:

1 - Season eggplant slices with salt and pepper, leave aside for 30 minutes and then dry them well.
2 - In a bowl, mix parsley with breadcrumbs, Italian seasoning, onion and garlic powder, salt and black pepper. Stir.
3 - In another bowl, mix milk with vegan mayo and also stir well.
4 - Brush eggplant slices with mayo mix. Dip them in breadcrumbs mix and place them on a lined baking sheet. Spray with cooking oil, introduce baking sheet in your air fryer's basket and cook them at 400° F for 15 minutes, flipping them halfway.
5 - Brush each bread slice with olive oil and arrange 2 of them on a working surface.
6 - Add baked eggplant slices, spread tomato sauce and basil. Top with the other bread slices, greased side down.
7 - Divide between plates and serve.

Nutrition: Calories: 324; Fat: 16 g; Fibers: 4 g; Carbs: 19 g; Proteins: 12 g.

33. Blueberry Muffins
Preparation time: 5 minutes
Cooking time: 25 minutes
Servings: 8

Ingredients:
- Almond milk – ½ cup
- Unsweetened applesauce – ½ cup
- Maple syrup – ½ cup
- Vanilla extract – 1 tsp.
- Whole-wheat flour – 2 cups
- Baking soda – ½ tsp.
- Blueberries – 1 cup

Directions:

1 - Preheat the oven to 375F.
2 - In a bowl, mix the applesauce, milk, maple syrup, and vanilla.
3 - Stir in the flour and baking soda until no dry flour is left, and the batter is smooth. Gently fold in the blueberries.
4 - In a muffin tin, fill 8 muffin cups (about ¾ full).
5 - Bake for 25 minutes.
6.   Cool and serve.
Nutrition: Calories: 200 Fat: 1g Carb: 45g Protein: 4g

34. Banana Bread

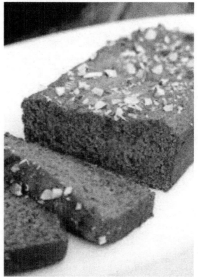

Preparation time: 5 minutes
Cooking time: 1 hour

Servings: 8

Ingredients:

- Ripe bananas – 4
- Maple syrup – ¼ cup
- Apple cider vinegar – 1 Tbsp.
- Vanilla extract – 1 tsp.
- Whole-wheat flour – 1 ½ cups
- Ground cinnamon – ½ tsp.
- Baking soda – ½ tsp.
- Walnut pieces – ¼ cup

Directions:

1 - Preheat the oven to 350F.
2 - Mash the bananas and stir in the maple syrup, apple cider vinegar, and vanilla.
3 - Stir in the flour, cinnamon, and baking soda. Fold in the walnut pieces.
4 - Pour the batter into a loaf pan (fill about ¾ full).
5 - Bake for 1 hour.
6 - Cool and slice.

Nutrition: Calories: 178 Fat: 1g Carb: 40g Protein: 4g

35. Pancakes
Preparation time: 5 minutes
Cooking time: 15 minutes
Servings: 8

Ingredients:

- Whole-wheat flour – 1 cup
- Baking powder – 1 tsp.
- Ground cinnamon – ½ tsp.
- Almond milk – 1 cup
- Unsweetened applesauce – ½ cup
- Maple syrup – ¼ cup
- Vanilla extract – 1 tsp.

Directions:

1 - Combine the flour, baking powder, and cinnamon.
2 - Stir in the milk, apple sauce, maple syrup, and vanilla until smooth.
3 - Heat a skillet and pour ¼ cup batter for each pancake. Cook about 2 minutes on each side.

4 - Repeat and serve.
Nutrition: Calories: 210 Fat: 2g Carb: 44g Protein: 5g

36. Granola
Preparation time: 5 minutes
Cooking time: 20 minutes
Servings: 4

Ingredients:

- Rolled oats – 1 ½ cups
- Pecan pieces – ¼ cup
- Maple syrup – ¼ cup
- Vanilla extract – 1 tsp.
- Ground cinnamon - ½ tsp.

Directions:

1 - Line a baking sheet with parchment paper. Preheat the oven to 300F.
2 - Combine the oats, pecan pieces, maple syrup, vanilla, and cinnamon. Stir to mix.
3 - Spread the mixture on the baking sheet.
4 - Bake for 20 minutes. Stirring once after 10 minutes.
5 - Cool, slice, and serve.

Nutrition: Calories: 220 Fat: 7g Carb: 35g Protein: 5g

37. Overnight Oatmeal
Preparation time: Overnight
Cooking time: 0 minutes
Servings: 2

Ingredients:

- Rolled oats – 2 cups
- Almond milk – 2 cups
- Diced mango – ½ cup
- Pineapple chunks – ½ cup
- Banana – 1, sliced
- Maple syrup – 1 Tbsp.
- Chia seeds – 1 Tbsp.

Directions:

1 - Mix the oats, milk, mango, pineapple, banana, maple syrup, and chia seeds.

2 - Cover and refrigerate overnight.

3 - Serve in the morning.

Nutrition: Calories: 510 Fat: 12g Carb: 93g Protein: 14g

38. Pumpkin Pie Oatmeal
Preparation time: 5 minutes
Cooking time: 35 minutes
Servings: 4

Ingredients:

- Almond milk – 3 cups
- Steel-cut oats – 1 cup
- Unsweetened pumpkin puree – 1 cup
- Maple syrup – 2 Tbsp.
- Ground cinnamon – 1 tsp.
- Ground cloves – 1/8 tsp.
- Ground nutmeg – 1/8 tsp.

Directions:

1 - In a pan, bring the milk to a boil. Then lower heat and stir in oats, pumpkin puree, maple syrup, cinnamon, cloves, and nutmeg.

2 - Cover and cook for 30 minutes. Stir from time to time.

Nutrition: Calories: 218 Fat: 5g Carb: 38g Protein: 7g

39. Chocolate And Peanut Butter Quinoa
Preparation time: 5 minutes
Cooking time: 10 minutes
Servings: 2

Ingredients:

- Almond milk – 1 cup
- Cooked quinoa – 2 cups
- Maple syrup – 1 Tbsp.
- Cocoa powder – 1 Tbsp.
- Defatted peanut powder – 1 tbsp.

Directions:

1 - Bring the milk to a boil in a saucepan.

2 - Then reduce the heat and stir in the quinoa, maple syrup, cocoa powder, and peanut powder.

3 - Cook and stir for 5 minutes.

Nutrition: Calories: 339 Fat: 8g Carb: 53g Protein: 14g

40. Breakfast Scramble
Preparation time: 5 minutes
Cooking time: 15 minutes
Servings: 2

Ingredients:

- Extra-firm tofu – 1 (14-ounce) package
- Mushrooms – 4 ounces, sliced
- Bell pepper – ½, diced
- Nutritional yeast – 2 Tbsp.
- Vegetable broth – 1 Tbsp.
- Garlic powder – ½ tsp.
- Onion powder – ½ tsp.
- Ground black pepper – 1/8 tsp.
- Fresh spinach – 1 cup

Directions:

1 - Heat a skillet over medium-low heat.

2 - Drain the tofu, and place it in the skillet. Mash with a spoon.

3 - Stir in bell pepper, mushrooms, nutritional yeast, garlic powder, onion powder, pepper, and broth.

4 - Cover and cook for 10 minutes. Stirring occasionally.

5 - Uncover and stir in the spinach.

6 - Cook for 5 minutes and serve.

Nutrition: Calories: 230 Fat: 10g Carb: 16g Protein: 27g

41. Sweet Potato Breakfast Skillet
Preparation time: 5 minutes
Cooking time: 15 minutes
Servings: 4

Ingredients:

- Sweet potatoes – 4-medium, chopped
- Mushrooms – 8 ounces, sliced
- Bell pepper – 1, diced
- Sweet onion – 1, diced
- Vegetable broth – 1 cup, plus more if needed
- Garlic powder – 1 tsp.
- Ground cumin – ½ tsp.
- Chili powder – ½ tsp.
- Ground black pepper – 1/8 tsp.

Directions:

1 - Heat a skillet over medium-low heat.
2 - Put the mushrooms, sweet potatoes, bell pepper, onion, broth, garlic powder, cumin, chili powder, and pepper in it and mix.
3 - Cover and cook for 10 minutes.
4 - Uncover and mix. Add more broth if needed.
5 - Cook, uncovered, for 5 minutes more. Stirring occasionally.

Nutrition: Calories: 158 Fat: 1g Carb: 34g Protein: 6g

42. Corn with Tofu
Preparation Time: 10 minutes
Cooking Time: 15 minutes
Servings: 1

Ingredients:

- 1 cups corn
- Salt and black pepper to the taste
- 1/2 tablespoon olive oil
- Juice of 1 lime
- 1 teaspoon smoked paprika
- 1/2 cup soft tofu, crumbled

Directions:

1 - In your air fryer, mix oil with corn, salt, pepper, lime juice and paprika. Toss well, cover and cook at 400° F for 15 minutes.
2 - Divide between plates. Sprinkle tofu crumbles all over, and serve hot.

Nutrition: Calories: 160; Fat: 2 g; Fibers: 2 g; Carbs: 12 g; Proteins: 4 g.

43. Cauliflower Oatmeal
Preparation Time: 15 minutes
Cooking Time: 15 minutes
Servings: 2

Ingredients:

- 1 cup cauliflower rice
- ½ cup unsweetened almond milk
- ½ teaspoon cinnamon
- 1 tablespoon maple syrup
- ½ tablespoon peanut butter
- 1 strawberry, sliced

Directions:
1 - Mix milk with cauliflower rice, maple syrup and cinnamon in a saucepan.
2 - Cook the rice mixture to a boil, then reduce the heat to low.
3 - Now cook the mixture for 10 minutes on a simmer.
4 - Allow the oatmeal to cool, then garnish it with a strawberry.

Nutrition: Calories: 234; Fat: 4.7 g; Sodium: 1 mg; Carbs: 18 g; Fiber: 7 g; Sugar: 3.3 g; Proteins: 6 g.

44. Pumpkin Oatmeal
Preparation Time: 15 minutes
Cooking Time: 45 minutes
Servings: 4
Ingredients:

- 2½ cups rolled oats
- 3 tablespoons chia seeds
- 1 teaspoon baking powder
- 1 teaspoon cinnamon
- ½ teaspoon cardamom
- ½ teaspoon salt
- 1 ¾ cups almond milk
- 1 (15-ounce) can pumpkin
- 1/3 cup maple syrup
- 1 tablespoon pure vanilla extract

Directions:

1 - Preheat your oven to 350° F. Layer an 8x8-inch baking dish with wax paper. Mix oats with salt, cardamom, cinnamon, baking powder, and chia seeds in a bowl.

2 - Now, stir the rest of the oatmeal ingredients and mix it well until smooth. Spread this batter in the baking dish and bake for 45 minutes. Allow the oatmeal to cool and serve.

Nutrition: Calories: 284; Fat: 7.9 g; Sodium: 704 mg; Carbs: 31 g; Fiber: 3.6 g; Sugar: 6 g; Proteins: 8 g.

45. Berry Cobbler

Preparation Time: 15 minutes
Cooking Time: 30 minutes
Servings: 4

Ingredients:

- 1 cup fresh blueberries
- 1 cup fresh blackberries
- 1 cup fresh raspberries
- 1 cup of water
- 3 tablespoons tapioca starch
- ½ teaspoon cinnamon
- ¼ cup coconut sugar
- Cobbler topping
- 1 cup rolled oats
- 2/3 cup whole wheat flour
- ¼ cup coconut sugar
- 1 tablespoon flaxseeds
- 1 tablespoon hemp seeds
- 1 tablespoon chia seeds
- 3 tablespoons coconut oil, melted
- 1/3 cup almond milk
- ¼ teaspoon pure vanilla extract
- ¼ teaspoon cinnamon
- ¾ teaspoon baking powder
- 1 pinch of pink salt

Directions:

1 - Preheat your oven to 375° F.
2 - Mix all the berries filling ingredients in a saucepan and cook on a simmer until it thickens.
3 - Remove the filling from the heat and spread it in a greased baking dish.

4 - Mix oats with coconut sugar with cinnamon, hemp shells, chia seeds, flour, flaxseeds, salt and baking powder in a large bowl.
5 - Stir in vanilla, milk and coconut oil, then mix well. Spread this batter on top of the filling.
6 - Bake the cobbler for 30 minutes at 375° F. Allow it to cool and serve.

Nutrition: Calories: 317; Fat: 13 g; Sodium: 114 mg; Carbs: 31 g; Fiber: 1 g; Sugar: 10 g; Proteins: 11 g.

46. Protein Bars

Preparation Time: 10 minutes
Cooking Time: 20 minutes
Servings: 6

Ingredients:

- 1½ cup quick-cooking oats
- ½ cup almond meal
- ½ cup flaxseed meal
- 2 teaspoons cinnamon
- ½ teaspoon salt
- 4 tablespoons vegan protein powder
- 1 teaspoon pure vanilla extract
- 2 bananas, ripe and mashed
- ½ cup applesauce
- ¼ cup creamy peanut butter
- 2 tablespoons maple syrup

Directions:

1 - Preheat your oven to 350° F. Layer an 8x8 square baking dish with cooking spray.
2 - Mix all the ingredients in a large bowl.
3 - Spread this mixture in the prepared pan.
4 - Bake the batter for 20 minutes in the oven.
5 - Allow the mixture to cool, then slice.

Nutrition: Calories: 248; Fat: 12 g; Sodium: 321 mg; Carbs: 26 g; Fiber: 4 g; Sugar: 8 g; Proteins: 7 g.

47. French Toast

Preparation Time: 5 minutes
Cooking Time: 12 minutes
Servings: 4

Ingredients:

- 4 slices of bread, whole-grain
- ½ cup rolled oats
- ½ cup pecans
- 1 tablespoon ground flax seed
- ½ teaspoon ground cinnamon
- 1/3 cup almond milk
- Maple syrup for serving
- Olive oil spray

Directions:

1 - Switch on the air fryer, insert the fryer basket, shut it with the lid, set the frying temperature 350º F, and preheat for 5 minutes.

2 - Meanwhile, prepare the topping. Place oats in a food processor; add flax seeds, pecans, and cinnamon it and pulse for 2 minutes until the mixture resembles breadcrumbs.

3 - Tip the mixture in a shallow dish; take another shallow dish and pour milk into it.

4 - Add bread slices, one at a time, and then let them soak for 15 seconds. Don't let it be mushy.

5 - Open the preheated fryer, place prepared bread slices in it in a single layer. Spray with olive oil, close the lid and cook for 6 minutes until golden brown, turning and spraying with oil halfway.

6. - When done, the air fryer will beep. Then open the lid and transfer the toast to a dish. Sprinkle the prepared topping on it, and cover with foil to keep it warm.

7 - Prepare the remaining toast in the same manner. Sprinkle with remaining topping, and serve straight away.

Nutrition: Calories: 102.2; Fat: 3.4 g; Carbs: 28.2 g; Proteins: 6.2 g; Fiber: 3.6 g.

48. Acai Bowl

Preparation time: 5 minutes
Cooking time: 5 minutes
Servings: 2

Ingredients:
For the toppings:
- 1 handful coconut flakes
- 1 handful pepitas
- 1/2 mango, diced
- 4 sliced strawberries

- 1 handful of blueberries

For the acai bowl:
- 1 cup pineapple chunks, frozen
- 1 large banana
- 1/2 mango
- 7 oz. acai pulp, frozen and unsweetened
- 1 tbsp lime juice
- 1/4 cup cold water

Directions:

1 - Start by freezing your serving bowls to help prevent the acai from melting once served.

2 - Next, start prepping the toppings by toasting the coconut flakes under medium heat in a small skillet, stirring often. Remove and transfer them to the frozen bowl.

For the acai:

3- Start by placing mango, banana, and pineapple in a high-speed blender. Blast until they are combined and chunky.

4 - Once done, thaw your acai pulp under lukewarm water until it breaks into smaller chunks, and then remove it from the packaging. Pour into the blender together with the lime juice and water. Blast on high for 2 minutes until smooth.

5 - Pour into the frozen bowls and top with the coconut, pepitas, mango, pineapple, banana, and berries.

6 - Serve immediately.

Nutrition: Calories: 78 Protein: 6 g Carbohydrates: 3.2 g Fat: 1 g

49. Banana Almond Granola

Preparation time: 10 minutes
Cooking time: 40 minutes
Servings: 6

Ingredients:

- 8 cups oats, rolled
- 2 cups dates, pitted and chopped
- 2 bananas, chopped
- 1 tsp almond extract
- 1 tsp salt
- 1 cup almonds, slivered and toasted (optional)

- 1 cup of water

Directions:

1. Preheat your oven to 275°F.
2. Put the oats in a large mixing bowl and set them aside.
3. In the meantime, line two baking sheets with parchment paper. I use the 13 × 18-inch.
4. Add 1 cup of water to the dates in a medium saucepan and boil over medium heat for 10 minutes.
5. Remove from the heat and transfer to a blender.
6. Add the almond extract, bananas, and salt. Blast on high for 2 minutes until smooth and creamy.
7. Pour the date mixture into the oats and mix well.
8. Equally, divide the almonds between the lined baking sheets and spread them out evenly.
9. Place in an oven and bake for 20 minutes, stirring occasionally, until crispy.
10 - Remove and allow it to cool for 10 minutes or more.
11 - Top with slivered almonds if you wish and enjoy.

Nutrition: Calories: 87 Protein: 18 g Carbohydrates: 9.7 g Fat: 2 g

50. Honeydew Smoothie
Preparation time: 5 minutes
Cooking time: 3 minutes
Servings: 2

Ingredients:

- 5 cups honeydew melon, diced
- 1/4 cup coconut milk
- 1/4 cup pineapple, frozen
- 1 tsp maple syrup
- 1/4 tsp vanilla extract
- A pinch kosher salts
- Mint leaves for garnishing

Directions:

1 - Place the diced honeydew melon in a blender and blend for 1 minute until smooth.

2 - Pour all the other remaining ingredients and continue blending for 2 more minutes.
3 - Pour into glasses, garnish, and enjoy.

Nutrition: Calories: 99 Protein: 13 g Carbohydrates: 6 g Fat: 3 g

51. Chocolate Blueberry Smoothie
Preparation time: 3 minutes
Cooking time: 2 minutes
Servings: 1

Ingredients:

- 1 banana, sliced
- 1 cup blueberries, frozen
- 1/2 cup almond milk
- 1 tbsp maple syrup
- 1/2 tsp vanilla extract
- 1 tbsp cocoa powder

Directions:

1 - Add all the ingredients into a high-powered blender and blend on high until smooth.

Nutrition: Calories: 107 Protein: 10 g Carbohydrates: 13.2 g Fat: 1.8 g

52. Chickpea Omelet
Preparation time: 5 minutes
Cooking time: 5 minutes
Servings: 3 omelets

Ingredients:

- 1 cup chickpea flour
- 3 medium green onions, chopped
- 4 oz. mushrooms, sautéed (optional)
- 1/2 tsp onion powder
- 1/2 tsp garlic powder
- 1/4 tsp white pepper
- 1/4 tsp black pepper, ground
- 1/3 cup nutritional yeast
- 1/2 tsp baking soda
- 1 cup of water

Directions:

1 - Combine all the dry ingredients in a medium bowl. Add 1 cup of water and stir until you have a smooth batter. Set aside.
2 - Heat a frying pan over medium heat and start pouring the batter as if you are making pancakes.
3 - As it cooks, sprinkle each omelet with onions and mushrooms.
4.   Serve and top with spinach, tomatoes, salsa, hot sauce, or any other plant-perfect fix you like.

Nutrition: Calories: 356 Protein: 27.2 g Carbohydrates: 5.2 g Fat: 8 g

53. Sweet Polenta with Pears

Preparation time: 5 minutes
Cooking time: 10 minutes
Servings: 3

Ingredients:

- 1/4 cup brown rice syrup
- 2 large pears, peeled, cored, and diced
- 1 cup fresh cranberries
- 1 tsp cinnamon, ground
- 1 batch Polenta, warm

Directions:

1 - Pour the rice syrup into a medium saucepan. Add the cranberries, pears, and cinnamon. Cook for 10 minutes stirring occasionally.
2 - Once the pears are tender, remove and pour on the polenta.

Nutrition: Calories: 226 Protein: 17.9 g Carbohydrates: 12 g Fat: 7 g.

54. Tropi-Kale Breeze

Preparation time: 5 minutes
Cooking time: 0 minutes
Servings: 4

Ingredients:

- 1 cup chopped pineapple (frozen or fresh)
- 1 cup chopped mango (frozen or fresh)

- 1/2 to 1 cup chopped kale
- 1/2 avocado
- 1/2 cup coconut milk
- 1 cup water, or coconut water
- 1 tsp Matcha green tea powder (optional)

Directions:

Preparing the ingredients.
1 - Purée everything in a blender until smooth, adding more water (or coconut milk) if needed.

Nutrition: Calories: 566 Protein: 8 g Fat: 36 g Saturated fat: 1 g Carbohydrates: 66 g Fiber: 12 g

55. Cinnamon Congee with Apricots and Dates

Preparation time: 8 minutes
Cooking time: 20 minutes
Servings: 4

Ingredients:

- 2 cups water
- 4 cups cooked brown rice
- 1/2 cup chopped unsulfured apricots
- 1/2 cup dates, pitted and chopped
- 1/4 tsp ground cloves
- 1 large cinnamon stick
- Salt, to taste (optional)

Directions:

1 - Bring the water to a boil in a large saucepan over medium heat.
2 - Once it starts to boil, add the remaining ingredients, except the salt, to the saucepan and stir well. Reduce the heat to medium-low and cook for 15 minutes, or until the mixture is thickened.
3 - Season to taste with salt, if desired. Remove the cinnamon stick before serving.

Nutrition: Calories: 313 Fat: 1.9 g Carbohydrates: 68.8 g Protein: 6.0 g Fiber: 6.2 g

56. Potato Medley

Preparation time: 15 minutes
Cooking time: 20 minutes
Servings: 4 to 6

Ingredients:

- 4 potatoes, peeled or unpeeled, cut into 3/4-inch cubes
- 1 onion, cut into cubes (separate the pieces)
- 1 green bell pepper, chopped into large pieces
- 4 garlic cloves, sliced
- 1 cup water, divided
- 2 cups thawed frozen or fresh corn
- 1 large tomato, diced

Directions:

1 - Combine the potatoes, onion, bell pepper, and garlic in a nonstick frying pan with 1/2 cup of water. Cook, stirring, over medium heat for 5 minutes.
2 - Add the remaining 1/2 cup of water to the pan. Cover and cook for an additional 10 minutes, stirring occasionally.
3 - Add the corn and tomato, stir, and cook for another 5 minutes.
4 - Serve warm.

Nutrition: Calories: 275 Fat: 0.7 g Carbohydrates: 60.1 g Protein: 7.5 g Fiber: 7.8 g

57. Orange French Toast
Preparation time: 10 minutes
Cooking time: 25 minutes
Servings: 3

Ingredients:

- 1 1/2 cup almond milk, unsweetened
- 1/2 cup almond flour
- 1 cup aquafaba
- 2 tbsp maple syrup
- 1/4 tsp cinnamon, ground
- 2 pinches of salt
- 1/2 tbsp orange zest
- 6 slices whole-grain bread
For the berry compote:

- 1 cup fresh blueberries
- 1/2 cup applesauce
- 1 tsp maple syrup

Directions:

1 - Preheat your oven to 400°F and place a wire rack over a baking sheet.
2 - Add the almond milk, almond flour, maple syrup, aquafaba, cinnamon, and salt to a bowl. Stir until you have a smooth mixture. Transfer the flour mixture to a shallow pan and pour in the orange zest. Mix well.
3 - In the meantime, start warming a nonstick skillet over medium heat. Immerse each bread slice into the flour mixture ensuring they are properly soaked on both sides. Place in the skillet and cook for 3 minutes on each side until golden brown.
4 - Repeat until all the toasts are done.
5 - Next, transfer them to the oven and bake for 15 minutes, until crisp.
Making the berry compote:
6 - Combine all the compote ingredients in a blender and blast on low for 30 seconds until you have a chunky consistency.
7 - Remove the toasts from the oven and serve with the berry compote.

Nutrition: Calories: 166 Protein: 12.4 g Carbohydrates: 26.8 g Fat: 13 g.

58. Almond Butter Banana Overnight Oats
Preparation Time: 5 minutes
Cooking Time: 10 minutes
Servings: 2

Ingredients:

- ½ cup rolled oats
- 1 cup almond milk
- 1 tablespoon chia seeds
- ¼ teaspoon vanilla extract
- ½ teaspoon ground cinnamon
- 1 tablespoon maple syrup
- 1 banana, sliced
- 2 tablespoons natural almond butter

Directions:

1 - Take a large bowl and add the oats, milk, chia seeds, vanilla, cinnamon, and maple syrup.
2 - Stir to combine then divide half of the mixture between two bowls.
3 - Top with the banana and peanut butter then add the remaining mixture.
4 - Cover then pop into the fridge overnight.
Nutrition: calories 227 fat 11 carbs 35 protein 7

59. Peach & Chia Seed Breakfast Parfait

Preparation Time: 5 minutes
Cooking Time: 10 minutes
Servings: 4

Ingredients:

- ¼ cup chia seeds
- 1 tablespoon pure maple syrup
- 1 cup of coconut milk
- 1 teaspoon ground cinnamon
- 3 medium peaches, diced small
- 2/3 cup granola

Directions:

1 - Find a small bowl and add the chia seeds, maple syrup, and coconut milk.
2 - Stir well then cover and pop into the fridge for at least one hour.
3 - Find another bowl, add the peaches and sprinkle with the cinnamon. Pop to one side.
4 - When it's time to serve, take two glasses, and pour the chia mixture between the two.
5 - Sprinkle the granola over the top, keeping a tiny amount to one side to use to decorate later.
6 - Top with the peaches and the reserved granola and serve.

Nutrition: calories 260 fat 13 carbs 22 protein 6

60. Blueberry Pancakes

Preparation time: 15 minutes
Cooking time: 20 minutes
Servings: 10 pancakes

Ingredients:

- 1 flax egg
- 1 cup almond flour
- 1 cup almond milk
- 1 cup fresh blueberries
- 2 tsp baking powder
- 1/4 tsp cinnamon
- 1/4 tsp kosher salt
- 1 tsp apple cider vinegar
- 1 tsp maple syrup, plus more for serving
- 2 tbsp vegetable oil
- A pinch turmeric (optional)

Directions:

1 - Flax egg recipe: 1 tbsp flaxseed meal + 3 tbsp water.
2 - Let the flax egg sit for at least 15 minutes.
3 - Meanwhile, whisk together the flour, salt, baking powder, and cinnamon in a mixing bowl.
4 - In a separate bowl, add the almond milk, vinegar, and oil. By now, the egg is done, add it into the mixture.
5 - Stir the dry ingredients into the wet ingredients with a pinch of turmeric.
6 - Heat a skillet over medium heat and lightly spray with vegetable oil. Pour the batter ensuring it forms small circles, and top with blueberries on top.
7 - Once the underside is cooked, flip and cook until golden brown.
8 - Serve immediately and top with maple syrup.

Nutrition: Calories: 137 Protein: 14.6 g Carbohydrates: 18 g Fat: 4.5 g

61. Apple Cinnamon Cut Oats

Preparation time: 5 minutes
Cooking time: 24 minutes
Servings: 6

Ingredients:

- 3 large apples, sliced
- 3 cups steel-cut oats
- 8 cups water
- 2 tsp vanilla extract

- 2 tsp cinnamon
- 1/4 tsp kosher salt

Toppings:
- Cashew butter
- Maple Syrup
- Milk
- Fruits of choice

Directions:

1 - Place all the ingredients into a pressure cooker except the toppings.
2 - Close the lid and seal the vent.
3 - Cook on high pressure: It will take around 10 minutes for your cooker to "preheat" and come up to pressure.
4 - Once ready, allow the pressure to naturally release for 10 minutes.
5 - Next, open the lid and stir the mixture to form a thick cream.
6 - Serve immediately and top with the milk, maple syrup, cashew butter, and fruits of choice.
Tip: You can store the leftovers refrigerated for up to 4 days.

Nutrition: Calories: 372 Protein: 18.3 g Carbohydrates: 30 g Fat: 11.2 g

62. Ful Medammes Breakfast

Preparation time: 10 hours
Cooking time: 2 hours 15 minutes
Servings: 6

Ingredients:

- 2 lb. dried fava beans, soaked for 10 hours
- 2 onions, diced
- 6 garlic cloves, minced
- 1 1/2 tsp cumin, ground
- Zest and juice of 2 lemons
- Salt to taste
- 1 medium lemon, quartered
- 4 inches of water

Directions:

1 - After soaking your fava bean for 10 hours, drain and rinse them.
2 - Transfer to a large cooking pot and cover with 4 inches of water.
3 - Bring to a boil over high heat and then reduce the heat to medium.
4 - Cover with a lid and continue cooking for 2 hours until tender.
5 - In the meantime, sauté your onions in a medium skillet over medium heat for 10 minutes.
6 - Toss in the garlic, cumin, and lemon juice, and zest. Continue cooking for 5 minutes. Set aside.
7 - By now, the beans are fully cooked. Drain the water in the cooking pot ensuring you leave 1 cup. Add the onion mixture and salt. Mix well.
8 - Serve and garnish with lemon quarters.

Nutrition: Calories: 95 Protein: 27.2 g Carbohydrates: 5 g Fat: 4 g.

Chapter 16.   Lunch

63. Cauliflower with Peas
Preparation Time: 15 minutes
Cooking Time: 15 minutes
Servings: 3

Ingredients:

- 2 medium tomatoes, chopped
- ¼ cup water
- 2 tablespoons olive oil
- 3 garlic cloves, minced
- ½ tablespoon fresh ginger, minced
- 1 teaspoon ground cumin
- 2 teaspoons ground coriander
- 1 teaspoon cayenne pepper
- ¼ teaspoon ground turmeric
- 2 cups cauliflower, chopped
- 1 cup fresh green peas, shelled
- Salt and ground black pepper, as required
- ½ cup warm water

Directions:

1 - In a blender, add tomato and ¼ cup of water and pulse until a smooth puree forms. Set aside.
2 - In a large skillet, heat the oil over medium heat and sauté the garlic, ginger, green chilies and spices for about 1 minute.
3 - Add the cauliflower, peas and tomato puree and cook, stirring for about 3-4 minutes.
4 - Add the warm water and bring to a boil.
5 - Now, lower the heat to medium-low and cook, covered for about 8-10 minutes or until vegetables are done completely.
6 - Serve hot.

Nutrition: Calories: 163 Fat: 10.1g Carbohydrates: 16.1g Dietary Fiber: 5.6g Sugar: 6.7g Protein: 6g

64. Banana Curry
Preparation Time: 15 minutes
Cooking Time: 15 minutes
Servings: 3

Ingredients:

- tablespoons olive oil
- 2 yellow onions, chopped
- 8 garlic cloves, minced
- 2 tablespoons curry powder
- 1 tablespoon ground ginger
- 1 tablespoon ground cumin
- 1 teaspoon ground turmeric
- 1 teaspoon ground cinnamon
- 1 teaspoon red chili powder
- Salt and ground black pepper, as required
- 2/3 cup soy yogurt
- 1 cup tomato puree
- 2 bananas, peeled and sliced
- 3 tomatoes, chopped finely
- ¼ cup unsweetened coconut flakes

Directions:

1 - In a large saucepan, heat the oil over medium heat and sauté onion for about 4-5 minutes.
2 - Add the garlic, curry powder and spices and sauté for about 1 minute.
3 - Add the soy yogurt and tomato sauce and bring to a gentle boil.
4 - Stir in the bananas and simmer for about 3 minutes.
5 - Stir in the tomatoes and simmer for about 1-2 minutes.
6 - Stir in the coconut flakes and immediately remove from the heat.
7 - Serve hot.

Nutrition: Calories: 382 Fat: 18.2g Carbohydrates: 53.4g Dietary Fiber: 11.3g Sugar: 24.8g Protein: 9g

65. Spiced Okra
Preparation Time: 15 minutes
Cooking Time: 13 minutes
Servings: 2

Ingredients:

- 1 tablespoon olive oil
- ½ teaspoon cumin seeds
- ¾ pound okra pods, trimmed and cut into 2-inch pieces

- ½ teaspoon curry powder
- ½ teaspoon red chili powder
- 1 teaspoon ground coriander
- Salt and ground black pepper, as required

Directions:

1 - In a large non-stick skillet, heat the oil over medium heat and sauté the cumin seeds for 30 seconds.
2 - Add the okra and stir fry for 1-1½ minutes.
3 - Now, lower the heat to low and cook, covered for 6-8 minutes, stirring occasionally.
4 - Uncover and increase the heat to medium.
5 - Stir in curry powder, red chili powder, and coriander and cook for 2-3 more minutes.
6 - Season with salt and remove from heat.
7 - Serve hot.

Nutrition: Calories: 134 Fat: 7.6g Carbohydrates: 13.6g Dietary Fiber: 5.9g Sugar: 2.6g Protein: 3.5g

66. Eggplant Curry
Preparation Time: 15 minutes
Cooking Time: 35 minutes
Servings: 3

Ingredients:

- 1 tablespoon coconut oil
- 1 medium onion, chopped finely
- 2 garlic cloves, minced
- ½ tablespoon fresh ginger, minced
- 1 Serrano pepper, seeded and minced
- 1 teaspoon curry powder
- ¼ teaspoon cayenne pepper
- Salt, as required
- 1 medium tomato, finely chopped
- 1 large eggplant, cubed
- 1 cup unsweetened coconut milk
- 2 tablespoons fresh cilantro, chopped

Directions:

1 - In a large non-stick skillet, melt the coconut oil over medium heat and sauté the onion for 8-9 minutes.

2 - Add the garlic, garlic, Serrano pepper, curry powder, cayenne pepper, and salt and sauté for 1 minute.
3 - Add the tomato and cook for 3-4 minutes, crushing with the back of spoon.
4 - Add the eggplant and salt and cook for 1 minute, stirring occasionally.
5 - Stir in the coconut milk and bring to a gentle boil.
6 - Now, lower the heat to medium-low and simmer, covered for 15-20 minutes or until done completely.
7 - Serve with a garnish of cilantro.

Nutrition: Calories: 124 Fat: 6.4g Carbohydrates: 16.6g Dietary Fiber: 7.5g Sugar: 7.4g Protein: 2.6g

67. Tofu with Broccoli
Preparation Time: 15 minutes
Cooking Time: 13 minutes
Servings: 4

Ingredients:

- 1 (14-ounce) package firm tofu, drained, pressed, and cut into 5 slices
- 2 tablespoons coconut oil, divided
- 2 cups small broccoli florets
- ¼ cup water
- ½ tablespoon garlic, minced
- ½ tablespoon fresh ginger, minced
- Ground black pepper, as required

Directions:

1 - In a large non-stick skillet, melt 1 tablespoon of the coconut oil over medium-high heat and cook the tofu for 4-5 minutes per side or until crispy
2 - With a slotted spoon, scoop the tofu slices onto a paper towel-lined plate to absorb any extra oil.
3 - Then, cut each tofu slice into equal sized pieces.
4 - Meanwhile, in a large microwave-safe bowl, add the broccoli florets and water.
5 - Cover the bowl and microwave on high for about 5 minutes.
6 - Remove from the microwave and drain the broccoli.
7 - In the same skillet, melt the remaining coconut oil over medium heat and sauté the garlic and ginger for about 1 minute.

8 - Add the tofu, broccoli and black pepper and cook for 2 minutes, tossing occasionally.

9 - Remove from the heat and serve hot.

Nutrition: Calories: 184 Fat: 14.1g Carbohydrates: 1.8g Dietary Fiber: 0.8g Sugar: 0.6g Protein: 10.2g

68. Tempeh with Bell Peppers

Preparation Time: 15 minutes
Cooking Time: 15 minutes
Servings: 3

Ingredients:

- 2 tablespoons balsamic vinegar
- 2 tablespoons low-sodium soy sauce
- 2 tablespoons tomato sauce
- 1 teaspoon maple syrup
- ½ teaspoon garlic powder
- 1/8 teaspoon red pepper flakes, crushed
- 1 tablespoon vegetable oil
- 8 ounces tempeh, cut into cubes
- 1 medium onion, chopped
- 2 large bell peppers, seeded and chopped

Directions:

1 - In a small bowl, add the vinegar, soy sauce, tomato sauce, maple syrup, garlic powder and red pepper flakes and beat until well combined. Set aside.

2 - Heat 1 tablespoon of oil in a large skillet over medium heat and cook the tempeh about 2-3 minutes per side.

3 - Add the onion and bell peppers and heat for about 2-3 minutes.

4 - Stir in the sauce mixture and cook for about 3-5 minutes, stirring frequently.

5 - Serve hot.

Nutrition: Calories: 241 Fat: 13g Carbohydrates: 19.7g Dietary Fiber: 2.1g Sugar: 8.1g Protein: 16.1g

69. Pasta with Asparagus

Preparation Time: 15 minutes
Cooking Time: 12 minutes
Servings: 4

Ingredients:

- ¼ cup olive oil
- 5 garlic cloves, minced
- ½ teaspoon red pepper flakes, crushed
- 1/8 teaspoon hot pepper sauce
- 1 pound asparagus, trimmed and cut into 1½-inch pieces
- Salt and ground black pepper, as required
- ½ pound cooked whole-wheat pasta, drained

Directions:

1 - In a large cast-iron skillet, heat the oil over medium heat and cook the garlic, red pepper flakes and hot pepper sauce for about 1 minute.

2 - Add the asparagus, salt and black pepper and cook for about 8-10 minutes, stirring occasionally.

3 - Place the hot pasta and toss to coat well.

4 - Serve immediately.

Nutrition: Calories: 326 Fat: 13.8g Carbohydrates: 39g Dietary Fiber: 8.5g Sugar: 2.2g Protein: 11.9g

70. Tofu Lettuce Wraps

Preparation Time: 20 minutes
Cooking Time: 6 minutes
Servings: 4

Ingredients:

For Wraps
- 1 tablespoon olive oil
- 14 ounces extra-firm tofu, drained, pressed and cut into cubes
- 1 teaspoon curry powder
- Salt, as required
- 8 lettuce leaves
- 1 small carrot, peeled and julienned
- ½ cup radishes, sliced
- ¼ cup peanuts, chopped
- 2 tablespoons fresh cilantro, chopped

For Sauce:
- ½ cup creamy peanut butter
- 2 tablespoons maple syrup
- 2 tablespoons low-sodium soy sauce
- 2 tablespoons fresh lime juice
- ¼ teaspoon red pepper flakes, crushed
- ¼ cup water

Directions:

1 - For tofu: in a skillet, heat the oil over medium heat and cook the tofu, curry powder and a little salt for about 5-6 minutes or until golden brown, stirring frequently.
2 - Remove from the heat and set aside to cool slightly.
3 - Meanwhile, for sauce: in a bowl, add all the ingredients and beat until smooth.
4 - Arrange the lettuce leaves onto serving plates.
5 - Divide the tofu, carrot, radish and peanuts over each leaf evenly.
6 - Garnish with cilantro and serve alongside the peanut sauce.

Nutrition: Calories: 381 Fat: 28.5g Carbohydrates: 19.2g Dietary Fiber: 4.4g Sugar: 11.4g Protein: 19.4g

71. Tofu & Oat Burgers

Preparation Time: 15 minutes
Cooking Time: 16 minutes
Servings: 4

Ingredients:

- 1 pound firm tofu, drained, pressed, and crumbled
- ¾ cup rolled oats
- ¼ cup flaxseeds
- 2 cups frozen spinach, thawed
- 1 medium onion, chopped finely
- 4 garlic cloves, minced
- 1 teaspoon ground cumin
- 1 teaspoon red pepper flakes, crushed
- Salt and ground black pepper, as required
- 2 tablespoons olive oil
- 6 cups fresh salad greens

Directions:

1 - In a bowl, add all the ingredients except for oil and salad greens and mix until well combined.
2 - Set aside for about 10 minutes.
3 - Make desired size patties from the mixture.
4 - In a non-stick frying pan, heat the oil over medium heat and cook the patties for 6-8 minutes per side.
5 - Serve these patties alongside the salad greens.

Nutrition: Calories: 185 Fat: 10.2g Carbohydrates: 14.6g Dietary Fiber: 5.1g Sugar: 2.8g Protein: 9.8g

72. Chickpea Lentil Burgers

Preparation Time: 20 minutes
Cooking Time: 10 minutes
Servings: 3

Ingredients:

For Burgers:
- 1 cup chickpea lentil
- 1 cup onion, chopped finely
- 2 green chilies, chopped finely
- 1 teaspoon garlic paste
- 1 teaspoon ginger paste
- Pinch of ground turmeric
- Salt, as required
- 2 tablespoons olive oil
  For Serving:
- 4 cups lettuce, torn

Directions:

1 - In a bowl of water, soak the chickpea lentil for at least 3-4 hours.
2 - Drain the lentils and rinse under cold running water.
3 - Through a strainer, strain the lentils completely.
4 - In the bowl of a food processor, place lentils and pulse until a coarse paste is formed.
5 - Transfer the lentils into a bowl.
6 - Add the onion, green chilies, garlic paste, ginger paste, turmeric and salt and mix until well combined.
7 - Make small equal-sized patties from the mixture.
8 - In a non-stick skillet, heat olive oil over medium heat and cook half of the patties for 5 minutes, flipping occasionally.
9 - Divide the lettuce onto serving plates and top each with patties.
10 - Serve immediately.

Nutrition: Calories: 204 Fat: 10.5g Carbohydrates: 24.7g Dietary Fiber: 4.9g Sugar: 2.4g Protein: 4.8g

73. Lentil Falafel

Preparation Time: 20 minutes

Cooking Time: 20 minutes
Servings: 4

Ingredients:

For Falafel:
• 4 tablespoons fresh parsley
• 1 small red onion, chopped roughly
• 2 garlic cloves, peeled
• 1 cup red lentils, soaked overnight
• 2 tablespoons chickpea flour
• 2 tablespoons fresh lemon juice
• 2 tablespoons olive oil
• ½ teaspoon ground cumin
• Salt and ground black pepper, as required
For Serving:
• 6 cups lettuce, torn

Directions:

1 - Preheat your oven to 400 °F.
2 - Line a baking sheet with parchment paper.
3 - For falafel: in a food processor, add the parsley, onion and garlic and pulse until finely chopped.
4 - Now, place the remaining ingredients and pulse until just combined.
5 - Make small-sized patties from the mixture.
6 - Arrange the patties onto the prepared baking sheet in a single layer.
7 - Bake for approximately 18-20 minutes or until patties become golden brown.
8 - For the dressing: in a bowl, add all the plates and serve immediately.

Nutrition: Calories: 265 Fat: 8g Carbohydrates: 35.6g Dietary Fiber: 16.1g Sugar: 3.1g Protein: 13.9g

74. Stuffed Avocados
Preparation Time: 15 minutes
Cooking Time: 0 minutes
Servings: 2

Ingredients:

• 1 large avocado, halved and pitted
• ¾ cup cooked chickpeas
• ¼ cup tomato, chopped
• ¼ cup cucumber, chopped
• ¼ cup onion, chopped
• 1 small garlic clove, minced
• 1 tablespoon fresh basil, chopped
• 1½ tablespoons fresh key lime juice
• ½ teaspoon olive oil

Directions:

1 - With a small spoon, scoop out the flesh from each avocado half.
2 - Then, cut half of the avocado flesh into equal-sized cubes.
3 - In a large bowl, add avocado cubes and remaining ingredients and toss to coat well.
4 - Stuff each avocado half with the chickpeas mixture evenly and serve immediately.

Nutrition: Calories: 337 Fat: 1.9g Carbohydrates: 32.2g Dietary Fiber: 4.4g Sugar: 1.9g Protein: 7g

75. Stuffed Bell Peppers
Preparation Time: 15 minutes
Cooking Time: 1 hour
Servings: 4

Ingredients:

• 1 tablespoon olive oil
• 1 medium onion, chopped
• 2 garlic cloves, minced
• ½ cup light coconut milk
• ½ cup green bell peppers, seeded and chopped
• 4 tablespoons tomatoes, crushed
• 2 tablespoons low-sodium soy sauce
• 1 tablespoon peanut butter
• ½ tablespoon curry powder
• ¼ teaspoon smoked paprika
• Salt and ground black pepper, as required
• 2 cups cooked rice
• 1 cup cooked black beans
• 4 bell peppers, tops removed and seeded

Directions:

1 - Preheat your oven 375 °F.

2 - Lightly, grease a baking dish.

3 - Heat the olive oil in a skillet over medium-low heat and sauté the onion and garlic for about 4-5 minutes.

4 - Add the chopped bell peppers, tomatoes, soy sauce, peanut butter, spices, salt, black pepper and coconut milk and simmer for about 5 minutes, stirring occasionally.

5 - Stir in the cooked rice and chickpeas and remove from heat.

6 - Set aside to cool slightly.

7 - Arrange the bell peppers onto the prepared baking dish.

8 - Stuff each bell pepper with rice mixture.

9 - Bake for approximately 30-45 minutes or until bell peppers are tender.

10 - Serve warm.

Nutrition: Calories: 315 Fat: 13.5g Carbohydrates: 42.4g Dietary Fiber: 8g Sugar: 6.3g Protein: 9.5g

76. Stuffed Sweet Potatoes

Preparation Time: 20 minutes
Cooking Time: 40 minutes
Servings: 2

Ingredients:

For Sweet Potatoes:
- 1 large sweet potato, halved
- ½ tablespoon olive oil
- Salt and ground black pepper, as required

For Filling:
- ½ tablespoon olive oil
- 1/3 cup canned chickpeas, rinsed and Drained
- 1 teaspoon curry powder
- 1/8 teaspoon garlic powder
- 1/3 cup cooked quinoa
- Salt and ground black pepper, as required
- 1 teaspoon fresh lime juice
- 1 teaspoon fresh cilantro, chopped
- 1 teaspoon sesame seeds

Directions:

1 - Preheat your oven to 375 °F.

2 - Rub each sweet potato half with oil evenly.

3 - Arrange the sweet potato halves onto a baking sheet, cut side down and sprinkle with salt and black pepper.

4 - Bake for 40 minutes or until sweet potato becomes tender.

5 - Meanwhile, for filling: in a skillet, heat the oil over medium heat and cook the chickpeas, curry powder and garlic powder for about 6-8 minutes, stirring frequently.

6 - Stir in the cooked quinoa, salt and black pepper and remove from the heat.

7 - Remove from the oven and arrange each sweet potato halves onto a plate.

8 - With a fork, fluff the flesh of each half slightly.

9 - Place chickpeas mixture in each half and drizzle with lime juice

10 - Serve immediately with the garnishing of cilantro and sesame seeds.

Nutrition: Calories: 340 Fat: 8.2g Carbohydrates: 50g Dietary Fiber: 10g Sugar: 8.8g Protein: 12.6g

77. Tangy Broccoli Salad

Preparation Time: 15 minutes
Cooking Time: 0 minutes
Servings: 4

Ingredients:

- 2 heads broccoli, stems, and florets chopped (about 5 cups)
- 3 scallions, thinly sliced
- ½ cup carrots, grated
- ¼ cup hemp hearts
- 2 tablespoons tahini
- 2 tablespoons apple cider vinegar
- 2 tablespoons water
- 2 teaspoons maple syrup
- 1 garlic clove
- ¼ teaspoon salt
- Freshly ground black pepper, to taste

Directions:

1 - Place the broccoli, scallions, carrots, and hemp hearts in a large bowl. Whisk the tahini, vinegar, water, maple syrup, garlic, and salt in a measuring cup or small bowl. Add as much pepper as you'd like.

2 - Put the dressing over the salad and mix until everything is well combined.

Nutrition: Calories: 189 Fat: 11 g Carbohydrates: 15 g Protein: 10 g

78. Summer Rolls with Peanut Sauce

Preparation Time: 15 minutes
Cooking Time: 0 minutes
Servings: 4-6
Ingredients:

- 6 to 8 Vietnamese/Thai round rice paper wraps
- 1 (13 ounces) package organic, extra-firm smoked or plain tofu, drained, cut into long, thin slices
- 1 cucumber, cored, cut into matchsticks (about 1 cup)
- 1 cup carrot, cut into matchsticks
- 1 cup mung bean or soybean sprouts
- 4 to 6 cups spinach
- 12 to 16 basil leaves
- 3 to 4 mint sprigs
- Sweet peanut dressing

Directions:

1 - Place the rice paper wrap under running water or in a large bowl of water for a moment, then set it on a plate or cutting board to absorb the water for 30 seconds. The wrap should be transparent and pliable.
2 - Place your desired amount of filling on each wrap, being careful not to overfill because they will be hard to close.
3 - Tightly fold the bottom of the wraps over the ingredients, and then fold in each side. Continue rolling each wrap onto itself to form the rolls. Enjoy your rolls dipped in sweet peanut dressing.

Nutrition: Calories: 216 Fat: 6 g Carbohydrates: 32 g Protein: 13 g

79. Cheesy White Bean Cauliflower Soup

Preparation Time: 15 minutes
Cooking Time: 35 minutes
Servings: 6

Ingredients:

- 1 tablespoon olive oil
- 1 onion, chopped
- 2 celery stalks, chopped
- 2 carrots, chopped
- 3 garlic cloves, minced
- 1 teaspoon turmeric
- 1 head cauliflower, chopped into florets (about 5 cups)
- 4 cups vegetable broth
- 1 cup unsweetened nondairy milk
- ¼ cup nutritional yeast
- 1 teaspoon onion powder
- ½ teaspoon salt
- ½ lemon juice
- 2 (14 ounces) cans white navy or cannellini beans, drained and rinsed
- Freshly ground black pepper, to taste

Directions:

1 - In a large stockpot, warm the oil over medium heat. Add the onion, celery, and carrots. Cook until the onions become slightly translucent, within 5 minutes. Add the garlic and turmeric and cook for 1 minute more.
2 - Add the cauliflower and broth. Cover and bring to a boil. Once boiling, reduce the heat and simmer, covered, until the cauliflower has softened, about 10 minutes. Pour in the milk, yeast, onion powder, and salt, then stir it.
3 - Remove the pot and either use an immersion blender to puree the soup or transfer it to a mixer and process it until smooth.
4 - Once a smooth consistency is reached, return the soup to heat and add the lemon juice and beans. Stir and taste it; add extra salt and black pepper, if desired. Enjoy this soup with hot sauce.

Nutrition: Calories: 238 Fat: 4 g Carbohydrates: 37 g Protein: 15 g

80. Split Pea Soup

Preparation Time: 15 minutes
Cooking Time: 60 minutes

Servings: 6

Ingredients:

- 2 tablespoons olive oil
- 1 medium onion, coarsely chopped
- 2 carrots, coarsely chopped
- 2 celery stalks, coarsely chopped
- 2 teaspoons plus a pinch salt, divided
- 2 cups yellow split peas, rinsed and drained
- 8 cups water
- 1 bay leaf
- 1 teaspoon paprika
- Freshly ground black pepper, to taste
- 6 cups spinach, chopped

Directions:

1 - In a large stockpot, warm the oil over medium heat. Add the onion, carrots, celery, and a pinch of salt and cook until the onions start to soften.
2 - Add the split peas, water, bay leaf, paprika, remaining 2 teaspoons of salt, and pepper. Bring to a boil.
3 - Adjust the heat to low, then simmer, occasionally stirring, until the split peas are soft and the soup is thick about 50 minutes.
4 - Remove and discard the bay leaf. Stir in the spinach and sausage (if using) and cook for a couple of minutes more, taste, adjust seasonings with salt and pepper.

Nutrition: Calories: 362 Fat: 10 g Carbohydrates: 46 g Protein: 25 g

81. Quinoa & Chickpea Tabbouleh

Preparation Time: 25 minutes
Cooking Time: 0 minutes
Servings: 6

Ingredients:

- 1 cup quinoa, cooked
- 1 cup tomato, chopped
- 1 cup cucumber, chopped
- 1 cup scallions, chopped
- 1 cup fresh parsley, chopped
- 1 (14 ounces) can chickpeas, drained and rinsed

- 2 garlic cloves, minced
- ¼ cup chopped mint/1 tablespoon dried mint
- 2 tablespoons olive oil
- 1 lemon juice
- ½ teaspoon salt
- Freshly ground black pepper, to taste

Directions:

1 - Mix the quinoa, tomato, cucumber, scallions, parsley, chickpeas, garlic, and mint in a large bowl.
2 - Pour the olive oil plus lemon juice over the quinoa mixture, then stir in the salt and as much pepper as you'd like. Stir until everything is well combined. Enjoy immediately.

Nutrition: Calories: 170 Fat: 6 g Carbohydrates: 25 g Protein: 6 g

82. Cauliflower Caesar Salad with Chickpea Croutons

Preparation Time: 15 minutes
Cooking Time: 40 minutes
Servings: 4

Ingredients:

- 1 head cauliflower, chopped (about 8 cups)
- 3 tablespoons oil, divided
- ¼ teaspoon plus a few pinches salt, divided
- 1 (14 ounces) can chickpeas, drained and rinsed
- 1 teaspoon oregano
- ¼ teaspoon garlic powder
- ¼ teaspoon onion powder
- 2 heads romaine lettuce, chopped
- Tofu Caesar dressing

Directions:

1 - Preheat the oven to 450°Fahrenheit. Prepare two baking sheets lined using parchment paper or silicone liners.
2 - Mix the cauliflower, 2 tablespoons of olive oil, and a few big pinches of salt in a large bowl. Blend to ensure the cauliflower is well coated with oil. Spread

the cauliflower out evenly on one of the baking sheets.

3 - In a medium bowl, combine the chickpeas, the remaining 1 tablespoon of olive oil, oregano, garlic powder, onion powder, and the remaining ¼ teaspoon of salt. Spread the chickpeas out evenly on the other baking sheet.

4 - Place the sheets in the oven and bake for 20 minutes; then give the sheet with the chickpeas a bit of a shake to ensure they aren't sticking or burning. Continue baking for 20 minutes more or until the cauliflower is soft and the chickpeas are crunchy.

5 - To serve, divide the lettuce among 4 bowls and top each with even portions of the cauliflower, chickpeas, and about ¼ cup of Caesar dressing.

Nutrition: Calories: 365 Fat: 20 g Carbohydrates: 37 g Protein: 16 g

83. Vegetable Rose Potato

Preparation Time: 15 minutes
Cooking Time: 20 minutes
Servings: 4

Ingredients:

* 4 red rose potatoes
* 6 leaves Lacinato kale, stemmed, chopped
* 2 tablespoons olive oil
* 1 onion, chopped
* 1 green bell pepper, diced
* Ground pepper and salt, to taste

Directions:

1 - Microwave your potatoes until done but still firm. Finely chop them when cool.

2 - Preheat oil in a skillet over medium heat. Sauté onions until translucent. Add potatoes and bell pepper and sauté, stirring constantly, over medium-high heat until golden brown.

3 - Stir in the kale and seasoning, then cook, stirring constantly until the mixture is a bit browned. Occasionally add water to prevent sticking if necessary. Sprinkle with pepper and salt to taste. Serve hot.

Nutrition: Calories: 337 Fat: 7.4 g Carbohydrates: 63 g Protein: 8 g

84. Rice Arugula Salad

Preparation Time: 15 minutes
Cooking Time: 8 minutes
Servings: 2

Ingredients:

* 1 cup wild rice, cooked
* 1 handful arugula, washed
* ¾ cup almonds
* 6 sun-dried tomatoes in oil, chopped
* 3 tablespoons olive oil
* 1 onion
* Pepper and salt, to taste

Directions:

1 - Put your frying pan over low heat and roast the almonds for 3 minutes. Transfer to a salad bowl.

2 - Sauté onions in olive oil for 3 minutes on low heat. Add dried tomatoes and cook for about 2 minutes. Transfer to a bowl.

3 - Add the remaining olive oil to the pan and fry the bread until crunchy. Sprinkle with pepper and salt. Set aside.

4 - Add arugula to the bowl containing sautéed tomato mixture. Add wild rice and toss to combine. Season with pepper and salt.

Nutrition: Calories: 688 Fat: 37.7 g Carbohydrates: 56 g Protein: 19 g

85. Tomato Salad

Preparation Time: 15 minutes
Cooking Time: 0 minutes
Servings: 4

Ingredients:

* 1 head romaine lettuce, washed, chopped
* 1 avocado, sliced
* 24 cherry tomatoes
* ½ cup cilantro, chopped
* Fresh lime juice, for dressing

Directions:

1 - Divide all the ingredients between 4 plates and drizzle with lime juice dressing.
2 - Toss well to combine.
3 - Enjoy immediately.

Nutrition: Calories: 203 Fat: 16.2 g Carbohydrates: 12 g Protein: 6 g

86. Kale Apple Roasted Root Vegetable Salad

Preparation Time: 15 minutes
Cooking Time: 25 minutes
Servings: 6

Ingredients:

- 1-½ cups parsnips, turnips, and red rose potatoes, diced
- 8 cups kale, chopped
- ½ cup apple chunks
- 2 tablespoons apple cider vinegar
- ½ teaspoon cinnamon
- ½ teaspoon turmeric
- 4 tablespoons olive oil, divided
- Salt and pepper, to taste

Directions:

1 - Place a skillet over medium heat. Add vinegar, apple, cinnamon, turmeric, and salt. Bring the mixture to a boil and set aside.
2 - Preheat the oven to 350°Fahrenheit. Preheat oil in a cast-iron pan over medium heat. Add parsnips, turnips and red rose potatoes then cook for about 5 minutes.
3 - Transfer to the oven and roast for about 10 minutes. Place a skillet over medium heat. Add the remaining olive oil. To the skillet add the kale and apples and cook for about 4 minutes.
4 - Add the parsnips, turnips, red rose potatoes, and vinegar mixture to the skillet. Cook for about 5 minutes. Add salt and pepper to taste. Serve while hot and enjoy!

Nutrition: Calories: 128 Fat: 16 g Carbohydrates: 32 g Protein: 3 g

87. Rice Arugula Salad with Sesame Garlic Dressing

Preparation Time: 15 minutes
Cooking Time: 0 minutes
Servings: 4

Ingredients:

- 1 cup wild rice, cooked
- 1 teaspoon cumin
- ½ bunch arugula, chopped
- 2 tablespoons parsley, chopped
- 2 tablespoons basil, chopped
- Salt and black pepper, to taste
  For the dressing:
- 1 head garlic, roasted and peeled
- ½ cup apple juice
- ¼ cup lemon juice
- ¼ cup tahini
- ¼ cup virgin olive oil
- Salt, to taste

Directions:

1 - Add the dressing ingredients to a blender and blend until the mixture is creamy and smooth. Set aside.
2 - Place a stockpot over medium-high heat. Season rice with cumin and salt. Pour half of the dressing on top and mix well. Set aside to chill for about 10 minutes.
3 - To the bowl, add arugula, parsley, basil, olives, salt, and pepper.
4 - Serve and enjoy!

Nutrition: Calories: 447 Fat: 44.4 g Carbohydrates: 43 g Protein: 19 g

88. Garden Pasta Salad

Preparation Time: 10 minutes
Cooking Time: 12 minutes
Servings: 4

Ingredients:

For the Salad:
- 1 cup chopped kale
- ¼ cup chopped basil

- 2 cups sliced yellow cherry tomatoes
- 16 ounces tri-colored pasta

For the Dressing:
- ½ teaspoon sea salt
- ¼ teaspoon ground black pepper
- 1 teaspoon dried Italian seasoning
- ½ cup white wine vinegar
- 3 tablespoons lemon juice
- 1 teaspoon olive oil

Directions:

1 - Cook the pasta. For this, take a large pot half full with salty water, place it over medium heat and bring it to a boil.
2 - Add pasta, cook within 10 to 12 minutes until tender, and then drain well into a colander.
3 - While pasta cooks, prepare the dressing. For this, take a small bowl, place all of its ingredients in it and whisk until combined.
4 - Transfer pasta into a large bowl. Add remaining ingredients for the salad; drizzle with prepared dressing and then toss until well combined.
5 - Serve straight away.

Nutrition: Calories: 424 Fat: 3 g Carbohydrates: 46 g Protein: 13 g

89. Roasted Vegetables and Tofu Salad

Preparation Time: 10 minutes
Cooking Time: 25 minutes
Servings: 4

Ingredients:

For the salad:
- 2 cups chopped tofu, firm, pressed, drained
- 2 cups cooked chickpeas
- 4 cups spinach
- 2 cups broccoli floret
- 2 cups chopped sweet potato, peeled
- 2 cups Brussel sprout, halved
- 4 teaspoons ground black pepper
- 4 teaspoons salt
- 4 tablespoons red chili powder
- 1 cup olive oil

For the dressing:
- 2 teaspoons salt

- 2 teaspoons ground black pepper
- 4 teaspoons dried thyme
- 4 tablespoons lemon juice
- 4 tablespoons olive oil
- 2 teaspoons water
- ½ cup hummus

Directions:

1 - Switch on the oven, then set it to 400°Fahrenheit and let it preheat.
2 - Take a large baking sheet, grease it with oil, and spread broccoli florets in one-fifth of the portion, reserving few florets for later use.
3 - Add sprouts, sweet potatoes, tofu, and chickpeas as an individual pile on the baking sheet, drizzle with oil, season with salt, black pepper, and red chili powder.
4 - Bake for 25 minutes until the tofu has turned nicely golden brown and vegetables are softened, tossing halfway.
5 - While vegetables, grains, and tofu are being roasted, prepare the dressing and for this, take a medium jar, add all of its ingredients in it, stir until well combined, and then divide the dressing among four large mason jars.
6 - When vegetables, grains, and tofu has been roasted, distribute evenly among four mason jars along with reserved cauliflower florets and shut with lid.
7 - When ready to eat, shake the Mason jar until the salad is coated with the dressing and then serve.

Nutrition: Calories: 477 Fat: 24 g Carbohydrates: 52 g Protein: 21 g

90. Roasted Lemon Asparagus Watercress Salad

Preparation Time: 15 minutes
Cooking Time: 5 minutes
Servings: 4

Ingredients:

- 2 cups asparagus, ends trimmed

- 2 cups baby spinach
- 1 lemon, sliced, seeded
- 1 onion, sliced
- 1 teaspoon cayenne
- 2 tablespoons olive oil
- Salt and pepper, to taste

Directions:

1 - Preheat 1 tablespoon oil in a skillet over medium heat. Add the asparagus and cook for about 5 minutes. Set aside. Return the skillet to medium-low heat. Add the remaining olive oil.
2 - Add onion and lemon slices and cook for about 5 minutes. Remove from heat and season with salt, cayenne and pepper.
3 - Add the baby spinach to a large bowl. Add cooked onion and lemon slices on top. Finally, add the asparagus. Serve and enjoy!

Nutrition: Calories: 129 Fat: 7 g Carbohydrates: 11 g Protein: 5 g

91. Pumpkin and Brussels Sprouts Mix

Preparation Time: 15 minutes
Cooking Time: 35-40 minutes
Servings: 8

Ingredients:

- 1 pound Brussels sprouts, halved
- 1 pumpkin, peeled, cubed
- 4 garlic cloves, sliced
- 2 tablespoons fresh parsley, chopped
- 1 cup olive oil
- Salt and pepper, to taste

Directions:

1 - Warm oven to 400°Fahrenheit. Prepare a baking dish and coat with cooking spray. Mix sprouts, pumpkin, and garlic in a bowl. Add oil and toss well to coat the vegetables.
2 - Transfer to the baking dish and cook for 35-40 minutes. Stir once halfway.
3 - Serve topped with parsley.

Nutrition: Calories: 152 Fat: 9 g Carbohydrate 17 g Protein: 4 g

92. Almond and Tomato Salad

Preparation Time: 15 minutes
Cooking Time: 10 minutes
Servings: 4

Ingredients:

- 1 cup arugula/rocket
- 7 ounce fresh tomatoes, sliced or chopped
- 2 teaspoons olive oil
- 2 cups kale
- ½ cup almonds

Directions:

1 - Put oil into your pan and heat it on medium heat. Add tomatoes into the pan and fry for about 10 minutes.
2 - Once cooked, allow it to cool. Combine all salad ingredients in a bowl and serve.

Nutrition: Calories: 355 Fat: 19.1 g Carbohydrates: 8.3 g Protein: 33 g

93. Best Avocado Zucchini Sushi

Preparation time: 10 minutes
Cooking time: 0 minutes
Serving: 3

Ingredients:

- 2 medium zucchinis, sliced into thin, flat strips
- 1 avocado, mashed
- ½ carrot, julienned
- ½ cucumber, julienned
- ¼ cup Rainbow Hummus
- ½ lime, juiced
- 1 tablespoon black sesame seeds

Directions:

1 - To assemble the sushi, lay the zucchini strips flat horizontally. Place the avocado, carrot, and cumber vertically on one side of the zucchini. On the other side, spread the Rainbow Hummus.

2 - Sprinkle the entire zucchini with lime juice.

3 - Roll up the sushi, starting with the vegetable side. Serve the sushi standing up vertically on plates, topped with the black sesame seeds.

Nutrition: Calories: 210 | fat: 14g | carbs: 18g | protein: 6g | fiber: 8g

94. Walnut Pesto Broiled Cauliflower

Preparation time: 5 minutes
Cooking time: 30 minutes
Serving: 4

Ingredients:

- 2 heads cauliflower, stems removed and sliced into 1-inch steaks/slices
- ¾ cup Spinach-Walnut Pesto

Directions:

1 - Preheat the oven to 400°F (204°C) Pesto-Baked Cauliflower Steaks. Line a baking sheet with parchment paper.

2 - Place the cauliflower steaks on the baking sheet in a single layer.

3 - Brush half of the pesto on top of steaks and bake for 15 minutes.

4 - Flip the steaks and brush on remaining half of the pesto over them and bake for 15 minutes more.

5 - Turn the oven to broil and broil for 1 to 2 minutes, or until as crisp as desired.

Nutrition: Calories: 316 | fat: 26g | protein: 9g | carbs: 39g | fiber: 8g

95. Garlic and Pepper Spiced Eggplant

Preparation time: 10 minutes
Cooking time: 10 minutes
Serving: 6

Ingredients:

- 1 tablespoon olive oil
- ½ yellow onion, diced
- 3 garlic cloves, minced
- 1 head broccoli, diced
- 1 to 2 eggplants cut to a 1-inch dice
- 1 teaspoon fresh grated ginger
- Salt, to taste
- Pepper, to taste
- 1 cup Sweet-and-Sour Sauce

Directions:

1 - In a large skillet, heat the oil over medium heat. Add the onion and garlic and cook for 3 to 5 minutes, or until the onion is translucent. Then add the broccoli and sauté until tender.

2 - Add the eggplant and grated ginger to the pan and cook until the eggplant softens, about 5 minutes.

3 - Add the sweet-and-sour sauce to the skillet and stir. Bring to a simmer and let cook for 5 minutes, or until the sauce has thickened.

Nutrition: Calories: 133 | fat: 1g | protein: 4g | carbs: 29g | fiber: 5g

96. Sesame with Bean Stir-Fry

Preparation time: 10 minutes
Cooking time: 20 minutes
Serving: 4

Ingredients:

- 1 (14-ounce) package extra-firm tofu
- 2 tablespoons canola oil
- 1-pound green beans, chopped
- 2 carrots, peeled and thinly sliced
- ½ cup Stir-Fry Sauce or store-bought lower-sodium stir-fry sauce
- 2 cups fluffy brown rice
- 2 scallions, thinly sliced
- 2 tablespoons sesame seeds

Directions:

1 - Remove the tofu from the package and place it on a plate lined with a kitchen towel. Place another

kitchen towel on top of the tofu and place a heavy pot on top, changing towels if they become soaked. Let sit for 15 minutes to remove the moisture. Cut the tofu into 1-inch cubes.

2 - Heat the canola oil in a large wok or skillet to medium-high heat. Add the tofu cubes and cook, flipping every 1 to 2 minutes so all sides become browned. Remove from the skillet and place the green beans and carrots in the hot oil. Stir-fry for 4 to 5 minutes, tossing occasionally, until crisp and slightly tender.

3 - While the vegetables are cooking, prepare the Stir-Fry Sauce (if using homemade).

4 - Place the tofu back in the skillet. Pour the sauce over the tofu and vegetables and let simmer for 2 to 3 minutes.

5 - Serve the stir-fry over rice and top with scallions and sesame seeds.

6 - For leftovers, divide the stir-fry evenly into microwaveable airtight containers and store in the refrigerator for up to 5 days. Reheat in the microwave on high for 2 to 3 minutes, until heated through.

Nutrition: Calories: 380 | Fat: 15g | Protein: 16g | carbs: 45g | Fiber: 8g

97. Ginger Garlic Spiced Chickpea Potato Curry

Preparation time: 8 minutes
Cooking time: 22 minutes
Serving: 4

Ingredients:

- 1 tablespoon olive oil
- 1 onion, cut into ¼-inch dice
- 1 (1-inch) piece ginger, peeled and grated
- 2 garlic cloves, minced
- 1 tablespoon curry powder
- 2 large potatoes, cut into ½-inch dice
- 3 carrots, cut into ¼-inch dice
- 1 cup chickpeas
- 1 (15-ounce/425 g) can tomatoes
- 1 cup fresh or frozen green peas
- 1 teaspoon garam masala

- 1 (13.5-ounce/ 383 g) can light coconut milk
- ¼ teaspoon sea salt

Directions:

1 - Heat the olive oil in a Dutch oven over medium heat. Add the onion, ginger, and garlic, and sauté for about 3 minutes, until the onion is translucent. Add the curry powder and stir until fragrant.

2 Add the potatoes and carrots and sauté for 6 minutes. Add the chickpeas, tomatoes, peas, and garam masala. Stir in and simmer for 3 minutes.

3 - Whisk the coconut milk and salt into the vegetables and simmer for about 10 minutes, or until the sauce starts to thicken.

4 - Divide among 4 bowls and serve.

Nutrition: Calories: 347 | fat: 9g | protein: 11g | carbs: 62g | fiber: 14g

98. Harvest Vegetable Sauté

Preparation time: 10 minutes
Cooking time: 14 minutes
Serving: 4

Ingredients:

- 2 cloves garlic, pressed
- 2 tablespoons soy sauce
- 1 teaspoon grated fresh ginger
- Dash of sesame oil (optional)
- 1 small onion, coarsely chopped
- ¼ pound (113 g) mushrooms, sliced
- 2 small zucchinis, sliced
- 1 small yellow crookneck squash, cut in half and sliced
- 1 cup small cauliflower florets
- 1 cup small broccoli florets
- Freshly ground black pepper, to taste
- 1 cup water, divided

Directions:

1 - In a pan over medium heat, combine the garlic, soy sauce, ginger, sesame oil (if desired) and ¼ cup of the water. Bring to a boil.

2 - Add the onion and cook for 2 minutes, or until softened, stirring constantly.

3 - Stir in the remaining vegetables. Cook for 5 minutes, stirring constantly, or until the vegetables are coated with sauce. Pour in the remaining ¾ cup of the water, cover and steam for 5 minutes. Uncover and cook for 2 more minutes, or until all the liquid has been absorbed, stirring constantly.

4 - Season with pepper and serve.

Nutrition: Calories: 192 | fat: 2.0g | carbs: 33.6g | protein: 15.8g | fiber: 5.6g

99. Provençal Summer Vegetables

Preparation time: 15 minutes
Cooking time: 15 minutes
Serving: 6

Ingredients:

- 2 small zucchinis
- 2 ripe tomatoes
- 2 small thin eggplants
- 1 medium green bell pepper
- 1 small red onion
- ¼ pound (113 g) mushrooms
- 1/3 cup water
- 1 clove garlic, minced
- 1 tablespoon unsweetened tomato purée
- Freshly ground pepper, to taste
- ¼ cup chopped fresh basil
- ¼ cup chopped fresh parsley
- 1 teaspoon minced fresh thyme
- ½ teaspoon minced fresh rosemary

Directions:

1 - Wash and trim all the vegetables and cut into ½-inch cubes.

2 - Place the water in a large, heavy pot. Add the garlic and tomato purée. Heat, stirring, until well mixed.

3 - Add all the vegetables. Cover and cook over low heat for about 15 minutes, or until the vegetables are softened but not mushy. Season with freshly ground pepper.

4 - Stir in the basil, parsley, thyme and rosemary. Serve warm or cold.

Nutrition: Calories: 121 | fat: 0.7g | carbs: 29.1g | protein: 4.5g | fiber: 8.7g

100. Stuffed Tomatoes with Bulgur

Preparation time: 10 minutes
Cooking time: 45 to 46 minutes
Serving: 4

Ingredients:

- 4 large tomatoes (about 2 pounds / 907 g)
- 2 leeks (white and light green parts), diced small and rinsed
- 1 clove garlic, peeled and minced
- 3 ears corn, kernels removed (about 1½ cups)
- 1 medium zucchini, diced small
- 1 cup bulgur, cooked in 2 cups low-sodium vegetable broth
- Zest and juice of 1 lemon
- ½ cup finely chopped basil
- Sea salt, to taste (optional)
- Freshly ground black pepper, to taste

Directions:

1 - Preheat the oven to 350°F (180°C).

2 - Cut the tops off the tomatoes and hollow out the flesh with a spoon, leaving a ½-inch wall. Set aside.

3 - Sauté the leeks in a large saucepan over medium heat for 7 to 8 minutes, stirring occasionally.

4 - Add the garlic and cook for another 3 minutes. Stir in the corn and zucchini and cook for an additional 5 minutes.

5 - Add the cooked bulgur, lemon zest, juice, and basil and stir well. Sprinkle with salt (if desired) and pepper.

6 - Remove from the heat. Spoon the bulgur mixture evenly into the tomatoes and transfer to a baking dish.

7 - Wrap the dish in aluminum foil and bake in the preheated oven for 30 minutes.

8 - Remove the foil and let cool for 5 to 8 minutes before serving.

Nutrition: Calories: 348 | fat: 3.6g | carbs: 69.3g | protein: 9.7g | fiber: 9.7g

101. Eggplant Stuffed with Rice and Herbs

Preparation time: 15 minutes
Cooking time: 1 hour 37 minutes
Serving: 4

Ingredients:

- 2 cups low-sodium vegetable broth
- 1 cup brown basmati rice
- 1 cinnamon stick
- 2 medium eggplants, stemmed and halved lengthwise
- 1 celery stalk, diced small
- 1 medium yellow onion, peeled and diced small
- 1 medium red bell pepper, seeded and diced small
- Water, as needed
- 2 cloves garlic, peeled and minced
- ¼ cup finely chopped cilantro
- ¼ cup finely chopped basil
- Sea salt, to taste (optional)
- Freshly ground black pepper, to taste

Directions:

1 - Pour the vegetable broth into a medium saucepan and bring to a boil.

2 - Stir in the rice and cinnamon stick and cook covered over medium heat for 45 minutes, or until the rice is soft. Set aside.

3 - Scoop out the eggplant flesh, leaving a ¼-inch-thick shell on each half. Chop the eggplant flesh and set it aside with the shells.

4 - Preheat the oven to 350°F (180°C).

5 - In a large saucepan, add the celery, onion, and red pepper and sauté over medium heat for 7 to 8 minutes, or until the veggies are lightly browned. Add water, 1 to 2 tablespoons at a time, to prevent sticking.

6 - Stir in the eggplant fresh and garlic and cook for an additional 5 minutes, or until the eggplant is softened.

7 - Turn off the heat. Add the cooked rice, cilantro, and basil to the eggplant mixture. Sprinkle with salt (if desired) and pepper.

8 - Spoon the filling into the eggplant shells and arrange the stuffed eggplants in a baking dish. Wrap the dish in aluminum foil and bake for 40 minutes, or until the eggplants are nicely browned.

9 - Remove from the oven and let cool for 5 minutes before serving.

Nutrition: Calories: 308 | fat: 2.5g | carbs: 62.9g | protein: 8.3g | fiber: 12.1g

102. Yam and Carrot Casserole

Preparation time: 5 minutes
Cooking time: 55 minutes
Serving: 6 to 8

Ingredients:

- 6 medium yams, peeled and coarsely chopped
- 1-pound (454 g) carrots, scrubbed and sliced 1-inch thick
- ¾ cup pitted prunes
- 1 cup freshly squeezed orange juice
- ½ cup maple syrup (optional)
- ½ teaspoon ground cinnamon

Directions:

6 - Preheat the oven to 350°F (180°C).

7 - Place the yams and carrots in a large pot and cover with water. Cook over medium heat for about 15 minutes, or until tender but still firm. Remove from the heat and drain.

8 - Place the vegetables in a covered casserole dish. Stir in the prunes.

9 - Whisk together the orange juice, maple syrup (if desired) and cinnamon in a bowl. Spread over the vegetables and fruit. Cover and bake in the oven for 30 minutes. Uncover, stir gently, and continue to bake, uncovered, for another 10 minutes.

10 - Serve hot.

Nutrition: Calories: 317 | fat: 0.5g | carbs: 77.1g | protein: 3.6g | fiber: 8.4g

103. Zucchini Noodles with Tomatoes

Preparation Time: 15 minutes
Cooking Time: 7 minutes
Servings: 3

Ingredients:

- 2 tablespoons avocado oil
- 2 medium zucchinis, spiralized with Blade C
- 1 garlic clove, minced
- 1 cup tomatoes, chopped
- Salt, as required

Directions:

1. In a skillet, heat avocado oil over medium heat and cook the zucchini for about 3 minutes.
2 - Add the garlic and cook for about 1 minute.
3 - Add the cherry tomatoes and salt and cook for about 2-3 minutes.
4 - Serve hot.
Nutrition: Calories: 46 Fat: 1.6g Carbohydrates: 7.6g Dietary Fiber: 2.6g Sugar: 3.9g Protein: 2.3g

104. Broccoli with Bell Pepper

Preparation Time: 15 minutes
Cooking Time: 10 minutes
Servings: 4

Ingredients:

- 2 tablespoons olive oil
- 4 garlic cloves, minced
- 1 large white onion, sliced
- 2 cups small broccoli florets
- 3 red bell peppers, seeded and sliced
- ¼ cup vegetable broth
- Salt and ground black pepper, as required

Directions:

1 - In a non-stick skillet, heat the oil over medium heat and sauté the garlic for about 1 minute.
2 - Add the onion, broccoli and bell peppers and stir fry for about 5 minutes.
3 - Add the broth and stir fry for about 4 minutes more.

Nutrition: Calories: 126 Fat: 7.5g Carbohydrates: 14.3g Dietary Fiber: 2.3g Sugar: 6.9g Protein: 3.1g

105. Mushrooms with Bell Peppers

Preparation Time: 15 minutes
Cooking Time: 10 minutes
Servings: 4
Ingredients:

- 1 tablespoon grapeseed oil
- 3 cups fresh button mushrooms, sliced
- ¾ cup red bell peppers, seeded and cut into long strips
- ¾ cup yellow bell peppers, seeded and cut into long strips
- 1½ cup white onions, cut into long strips
- 2 teaspoons fresh sweet basil
- 2 teaspoons fresh oregano
- ½ teaspoon cayenne powder
- Salt, as required

Directions:

1 - In a cast-iron skillet, heat the grapeseed oil over medium-high heat and sauté the mushrooms, bell peppers and onion for about 5-6 minutes.
2 - Add in the herbs, cayenne pepper and salt and cook for about 2-3 minutes.
3 - Add in the lime juice and remove the skillet of veggies from heat.
4 - Serve hot.

Nutrition: Calories: 76 Fat: 3.8g Carbohydrates: 8.8g Dietary Fiber: 2.4g Sugar: 5g Protein: 2.7g

106. Tomato Soup

Preparation Time: 10 minutes
Cooking Time: 45 minutes
Servings: 4

Ingredients:

- 2 tablespoons coconut oil
- 2 carrots, peeled and chopped roughly
- 1 large white onion, chopped roughly
- 3 garlic cloves, minced
- 5 large tomatoes, chopped roughly
- ¼ cup fresh basil, chopped
- 1 tablespoon tomato paste
- 3 cups vegetable broth
- ¼ cup coconut milk
- Salt and ground black pepper, as required

Directions:

1 - In a large saucepan, melt the coconut oil over medium heat and cook the carrot and onion for about 10 minutes, stirring frequently.
2 - Add the garlic and cook for 1-2 minutes.
3 - Stir in the tomatoes, basil, tomato paste, and broth and bring to a boil.
4 - Now, lower the heat to low and simmer for about 30 minutes.
5 - Stir in the coconut milk, salt, and black pepper and remove from the heat.
6 - With an immersion blender, blend the soup until smooth.
7 - Serve hot.

Nutrition: Calories: 197 Fat: 12g Carbohydrates: 18.4g Dietary Fiber: 4.8g Sugar: 10.6g Protein: 7g

107. Harvest Bowl
Preparation Time: 15 minutes
Cooking Time: 35 minutes
Servings: 4

Ingredients:

- 1 tablespoon olive oil
- 2 small sweet potatoes, chopped (about 2 cups)
- ½ teaspoon cinnamon
- ¼ teaspoon salt
- 2 cups wild rice, cooked
- 1 (14 ounces) can lentils, drained and rinsed
- 1 (14 ounces) can chickpeas, drained and rinsed
- 4 cups kale, thinly sliced and gently massaged
- 1 cup grated or shredded carrots
- ¼ cup hemp hearts
- ¼ cup raw sauerkraut (optional)
- 3 tablespoons tahini apple cider vinaigrette

Directions:

1 - Warm oven to 400° Fahrenheit and lines a baking sheet with parchment paper. In a small bowl, mix the oil, potatoes, cinnamon, and salt.
2 - Place the potatoes on the baking sheet and bake for 35 minutes or until the potatoes are nice and soft.
3 - In each of the 4 food storage containers, put ½ cup of rice, ¼ cup of lentils, ¼ cup of chickpeas, ¼ of the sweet potatoes, 1 cup of kale, and ¼ cup of carrots.
4 - Garnish it with 1 tablespoon of hemp hearts and 1 tablespoon of sauerkraut (if using).
5 - Finally, top it with 3 tablespoons of tahini vinaigrette. Cover the remaining containers with airtight lids and store them in the refrigerator.

Nutrition: Calories: 563 Fat: 19 g Carbohydrates: 75 g Protein: 24 g

108. Cauliflower Fried Rice
Preparation Time: 15 minutes
Cooking Time: 15 minutes
Servings: 6

Ingredients:

- 1 head cauliflower
- 1 tablespoon sesame oil
- 1 white onion, finely chopped
- 1 large carrot, finely chopped
- 4 garlic cloves, minced
- 2 cups frozen edamame or peas
- 3 scallions, sliced
- 3 tablespoons Bragg liquid aminos or tamari
- Salt to taste
- Freshly ground black pepper, to taste

Directions:

1 - Cut the cauliflower into florets and transfer them to a food processor. Process the cauliflower using the

chopping blade and pulsing until the cauliflower gets the consistency of rice. Set aside.

2 - Warm a large skillet or wok over medium-high heat. Drizzle in the sesame oil and then add the onion and carrot, cooking until the carrots begin to soften for about 5 minutes. Stir in the garlic and cook within another minute.

3 - Add the cauliflower and edamame or peas. Heat until the cauliflower softens and the edamame or peas cook for about 5 minutes. Then add the scallions and liquid aminos or tamari. Combine well. Add in black pepper if desired.

Nutrition: Calories: 117 Fat: 3 g Carbohydrates: 19 g Protein: 7 g

109.   Curried Quinoa Salad

Preparation Time: 15 minutes
Cooking Time: 15 minutes
Servings: 6

Ingredients:

- 1 tablespoon olive oil
- 1 garlic clove, minced
- 1 teaspoon-sized piece ginger, minced
- 2 teaspoons curry powder
- 1 cup quinoa, rinsed under cold water using a fine-mesh strainer
- 1-½ cups vegetable broth
- 1 (14 ounces) can chickpeas, drained and rinsed
- 2 celery stalks, finely chopped
- 1 cup carrots, shredded
- ¾ cup raisins
- 1 cup cilantro, chopped
- 3 tablespoons olive oil
- 3 tablespoons apple cider vinegar
- ½ teaspoon salt
- Freshly ground black pepper, to taste

Directions:

1 - Warm up oil over medium heat in a small saucepan. Add the garlic and ginger; then cook for 1 minute. Add the curry powder and stir.

2 - Next, add the quinoa and toast it for about 5 minutes, stirring regularly. Then pour in the broth, turn the heat to high, and boil.

3 - Adjust your heat to simmer, cover the saucepan, and cook for about 15 minutes or until the quinoa is light and fluffy.

4 - Meanwhile, in a medium bowl, combine the chickpeas, celery, carrots, raisins, and cilantro. Once the quinoa is cooked, add it to the bowl as well. Then dress it with olive oil, vinegar, salt, and as much pepper as you'd like. Blend until well combined.

Nutrition: Calories: 327 Fat: 12 g Carbohydrates: 50 g Protein: 8 g

110.   Lettuce Wraps with Smoked Tofu

Preparation Time: 15 minutes
Cooking Time: 25 minutes
Servings: 4

Ingredients:

- 1 (13 ounces) package organic, extra-firm smoked tofu, drained and cubed
- 1 tablespoon coconut oil
- ½ cup yellow onion, finely chopped
- 3 celery stalks, finely chopped
- 1 red bell pepper, chopped
- A pinch salt
- 1 cup Cremini mushrooms, finely chopped
- 1 garlic clove, minced
- ½ teaspoon ginger, minced
- 3 tablespoons Bragg liquid aminos, coconut aminos, or tamari
- ½ teaspoon red pepper flakes
- Freshly ground black pepper, to taste
- 8 to 10 large romaine leaves, washed and patted dry

Directions:

1 - Preheat the oven to 350°Fahrenheit. Prepare a baking sheet lined using parchment paper or a silicone liner; then place the tofu cubes in a single layer. Bake the tofu cubes for 25 minutes, flipping them after 10 to 15 minutes. Set aside.

2 - Meanwhile, warm the coconut oil in a non-stick sauté pan over medium-high heat. Add the onion, celery, bell pepper, and salt and cook for about 5 minutes or until the onions are slightly translucent.

3 - Add the mushrooms, garlic, and ginger and sauté for about 5 minutes more or until the mushrooms begin to release water. Adjust the heat to medium; then put the aminos or tamari and the red pepper flakes.

4 - Add the baked tofu cubes to the pan and sprinkle with pepper. Sauté for a few minutes more, until the tofu is coated with sauce and the veggies are tender.

5 - To serve, scoop as much of the veggie and tofu mixture into each romaine leaf as you'd like.

Nutrition: Calories: 160 Fat: 8 g Carbohydrates: 6 g Protein: 14 g

111. Brussels Sprouts & Cranberries Salad

Preparation Time: 10 minutes
Cooking Time: 0 minutes
Servings: 6

Ingredients:

- 3 tablespoons lemon juice
- ¼ cup olive oil
- Salt and pepper to taste
- 1 pound Brussels sprouts, sliced thinly
- ¼ cup dried cranberries, chopped
- ½ cup pecans, toasted and chopped
- ½ cup parmesan cheese shaved

Directions:

1 - Mix the lemon juice, olive oil, salt, and pepper in a bowl. Toss the Brussels sprouts, cranberries, and pecans in this mixture. Sprinkle the parmesan cheese on top.

Nutrition: Calories: 245 Fat: 18.9 g Carbohydrates: 15.9 g Protein: 6.4 g

112. Quinoa Avocado Salad

Preparation Time: 15 minutes
Cooking Time: 4 minutes
Servings: 4

Ingredients:

- 2 tablespoons balsamic vinegar
- ¼ cup cream
- 5 tablespoons freshly squeezed lemon juice, divided
- 1 garlic clove, grated
- 2 tablespoons shallot, minced
- Salt and pepper to taste
- 2 tablespoons avocado oil, divided
- 1-¼ cups quinoa, cooked
- 2 heads endive, sliced
- 2 firm pears, sliced thinly
- 2 avocados, sliced
- ¼ cup fresh dill, chopped

Directions:

1 - Combine the vinegar, cream, 1 tablespoon of lemon juice, garlic, shallot, salt, and pepper in a bowl. Pour 1 tablespoon of oil into a pan over medium heat. Heat the quinoa for 4 minutes.

2 - Transfer quinoa to a plate. Toss the endive and pears in a mixture of remaining oil, remaining lemon juice, salt, and pepper. Transfer to a plate.

3 - Toss the avocado in the reserved dressing. Add to the plate. Top with the dill and quinoa.

Nutrition: Calories: 431 Fat: 28.5 g Carbohydrates: 42.7 g Protein: 6.6 g

113. Roasted Sweet Potatoes

Preparation Time: 20 minutes
Cooking Time: 20 minutes
Servings: 4

Ingredients:

- 2 potatoes, sliced into wedges
- 2 tablespoons olive oil, divided
- Salt and pepper to taste
- 1 red bell pepper, chopped
- ¼ cup fresh cilantro, chopped
- 1 garlic, minced
- 2 tablespoons almonds, toasted and sliced
- 1 tablespoon lime juice

Directions:

1 - Warm your oven to 425°Fahrenheit. Toss the sweet potatoes in oil and salt. Transfer to a baking pan. Roast for 20 minutes.

2 - In a bowl, combine the red bell pepper, cilantro, garlic, and almonds. In another bowl, mix the lime juice, remaining oil, salt, and pepper.

3 - Drizzle this mixture over the red bell pepper mixture. Serve sweet potatoes with the red bell pepper mixture.

Nutrition: Calories: 146 Fat: 8.6 g Carbohydrates: 16 g Protein: 2.3 g

114.   Greek Zoodle Bowl

Preparation Time: 10 minutes
Cooking Time: 0 minutes
Servings: 4

Ingredients:

- ½ cup chopped artichokes
- 14 cherry tomatoes, chopped
- 1 medium red bell peppers, cored, chopped
- 4 medium zucchinis
- 1 medium yellow bell pepper, cored, chopped
- 6 tablespoons hemp hearts
- 1 English cucumber
- 6 tablespoons chopped red onion
- 2 tablespoons chopped parsley leaves
- 2 tablespoons chopped mint

For the Greek Dressing:
- 2 tablespoons chopped mint
- 1 teaspoon garlic powder
- ½ teaspoon salt
- ¼ teaspoon dried oregano
- 2 teaspoons Italian seasoning
- 3 tablespoons red wine vinegar
- 1 tablespoon olive oil

Directions:

1 - Prepare zucchini and cucumber noodles, spiralize them using a spiralizer or vegetable peeler and then divide evenly among four bowls.

2 - Top zucchini and cucumber noodles with artichokes, tomato, bell pepper, hemp hearts, onion, parsley, and mint. Then set aside until required.

3 - Prepare the dressing: take a small bowl and add all the ingredients for the dressing. Whisk until combined.

4 - Add the prepared dressing evenly into each bowl. Then toss until the vegetables are well coated with the dressing and serve.

Nutrition: Calories: 250 Fat: 14 g Carbohydrates: 19 g Protein: 13 g

115.   Vegetable Burritos

Preparation time: 10 minutes
Cooking time: 7 to 8 minutes
Serving: 4

Ingredients:

- 1 bunch scallions, cut into 1-inch pieces
- 1 red bell pepper, sliced into strips
- 1 green bell pepper, sliced into strips
- ½ cup water
- 1 cup frozen corn kernels, thawed
- 1 cup salsa
- 2 teaspoons cornstarch
- 12 cherry tomatoes, cut in half
- 4 large whole-wheat tortillas
- Fresh cilantro sprigs (optional)

Directions:

1 - In a pan over medium heat, sauté the scallions and peppers in the water for 2 minutes. Add the corn and cook for another 2 to 3 minutes.

2 - Stir together the salsa and cornstarch in a small bowl. Pour over the vegetables. Cook for 2 minutes, stirring, or until thickened. Add the tomatoes and cook for 1 more minute.

3 - Place a line of the vegetable mixture down the center of a tortilla, and top with sprigs of cilantro, if desired. Roll up and serve.

Nutrition: Calories: 228 | fat: 4.9g | carbs: 40.2g | protein: 7.7g | fiber: 8.2g

116.   Twice-Baked Potatoes

Preparation time: 15 minutes
Cooking time: 1 hour 30 minutes
Serving: 6

Ingredients:

- 6 large russet potatoes, scrubbed
- 1 medium yellow onion, peeled and diced small
- 1 red bell pepper, deseeded and diced small
- 1 jalapeño pepper, deseeded and minced
- 2 cloves garlic, peeled and minced
- 1 tablespoon toasted and ground cumin seeds
- 2 teaspoons ancho chile powder
- 3 ears corn, kernels removed
- 2 cups cooked black beans
- 1 teaspoon salt (optional)
- ½ cup chopped cilantro
- 1 (12 ounce / 340-g) package extra firm silken tofu, drained
- ½ cup chopped green onion, white and green parts

Directions:

1 - Preheat the oven to 350°F (180°C).
2 - Pierce each potato with a fork a few times so that it will release steam during baking. Place the potatoes on a baking sheet and bake for 60 to 75 minutes, or until tender. Let cool until safe to handle.
3 - Place the onion and red pepper in a large skillet and sauté over medium heat for 7 to 8 minutes, or until the onion starts to brown. Add water 1 to 2 tablespoons at a time to keep the vegetables from sticking to the pan. Add the jalapeño pepper, garlic, cumin, and chile powder and sauté for another minute. Add the corn, black beans, salt (if desired) and cilantro and mix well. Remove from the heat.
4 - Puree the silken tofu in the blender. Add the pureed tofu to the vegetable mixture in the pan and mix well.
5 - Halve each potato lengthwise, and scoop out the flesh, leaving a ¼-inch-thick shell. Reserve the flesh for another use. Divide the vegetable filling evenly among the potato halves. Place the filled potatoes on a baking sheet and bake for 30 minutes.
6 - Serve garnished with the chopped green onion.

Nutrition: Calories: 503 | fat: 5.2g | carbs: 99.3g | protein: 21.8g | fiber: 13.3g

117.   Creamy Mushroom Stroganoff

Preparation time: 10 minutes
Cooking time: 25 to 26 minutes
Serving: 6 to 8

Ingredients:

- 1 large onion, chopped
- 1-pound (454 g) mushrooms, sliced
- 1 cup low-sodium vegetable broth
- 1 cup unsweetened soy milk
- 2 tablespoons sherry
- 2 tablespoons soy sauce
- Dash of cayenne
- 2 cups sliced seitan
- 2 tablespoons cornstarch, mixed with 1/3 cup cold water

Directions:

1 - In a saucepan over medium, heat a small amount of water. Add the onion and sauté for 2 to 3 minutes.
2 - Add the mushrooms and sauté for 3 minutes, or until the mushrooms are slightly limp.
3 - Stir in the vegetable broth, soy milk, sherry, soy sauce and cayenne. Mix in the seitan. Cover and cook over low heat for 20 minutes.
4 - Add the cornstarch mixture to the pan and stir until thickened.

Nutrition: Calories: 308 | fat: 3.7g | carbs: 52.4g | protein: 21.2g | fiber: 7.1g

118.   Carrot Pesto Chili

Preparation time: 10 minutes
Cooking time: 8 minutes
Serving: 4

Ingredients:

- ¼ cup olive oil, divided
- 2 medium carrots, peeled diced
- 1 small yellow onion, chopped
- 1 (15-ounce /425g) can diced tomatoes

- 1 teaspoon salt
- 1 teaspoon freshly ground black pepper
- 2 cups water
- 1 (15-ounce/425g) can chickpeas, drained and rinsed
- 1 (15-ounce/425g) can cannellini beans, drained and rinsed
- 1 (15-ounce/425g) can kidney beans, drained and rinsed
- ½ cup pesto

Directions:

1 - Add 1 tablespoon oil, carrots, and onion to a large saucepan over high heat and cook 3 to 5 minutes or until carrots are tender.

2 - Stir in tomatoes, salt, pepper, and water and bring to a boil. Add chickpeas and other cans of beans, cooking until heated through (about 3 minutes).

3 - Divide into 4 equal portions, top with pesto, and serve.

Nutrition: Calories: 537 | Fat: 39 g | Carbs: 37 g | Protein: 11 g | Fiber: 12 g

119. Spicy Chickpeas

Preparation Time: 15 minutes
Cooking Time: 20 minutes
Servings: 8

Ingredients:

- 1 tablespoon extra-virgin olive oil
- 1 yellow onion, diced
- 1 teaspoon curry
- ¼ teaspoon allspice
- 1 can diced tomatoes
- 2 cans chickpeas, rinsed, drained
- Salt and cayenne pepper, to taste

Directions:

1 - Simmer onions in 1 tablespoon oil for 4 minutes. Add allspice and pepper, cook for 2 minutes. Stir in tomatoes, and cook for another 2 minutes.

2 - Add chickpeas, and simmer for 10 minutes. Season with salt, and serve.

Nutrition: Calories: 146 Carbohydrates: 25 g Fat: 3 g Protein: 5 g

120. Farro with Pistachios & Herbs

Preparation Time: 20 minutes
Cooking Time: 45 minutes
Servings: 10

Ingredients:

- 2 cups farro
- 4 cups water
- 1 teaspoon kosher salt, divided
- 2-½ tablespoons extra-virgin olive oil
- 1 onion, chopped
- 2 garlic cloves, minced
- ½ teaspoon ground pepper, divided
- ½ cup parsley, chopped
- 4 ounces salted shelled pistachios, toasted, chopped

Directions:

1 - Combine farro, water, and ¾ teaspoon salt, simmer for 40 minutes. Cook onion plus garlic in 2 tablespoon oil for 5 minutes.

2 - Combine ½ teaspoon oil, ¼ teaspoon pepper, parsley, pistachios, and toss well. Combine all. Season with salt and pepper.

Nutrition: Calories: 220 Carbohydrates: 30 g Fat: 9 g Protein: 8 g

121. Broccoli Soup

Preparation Time: 15 minutes
Cooking Time: 45 minutes
Servings: 4

Ingredients:

- 2 tablespoons olive oil
- ½ cup onion, chopped
- 1 garlic clove, minced
- 1 tablespoon fresh thyme, chopped
- ¼ teaspoon ground cumin
- ¼ teaspoon red pepper flakes, crushed

- 2 medium heads broccoli, cut into florets
- 4 cups vegetable broth
- 1 avocado, peeled, pitted and chopped

Directions:

1 - In a large soup pan, heat the oil over medium heat and sauté the onion for about 4-5 minutes.
2 - Add the garlic, thyme and spices and sauté for about 1 minute more.
3 - Add the broccoli and cook for about 3-4 minutes.
4 - Stir in the broth and bring to a boil over high heat.
5 - Now, lower the heat to medium-low.
6 - Cover the soup pan and cook for about 32-35 minutes.
7 - Remove from the heat and set aside to cool slightly.
8 - In a blender, place the mixture in batches with avocado and pulse until smooth.
9 - Serve immediately.

Nutrition: Calories: 254 Fat: 18.7g Carbohydrates: 15.8g Dietary Fiber: 7.3g Sugar: 3.8g Protein: 9.7g

122.   Pumpkin Soup

Preparation Time: 15 minutes
Cooking Time: 25 minutes
Servings: 4

Ingredients:

- 2 teaspoons olive oil
- 1 onion, chopped
- 1 teaspoon fresh ginger, chopped
- 2 garlic cloves, chopped
- ¼ teaspoon ground coriander
- ¼ teaspoon ground cumin
- 2 tablespoons fresh cilantro, chopped
- 3 cups pumpkin, peeled and cubed
- 4¼ cups vegetable broth
- Salt and ground black pepper, as required
- ½ cup coconut cream
- 2 tablespoons fresh lime juice

Directions:

1 - In a large soup pan, heat oil over medium heat and sauté the onion, turmeric, ginger, garlic, spices and cilantro for about 3-4 minutes.
2 - Add the pumpkin and broth and bring to a boil
3 - Turn the heat to low and simmer, covered for about 15 minutes.
4 - Remove from heat and set aside to cool slightly.
5 - Transfer the mixture into a high-powered blender in batches and pulse until smooth.
6 - Return the soup into the same pan over medium heat and cook for about 3 minutes or until heated through.
7 - Serve hot.

Nutrition: Calories: 208 Fat: 11.5g Carbohydrates: 21g Dietary Fiber: 6.7g Sugar: 9g Protein: 8.3g

Chapter 17. Dinner

123. Summer Bell Peppers Mix

Preparation time: 10 minutes
Cooking time: 15 minutes
Servings: 6

Ingredients:

- Roasted bell peppers – 12 ounces, cut into strips
- Olive oil – 2 tbsp.
- Garlic – 2 cloves, minced
- Salt and black pepper to taste
- Coconut cream – 2/3 cup
- Yellow onion – 1, chopped
- Cashew cheese – ¼ cup, grated
- Celery stalks – 2, chopped

Directions:

1 - Heat oil in a pot. Add garlic, onion, celery, salt, and pepper. Stir and cook for 10 minutes.
2 - Add the bell peppers, toss and cover. Lower heat and cook for five minutes more.
3 - Add the cream and cashew cheese. Mix and serve.

Nutrition: Calories: 216 Fat: 13g Carb: 14g Protein: 8g

124. Cabbage Skillet

Preparation time: 10 minutes
Cooking time: 15 minutes
Servings: 8

Ingredients:

- Garlic – 1 clove, minced
- Olive oil – 2 tsp.
- Green cabbage head – 1, shredded
- Yellow onion – 1, chopped
- Cumin powder – 1 tsp.
- Salt and black pepper to taste
- Canned tomatoes and green chilies – 10 ounces, chopped
- Veggie stock – ½ cup

Directions:

1 - Heat oil in a pan. Add garlic and onion. Stir-fry for 4 minutes.
2 - Add the cumin, cabbage, salt, pepper, tomatoes, and stock. Mix and cook for 10 minutes.

Nutrition: Calories: 190 Fat: 4g Carb: 11g Protein: 8g

125. Creamy Brussels Sprouts Mix

Preparation time: 10 minutes
Cooking time: 30 minutes
Servings: 4

Ingredients:

- Yellow onions – 2 ounces, chopped
- Garlic – 1 tsp. minced
- Brussels sprouts – 6 ounces, halved
- Olive oil – 2 tbsp.
- Coconut aminos – 1 tbsp.
- Salt and black pepper to taste
- Cashew cheese – 2.5 ounces, grated
- Coconut cream – ½ cup
- Turmeric powder – ¼ tsp.
- Sweet paprika – ¼ tsp.

Directions:

1 - Heat a pan with oil. Add onion and garlic. Stir-fry for 5 minutes.
2 - Add the salt, pepper, sprouts, coconut aminos, turmeric, and paprika. Toss and cook for 20 minutes.
3 - Add the cashew cheese and the cream. Toss and cook for 5 minutes more.

Nutrition: Calories: 270 Fat: 10g Carb: 8g Protein: 6g

126. Zucchini-Rice Casserole

Preparation time: 10 minutes
Cooking time: 35 minutes
Servings: 4

Ingredients:

- Extra-virgin olive oil – 1 tbsp.
- Zucchini – 1 ½ pounds, cut into ½ inch cubes

- Chopped onion – 1 cup
- Garlic – 2 large cloves, finely chopped
- Salt – ½ tsp.
- Ground cumin – ½ tsp.
- Dried oregano – ½ tsp.
- Cayenne pepper – 1/8 tsp.
- Freshly ground black pepper to taste
- Kidney beans – 1 (15-ounce) can, rinsed and drained
- Mild or medium salsa – 1 ¼ cups
- Cooked long-grain white rice – 1 cup
- Crushed taco shell – 1

Directions:

1 - Preheat the oven to 350F. Lightly grease a baking dish and set aside.
2 - In a large nonstick skillet, heat the oil over medium heat.
3 - Add the zucchini and onion. Cook and stir for 8 minutes or until tender.
4 - Add the oregano, cumin, salt, garlic, cayenne, and black pepper the last few minutes of the cooking.
5 - Except for the crushed taco shell, add the remaining ingredients. Cook and stir for 3 minutes.
6 - Transfer to the baking dish. Then cover with foil.
7 - Bake heated through the center, about 20 minutes.
8 - Uncover and sprinkle with the crushed taco shell.
9 - Bake for 5 minutes or until lightly browned.
10 - Serve warm.

Nutrition: Calories: 251 Fat: 5g Carb: 44g Protein: 10g

127.   Vegetable Casserole
Preparation time: 10 minutes
Cooking time: 45 minutes
Servings: 6

Ingredients:

- Extra-virgin olive oil – 2 tbsp.
- Chopped onion – 1 cup
- Chopped green bell pepper – 1 cup
- Frozen yellow corn – 1 cup, thawed
- Ground cumin – 1 tbsp.
- Salt – ¼ tsp.
- Freshly ground black pepper to taste

- Cut sweet potatoes – 1 (15-ounce) can, well-drained
- Black beans – 1 (15-ounce) can, rinsed and drained
- Diced tomatoes with green chilies– 1 (14.5-ounce) can, briefly drained
- Hickory-smoked barbecue sauce – 1 cup
- Cayenne pepper or hot sauce to taste
- Crushed taco shell – 1

Directions:

1 - Preheat the oven to 350F. Lightly grease a 2 ½-quart casserole with a lid and set aside.
2 - Heat the oil in a skillet.
3 - Add the corn, bell pepper, and onion. Cook and stir for about 7 minutes.
4 - Add the black pepper, salt, and cumin. Cook and stir for 1 minute.
5 - Add the rest of the ingredients, except for the crushed taco shell. Stir well to mix.
6 - Remove from the heat. Then transfer to the prepared casserole.
7 - Bake, covered, 30 minutes.
8 - Remove cover and sprinkle with the crushed taco shell.
9 - Bake for 5 minutes more.
10 - Serve warm.
Nutrition: Calories: 336 Fat: 9g Carb: 57g Protein: 10g

128.   Three-Bean Barley Chili
Preparation time: 10 minutes
Cooking time: 50 minutes
Servings: 8

Ingredients:

- Water – 4 cups
- Mild or medium salsa – 2 cups
- Diced tomatoes with jalapeno chilies – 1 (14.5-ounce) can, juiced included
- Low-sodium vegetable broth – 1 (14-ounce) can
- Pearl barley – 1 cup
- Extra-virgin olive oil – 2 tbsp.
- Chili powder – 1 ½ tbsp.
- Ground cumin – ½ tbsp.

- Salt – ½ tsp.
- Freshly ground black pepper to taste
- Cayenne pepper to taste
- Red kidney beans – 1 (19-ounce) can, rinsed and drained
- Black beans – 1 (15-ounce) can, rinsed and drained
- Great Northern or navy or other white beans – 1 (15-ounce) can, rinsed and drained
- Frozen yellow corn – 1 cup, partially thawed
- Chopped onion

Directions:

1 - Combine the tomatoes with liquids, salsa, water, broth, barley, oil, chili powder, cumin, salt, black pepper, and cayenne in a stockpot.
2 - Bring to a boil over high heat. Stirring occasionally.
3 - Reduce the heat to low. Cover, and simmer for 40 minutes or until barley is just tender. Stirring occasionally.
4 - Add the corn and beans and return to a boil over high heat.
5 - Lower the heat and simmer, uncovered for 5 minutes or until the barley is tender. Stirring occasionally.
6 - Serve warm garnished with onion.

Nutrition: Calories: 297 Fat: 5g Carb: 51g Protein: 16g

129. Peppery Black Beans

Preparation time: 10 minutes
Cooking time: 33 to 34 minutes
Serving: 4

Ingredients:

- 1 red bell pepper, deseeded and chopped
- 1 medium yellow onion, peeled and chopped
- 2 jalapeño peppers, deseeded and minced
- 4 cloves garlic, peeled and minced
- 1 tablespoon thyme
- 1 tablespoon curry powder
- 1½ Teaspoon's ground allspice
- 1 teaspoon freshly ground black pepper
- 1 (15-ounce / 425-g) can diced tomatoes

- 4 cups cooked black beans

Directions:

1 - Add the red bell pepper and onion to a saucepan and sauté over medium heat for 10 minutes, or until the onion is softened. Add water 1 to 2 tablespoons at a time to keep the vegetables from sticking to the pan.
2 - Stir in the jalapeño peppers, garlic, thyme, curry powder, allspice and black pepper. Cook for 3 to 4 minutes, then add the tomatoes and black beans. Cook over medium heat for 20 minutes, covered.
Nutrition: Calories: 283 | fat: 1.7g | carbs: 52.8g | protein: 17.4g | fiber: 19.8g

130. Walnut, Coconut, and Oat Granola

Preparation time: 15 minutes
Cooking time: 1 hour 40 minutes
Serving: 4¼ cups

Ingredients:

- 1 cup chopped walnuts
- 1 cup unsweetened, shredded coconut
- 2 cups rolled oats
- 1 teaspoon ground cinnamon
- 2 tablespoons hemp seeds
- 2 tablespoons ground flaxseeds
- 2 tablespoons chia seeds
- ¾ teaspoon salt (optional)
- ¼ cup maple syrup
- ¼ cup water
- 1 teaspoon vanilla extract
- ½ cup dried cranberries

Directions:

1 - Preheat the oven to 250ºF (120ºC). Line a baking sheet with parchment paper.
2 - Mix the walnuts, coconut, rolled oats, cinnamon, hemp seeds, flaxseeds, chia seeds, and salt (if desired) in a bowl.

3 - Combine the maple syrup and water in a saucepan. Bring to a boil over medium heat, then pour in the bowl of walnut mixture.

4 - Add the vanilla extract to the bowl of mixture. Stir to mix well. Pour the mixture in the baking sheet, then level with a spatula so the mixture coats the bottom evenly.

5 - Place the baking sheet in the preheated oven and bake for 90 minutes or until browned and crispy. Stir the mixture every 15 minutes.

6 - Remove the baking sheet from the oven. Allow to cool for 10 minutes, then serve with dried cranberries on top.

Nutrition: Calories: 1870 | fat: 115.8g | carbs: 238.0g | protein: 59.8g | fiber: 68.9g

131.   Ritzy Fava Bean Ratatouille

Preparation time: 15 minutes
Cooking time: 40 minutes
Serving: 4

Ingredients:

- 1 medium red onion, peeled and thinly sliced
- 2 tablespoons low-sodium vegetable broth
- 1 large eggplant, stemmed and cut into ½-inch dice
- 1 red bell pepper, seeded and diced
- 2 cups cooked fava beans
- 2 Roma tomatoes, chopped
- 1 medium zucchini, diced
- 2 cloves garlic, peeled and finely chopped
- ¼ cup finely chopped basil
- Salt, to taste (optional)
- Ground black pepper, to taste

Directions:

1 - Add the onion to a saucepan and sauté for 7 minutes or until caramelized.

2 - Add the vegetable broth, eggplant and red bell pepper to the pan and sauté for 10 more minutes.

3 - Add the fava beans, tomatoes, zucchini, and garlic to the pan and sauté for an additional 5 minutes.

4 - Reduce the heat to medium-low. Put the pan lid on and cook for 15 minutes or until the vegetables are soft. Stir the vegetables halfway through.

5 - Transfer them onto a large serving plate. Sprinkle with basil, salt (if desired), and black pepper before serving.

Nutrition: Calories: 114 | fat: 1.0g | carbs: 24.2g | protein: 7.4g | fiber: 10.3g

132.   Mashed White Beans, Potatoes, and Kale

Preparation time: 10 minutes
Cooking time: 30 minutes
Serving: 4

Ingredients:

- 2 large Russet potatoes, rinsed, quartered, then halve each quarter
- ½ cup low-sodium vegetable soup
- 1 (14.5-ounce / 411-g) can great northern beans or other white beans, rinsed and drained
- 6 ounces (170 g) kale, torn into bite-size pieces
- Salt, to taste (optional)
- ¼ teaspoon freshly ground black pepper

Directions:

1 - Put the potato pieces in a pot, and then pour in enough water to cover. Bring to a boil over medium-high heat. Reduce the heat to medium, cover, and simmer for 20 minutes or until soft.

2 - Transfer the potatoes in a colander and rinse under running water. Drain the potatoes and put them back to the pot. Pour the vegetable soup over.

3 - Add the beans and kale to the pot, cover and simmer over low heat for 5 minutes or until the kale is wilted.

4 - Pour the mixture into a food processor. Sprinkle with salt (if desired) and pepper and pulse until creamy and smooth.

Nutrition: Calories: 255 | fat: 1.0g | carbs: 53.0g | protein: 12.0g | fiber: 11.0g

133. Spicy Chickpea Curry with Mango

Preparation time: 5 minutes
Cooking time: 15 minutes
Serving: 6

Ingredients:

- 3 cups chickpeas, cooked
- 2 cups fresh mango chunks
- 2 cups unsweetened coconut milk
- 2 tablespoons maple syrup (optional)
- 1 tablespoon ground ginger
- 1 tablespoon curry powder
- 1 teaspoon garlic powder
- 1 teaspoon onion powder
- 1 teaspoon ground coriander
- 1/8 Teaspoon ground cinnamon

Directions:

1 - Heat a saucepan over medium heat. Add all the ingredients to the saucepan and stir well. Cook for 10 minutes, covered, stirring halfway through to avoid sticking.
2 - Uncover and cook for another 5 minutes, stirring constantly.
3 - Serve hot.

Nutrition: Calories: 218 | fat: 13.9g | carbs: 7.8g | protein: 8.1g | fiber: 9.2g

134. Red Jerk Beans

Preparation time: 5 minutes
Cooking time: 15 minutes
Serving: 2 to 4

Ingredients:

- ¼ cup low-sodium vegetable soup
- 1 large yellow onion, diced
- 2 tablespoons Jerk spices (no salt or sugar added)
- 1 (14.5-ounce / 411-g) can diced tomatoes with juice
- 1 (15-ounce / 425-g) can red kidney beans, drained and rinsed
- 1 (14.5-ounce / 411-g) can unsweetened tomato sauce

Directions:

1 - Heat the soup in a saucepan over medium-high heat.
2 - Add the onion and sauté for 5 minutes or until translucent. Sprinkle with Jerk spices and sauté for a minute more.
3 - Add the tomatoes with juice, beans, then pour the tomato sauce over. Bring to a simmer. Cover the pan and cook for another 10 minutes. Stir periodically.
4 - Serve immediately.

Nutrition: Calories: 136 | fat: 4.4g | carbs: 20.7g | protein: 5.2g | fiber: 5.4g

135. Easy Tahini Green Beans

Preparation time: 10 minutes
Cooking time: 5 minutes
Serving: 2

Ingredients:

- ¼ cup water
- 1 pound (454 g) green beans, rinsed and trimmed
- 2 tablespoons organic tahini
- Zest and juice of 1 lemon
- 1 garlic clove, minced
- Salt and ground black pepper, to taste (optional)
- 1 teaspoon toasted black or white sesame seeds

Directions:

1 - Pour the water in a saucepan, and then add the green beans and steam over medium-high heat for 5 minutes or until the green beans are tender.
2 - Remove the green beans from the pan and reserve about ¼ cup of juice remains in the pan.
3 - Combine the tahini, lemon zest and juice, garlic, salt (if desired), and pepper in a large bowl. Thin with the reserved juice as needed.
4 - Toss the green beans with the tahini mixture and sprinkle with sesame seeds to serve.

Nutrition: Calories: 154 | fat: 9.8g | carbs: 15.5g | protein: 5.5g | fiber: 6.0g

136. Red Beans with Cauliflower Rice

Preparation time: 15 minutes
Cooking time: 17 minutes
Serving: 4

Ingredients:

- 1 large head cauliflower
- 2 tablespoons avocado oil (optional)
- ½ cup diced celery ribs
- ½ cup chopped green bell pepper
- ½ cup chopped sweet onion
- 1½ cups cooked red beans
- 1 cup cooked brown rice
- 2 teaspoons cumin
- 1 tablespoon minced garlic
- 1 teaspoon chili powder
- ½ teaspoon basil
- ½ teaspoon chopped fresh parsley
- 1 teaspoon paprika
- ½ teaspoon ground black pepper
- 2 cups water
-

Directions:

1 - Pulse the cauliflower in a food processor to make the cauliflower rice. Set aside.
2 - Heat the avocado oil (if desired) in a skillet over medium-high heat.
3 - Add the celery, green pepper, and onion to the skillet and sauté for 7 minutes or until tender.
4 - Add the remaining ingredients to the skillet and sauté for 10 minutes until well combined and the cauliflower rice is soft.
5 - Serve immediately.

Nutrition: Calories: 278 | fat: 8.9g | carbs: 41.9g | protein: 12.0g | fiber: 11.4g

137. Gold Chickpea Poppers

Preparation time: 15 minutes
Cooking time: 25 minutes
Serving: 3

Ingredients:

- 2 cups cooked chickpeas
- ½ teaspoon garlic powder
- ¼ teaspoon onion powder
- ½ teaspoon salt (optional)
- 1 tablespoon coconut oil (optional)
- ½ teaspoon chili powder
- ¼ teaspoon cumin
- ¼ teaspoon ground cayenne pepper
- ¼ teaspoon paprika

Directions:

1 - Preheat the oven to 400°F (205°C). Line a baking pan with parchment paper.
2 - Pour the chickpeas on the baking pan and top with the garlic powder, onion powder, salt (if desired), and coconut oil (if desired). Toss to combine well.
3 - Bake in the preheated oven for 25 minutes or until the chickpeas are golden and crispy. Stir the chickpeas every 5 minutes.
4 - Transfer the toasted chickpeas to a large bowl and allow to cool for 10 minutes. Sprinkle with remaining spices and serve.

Nutrition: Calories: 192 | fat: 7.8g | carbs: 21.5g | protein: 9.1g | fiber: 12.8g

138. Black Beans and Avocado on Toast

Preparation time: 5 minutes
Cooking time: 3 minutes
Serving: 4

Ingredients:

- 4 (½-inch-thick) slices whole-wheat crusty bread
- 4 ounces (113 g) cherry tomatoes, quartered
- 4 Teaspoons avocado oil, divided (optional)
- Salt and ground black pepper, to taste (optional)
- 1 (15-ounce / 425-g) can black beans, rinsed and drained
- ½ teaspoon lime zest

- 1 tablespoon lime juice
- ¼ cup boiling water
- 1 ripe avocado, halved, pitted, and sliced thinly
- ¼ cup fresh cilantro leaves

Directions:

1 - Set the oven to boil and line a baking pan with parchment paper.
2 - Arrange the bread slices on the baking pan and toast in the oven for 3 minutes or until golden brown on both sides. Flip the bread halfway through.
3 - Meanwhile, put the cherry tomatoes in a large bowl. Drizzle with 1 teaspoon avocado oil (if desired) and sprinkle with salt (if desired) and black pepper. Toss to combine well.
4 - Combine the black beans with lime zest and juice in a food processor. Pour in the boiling water. Drizzle with 1 tablespoon of avocado oil (if desired) and sprinkle with salt (if desired) and pepper. Pulse to mix well and leave some beans intact.
5 - Transfer the toasted bread on a plate, then spread with mashed bean mixture on top. Place the avocado over the bean mixture and top the avocado with cherry tomatoes and cilantro leaves.
6 - Serve immediately.

Nutrition: Calories: 513 | fat: 14.2g | carbs: 75.3g | protein: 25.0g | fiber: 20.1g

139. Hummus Pizza with Tomatoes and Olives

Preparation time: 10 minutes
Cooking time: 20 minutes
Servings: 4

Ingredients:

- Prepared plain hummus – 1 ¼ cups
- Garlic – 1 to 2 cloves, chopped
- Refrigerated pizza dough – 1 (10 or 13-ounce) can
- Julienned, oil-packed sun-dried tomatoes – 1/3 cup (keep 1 tbsp. marinade reserved)
- Pitted Kalamata olives – 6, halved

Directions:

1 - Preheat the oven to 350F.

2 - Lightly grease a baking sheet and set aside.
3 - In a bowl, mix together the garlic and hummus until mixed well. Set aside.
4 - Unfold the pizza dough.
5 - Then press the dough onto the baking sheet to fit.
6 - Brush sun-dried tomatoes over the dough.
7 - Then use a fork to prick in a few places.
8 - Bake in the oven until very lightly browned, about 12 to 15 minutes.
9 - Remove and spread evenly with the hummus-garlic mixture.
10 - Top evenly with olives and sun-dried tomatoes.
11 - Place on the bottom rack and bake 5 minutes, until the edges are nicely browned.
12 - Cut into wedges and serve.

Nutrition: Calories: 383 Fat: 13g Carb: 57g Protein: 10g

140. Sloppy Joe Sandwiches

Preparation time: 10 minutes
Cooking time: 15 minutes
Servings: 6

Ingredients:

- Extra-virgin olive oil – 1 tbsp.
- Chopped onion – 1 cup
- Chopped green bell pepper – ½ cup
- Garlic – 2 cloves, chopped
- Pinto beans – 1 (15-ounce) can, rinsed and drained
- Tomato paste – 1 (6-ounce) can
- Water – ¾ cup
- Wheat germ – ½ cup
- Molasses – ¼ cup
- Chili powder – to taste
- Liquid smoke – 1 tsp.
- Ground black pepper to taste
- Hamburger buns – 6
- Hot sauce to taste
- Salt to taste

Directions:

1 - Heat the oil in a skillet.
2 - Add onion and bell pepper. Cook for 3 minutes.
3 - Add the garlic. Cook for 1 minute.

4 - Add the remaining ingredients (except for the buns).

5 - Bring to a gentle simmer, stirring occasionally.

6 - Lower heat and simmer for 10 minutes. Stirring occasionally. Then mash the beans with a spoon.

7 - Spoon bean mixture on each hamburger buns and serve.

Nutrition: Calories: 292 Fat: 6g Carb: 52g Protein: 11g

141.   Gnocchi With Sauce
Preparation time: 10 minutes
Cooking time: 15 minutes
Servings: 4

Ingredients:

- Gnocchi – 1 (16-ounce) package
- Roasted red bell peppers – 1 (12-ounce) jar
- Olive oil – 2 tbsp.
- Garlic – 3 cloves, chopped
- Lemon juice – 2 tsp.
- Salt – ½ tsp.
- Ground black pepper to taste
- Fresh basil – ¼ cup, chopped

Directions:

1 - Cook the gnocchi and drain.

2 - Meanwhile, in a food processor, process the bell peppers, oil, garlic, lemon juice, salt, and black pepper until pureed. Set aside.

3 - Transfer the bell pepper mixture to a stockpot and bring to a simmer. Stirring frequently.

4 - Add the drained gnocchi and basil. Mix and serve.

Nutrition: Calories: 412 Fat: 8g Carb: 72g Protein: 12g

142.   Minestrone Soup
Preparation time: 10 minutes
Cooking time: 30 minutes
Servings:4
Ingredients:

- Carrots – 3, chopped
- Yellow onion – 1, chopped
- Celery – 4 sticks, chopped
- Garlic – 2 cloves, minced
- Olive oil – 1 tbsp.
- Potatoes – 2, cubed
- Veggie stock – 2 quarts
- Tomato puree – 2 tbsp.
- Canned tomatoes – 10 ounces, chopped
- Canned cannellini beans – 10 ounces, drained
- Savory cabbage – ½ head, shredded

Directions:

1 - Heat a pot with oil over medium heat.

2 - Add the onion and garlic and stir-fry for 4 minutes.

3 - Add the carrots, celery, potatoes, tomato puree, stock, and tomatoes, Sir, bring to a simmer and cook for 15 minutes.

4 - Add the cabbage and beans. Stir and cook for 10 minutes.

Nutrition: Calories: 256 Fat: 8g Carb: 15g Protein: 7g

143.   Tomato And Spaghetti Soup
Preparation time: 10 minutes
Cooking time: 35 minutes
Servings: 4

Ingredients:

- Olive oil – 1 tbsp.
- Red onion – 1, chopped
- Red chili – 1, chopped
- Tomatoes – 1 ½ pound, chopped
- Veggie stock – 1 quart
- Spaghetti – 3 ounces
- Black olives – 4 tbsp. pitted and sliced
- Capers – 2 tbsp. chopped
- Basil – 1 handful, chopped

Directions:

1 - Heat oil in a pot.

2 - Add chili and onion and stir-fry for 10 minutes.

3 - Add the tomatoes and stock. Stir, bring to a boil and simmer for 6 minutes.

4 - Add the spaghetti, stir and cook for 5 minutes more.

5 - Add the olives, capers, and basil.

6 - Stir and serve.

Nutrition: Calories: 200 Fat: 6g Carb: 20g Protein: 6g

144. Asparagus Cream Soup

Preparation time: 5 minutes
Cooking time: 0 minutes
Servings: 2

Ingredients:

- White mushrooms – 8 ounces
- Asparagus spears – 12, trimmed
- Avocado – 1, pitted and peeled
- A pinch of salt and white pepper
- Yellow onion – 1, peeled and chopped
- Veggie stock – 3 cups

Directions:

1 - In a blender, mix the mushrooms with avocado, asparagus, onion, water, salt, and pepper and puree very well.
2 - Divide into bowls and serve.

Nutrition: Calories: 200 Fat: 4g Carb: 15g Protein: 6g

145. Arugula Salad

Preparation time: 10 minutes
Cooking time: 0 minutes
Servings: 4

Ingredients:

- Arugula leaves – 5 ounces
- Strawberries – 1 pound, sliced
- Basil – ½ cup, chopped
- Red onion – 1 cup, chopped
- Avocado – 1, cubed
- Sunflower seeds – ½ cup, roasted
- Radishes – ½ cup, sliced
- Jalapeno – 1, chopped
- Olive oil – ¼ cup
- Balsamic vinegar – 1 ½ Tbsp.
- Mustard – 1 tbsp.
- Stevia – ½ tbsp.
- Garlic – 1 clove, minced
- A pinch of salt and black pepper

Directions:

1 - In a bowl, mix the arugula with basil, strawberries, onion, avocado, sunflower seeds, radishes, and the jalapeno and toss.
2 - In another bowl, mix the oil with the mustard, vinegar, stevia, garlic, salt, and pepper and mix well.
3 - Add this to salad, mix and serve.

Nutrition: Calories: 200 Fat: 11g Carb: 20g Protein: 12g

146. Smoky Tofu and Bean Bowls

Preparation time: 10 minutes
Cooking time: 10 minutes
Serving: 4

Ingredients:

- ¼ cup water
- 7 ounces (198 g) smoked tofu, cubed
- 2 cups fresh tomato, cubed
- 2 cups cooked black beans
- 1 cup cooked brown rice
- 1 tablespoon no-salt-added Cajun seasoning

Directions:

1 - Heat the water in a saucepan over medium-high heat.
2 - Add the tofu and tomato cubes to the pan and sauté for 3 minutes or until the tomatoes are tender.
3 - Add the beans and rice, then sprinkle with Cajun seasoning. Reduce the heat to low and stir to mix for 5 minutes until heated through.
4 - Divide them among 4 bowls
and serve immediately.

Nutrition: Calories: 371 | fat: 5.0g | carbs: 60.6g | protein: 19.6g | fiber: 11.9g

147. Sloppy Black Bean Burgers

Preparation time: 20 minutes
Cooking time: 5 minutes
Serving: 4

Ingredients:

- ¼ cup low-sodium vegetable soup
- 1 cup fresh tomato, cubed
- 1 (7-ounce / 198-g) pack textured soya mince
- 1 cup cooked black beans
- ¼ cup no-salt-added taco seasoning
- 4 whole-wheat buns, split in half
- 1 medium red onion, chopped
- 2 tablespoons tahini

Directions:

1 - Heat the vegetable soup in a saucepan over medium-high heat.

2 - Add the tomato cubes and soya mince and sauté for 3 minutes or until the tomatoes are tender.

3 - Add the beans and sprinkle with taco seasoning. Sauté for 2 more minutes.

4 - Remove the pan from the heat and allow to cool for 5 minutes, then divide the bean mix over 4 bun halves.

5 - Spread the onion and tahini on top of the bean mix and place the remaining halves over to make 4 burgers.

Nutrition: Calories: 483 | fat: 22.0g | carbs: 62.5g | protein: 10.3g | fiber: 8.5g

148. Super Three-Bean and Grains Bowl

Preparation time: 30 minutes
Cooking time: 50 minutes
Serving: 8

Ingredients:

- 2 tablespoons water
- 1 medium onion, chopped
- 1 (15-ounce / 425-g) can black beans, drained and rinsed
- 1 (15-ounce / 425-g) can kidney beans, drained and rinsed
- 1 (15-ounce / 425-g) can garbanzo beans, drained and rinsed
- 2 cups long-grain brown rice
- 1 (15-ounce / 425-g) can stewed tomatoes
- 4 cups low-sodium vegetable soup

- 2 cups frozen corn kernels
- 1 (4-ounce / 113-g) can chopped green chilies

Directions:

1 - Heat the water in a saucepan over medium-high heat.

2 - Add the onion and sauté for 3 minutes or until translucent.

3 - Add the beans, rice, and tomatoes. Pour in the vegetable soup. Bring to a boil. Keep stirring.

4 - Reduce the heat to low. Cover the pan and simmer for 30 minutes or until the beans and rice are soft. Stir periodically.

5 - Add the corn and chilies, simmer for 15 more minutes. Stir periodically.

6 - Allow to cool for 15 minutes before serving.

Nutrition: Calories: 688 | fat: 5.5g | carbs: 130.1g | protein: 32.1g | fiber: 27.8g

149. Quick and Easy Veggie Pasta Soup

Preparation time: 15 minutes
Cooking time: 30 minutes
Serving: 8 Cups

Ingredients:

- 1 cup chopped onion
- 1 cup chopped celery
- 1 cup chopped carrots
- 6 cups vegetable stock
- 1 teaspoon low-sodium tamari or soy sauce
- ½ teaspoon dried marjoram, crushed
- ½ teaspoon dried sage, crushed
- ¼ teaspoon dried thyme, crushed
- Freshly ground black pepper, to taste
- 3 cups whole-wheat pasta, broken

Directions:

1 - Combine the onion, celery, carrots, stock, tamari, marjoram, sage, thyme, and pepper in a 4-quart Dutch oven.

2 - Bring to a boil over high heat. Reduce heat to medium-low; cover and simmer for 20 minutes.

3 - Stir in the noodles; return to a boil. Cook for 10 minutes more or until noodles are tender.

Nutrition: Calories: 1298| fat: 5.5g | carbs: 261g | protein: 49.57g | fiber: 33.1g

150. Homemade Garlic Black Bean Burgers

Preparation time: 20 minutes
Cooking time: 30 minutes
Serving: 6 burgers

Ingredients:

- 1 cup cooked brown rice
- 1 (15-ounce/425 g) can black beans
- ½ onion, diced
- ¼ cup corn
- 1 teaspoon cumin
- 1 teaspoon garlic powder
- ¼ teaspoon chili powder
- ¼ cup cornmeal
- 2 tablespoons salsa

Directions:

1 - To cook the brown rice, bring ½ cup of rice and 1 cup of water to a boil in a pot. Once boiling, reduce heat to simmer. Once water is absorbed, taste rice to see if fully cooked. If not, add a little more water and let simmer until it's ready.

2 - Boil beans until soft or drain canned beans. Pour beans in a medium size bowl and mash them with your hands, potato masher, or fork.

3 - Preheat oven to 350° F (177 ° C). Lay a piece of parchment paper on sheet pan.

4 - Sweat the onion in a sauté pan. Sweat means the moisture comes from the veggies so no oil is needed. If the onions do start to stick, add a little bit of water. When onions become translucent add corn and spices. Cook for a few more minutes.

5 - Add cornmeal, salsa, veggies, and rice to bean bowl. Mix everything together so there is an even consistency. Feel free to do this with your hands.

6 - Then form mixture into patties. A good thickness is about ½ inch and I like to make mine around 3 inches in diameter.

7 - Place patties onto parchment paper and bake for 15 minutes at 350ºF (177 ° C).

8 - Flip the patties and bake for another 15 minutes.

9 - Serve between two leaves of romaine lettuce with tomato, onion, ketchup, and mustard. Or try putting the burger on a bed of fresh spinach instead of the bun…delicious!

Nutrition: Calories: 1128| fat: 10.7g | carbs: 234.4g | protein: 28.3g | fiber: 21.4

151. Delicious Worcestershire Lentil Sloppy Joes

Preparation time: 10 minutes
Cooking time: 60 minutes
Serving: 6 Burgers

Ingredients:

- 3 1/3 cups water or low-sodium vegetable stock
- 1 onion, chopped
- 1 red bell pepper, chopped
- 1 tablespoon chili powder
- 1 ½ cups dried brown lentil
- 1 (15-ounce/ 425 g) can diced fire roasted tomatoes
- 2 tablespoons soy sauce
- 2 tablespoons Dijon mustard
- 2 tablespoons brown sugar
- 1 teaspoon rice vinegar
- 1 teaspoon vegetarian Worcestershire sauce
- Salt to taste

Directions:

1 - Place 1 cup of the water or stock in a large pot.

2 - Add the onions and bell pepper and cook, stirring occasionally until onions soften slightly, about 5 minutes.

3 - Add the chili powder and mix in well. Add the remaining liquid, lentils, tomatoes, and the rest of the seasonings. Mix well, bring to a boil, reduce heat,

cover and cook over low heat for one hour, stirring occasionally.

4 - Serve on whole-wheat buns, or fresh baked bread, with the trimmings of your choice.

Nutrition: Calories: 1008| fat: 26g | carbs: 155g | protein: 61.2g | fiber: 20.2g

152. Appetizing Veggie Chili with Onion Toppings

Preparation time: 15 minutes
Cooking time: 60 minutes
Serving: 6

Ingredients:

- 2 cups dried pinto beans, rinsed and drained
- 1 (14.5-ounce/411 g) can no-salt-added fire-roasted diced tomatoes, undrained
- 1 cup chopped red onion
- 1 (1-ounce/28 g) packet vegetarian chili seasoning, such as Simply Organic, or chili seasonings of your choice
- 6 cloves garlic, minced
- 4 cups unsalted vegetable stock
- 2 cups water
- 1 cup fresh or frozen whole kernel corn
- Toppings such as chopped bell pepper, sliced green onions, and/or snipped fresh cilantro

Directions:

1 - In a cooker, combine the beans, tomatoes, onion, seasoning, and garlic. Add the stock and water.
2 - Cover and cook on high heat for 60 minutes; stir in the corn for the last 15 minutes. Serve with toppings.
Nutrition: Calories: 1742| fat: 7.49g | carbs: 318.6g | protein: 96g | fiber: 78.3g

153. Authentic Italian Zucchini Onion Sauté

Preparation time: 25 minutes
Cooking time: 25 minutes
Serving: 6 cups

Ingredients:

- 1 onion, chopped (1 cup)
- 1 large red bell pepper, chopped (1 cup)
- 6 cloves garlic, minced
- 1 teaspoon dried oregano
- ½ teaspoon dried thyme
- 3 medium zucchinis, halved lengthwise and cut into ¼-inch slices (4 cups)
- 1 (15-oz./28 g) can chickpeas, rinsed and drained (1½ cups)
- 1 cup oil-free marinara sauce
- 1 tablespoon white wine vinegar
- Sea salt and freshly ground black pepper, to taste
- 8 to 10 fresh basil leaves, chopped

Directions:

1 - Heat an extra-large skillet over medium.
2 - Add the first five ingredients (through thyme); cook 10 minutes, stirring often and adding water, 1 to 2 Tbsp. at a time, as needed to prevent sticking.
3 - Add zucchini; cook 10 minutes more or until zucchini is tender. Stir in chickpeas, marinara sauce, and vinegar.
4 - Season with salt and black pepper. Heat through. Serve immediately garnished with basil.

Nutrition: Calories: 973| fat: 11.8g | carbs: 173g | protein: 41.1g | fiber: 46.7g

154. Mushroom Halloumi Fajitas

Preparation time: 10 minutes
Cooking time: 20 minutes
Serving: 4

Ingredients:
- 1 green bell pepper, seeded and cut into slices
- 1 cup sliced grape tomatoes, divided
- ½ cup sliced mushrooms
- 1/3 small white onion, thinly sliced
- 7 ounces (198g) Halloumi, cut into strips
- ½ tablespoon olive oil
- 1 tablespoon fajita seasoning
- 8 (6-inch/98g) corn tortillas
- 2 cups shredded lettuce

Directions:

1 - Preheat the oven to 450°F (235°C), line a large baking sheet with parchment paper, and set aside.

2 - In a large bowl, add the bell pepper, ½ cup of tomatoes, mushrooms, onion, Halloumi, and olive oil and mix well. Sprinkle with the fajita seasoning, mix again, then arrange on the parchment paper, ensuring it is not overcrowded.

3 - Bake in the oven for 12 to 15 minutes, or until golden brown. Remove the cooked Halloumi and continue to cook the vegetables for 5 minutes or until slightly tender.

4 - To assemble, evenly divide the filling mixture into the tortillas and top with lettuce and the remaining ½ cup of tomatoes.

Nutrition: Calories: 346 | Fat: 17 g | Carbs: 18 g | Protein: 18 g | Fiber: 4 g

155. Rice with Sweet Crispy Tofu Bowl

Preparation time: 15 minutes
Cooking time: 15 minutes
Serving: 4

Ingredients:

- 1 (14-ounce/397g) package extra-firm tofu, drained
- 1½ cups quick brown rice
- 2 cups frozen shelled edamame
- 2 tablespoons low-sodium soy sauce
- 2 tablespoons reduced-sugar ketchup
- 2 teaspoons sriracha
- 1 tablespoon olive oil, divided
- 2 tablespoons cornstarch
- 1 small cucumber, thinly sliced
- 1 cup mango chunks

Directions:

1 - To press the tofu, wrap it in several layers of paper towel and place it between 2 plates. Place a weight on top and let it sit for at least 20 minutes. Cut the tofu into ½-inch (8g) cubes.

2 - Cook the rice according to the package instructions.

3 - In a medium pot, combine the edamame and enough water to cover and bring to a boil over medium-high heat. Cook until tender, 3 to 5 minutes. In a small bowl, mix the soy sauce, ketchup, and sriracha. Set aside.

4 - In a large bowl, toss the tofu with ½ tablespoon of olive oil. Add the cornstarch and toss until evenly coated.

5 - Heat the remaining ½ tablespoon of olive oil in a large nonstick skillet over medium-high heat. Add the tofu and cook, flipping the tofu over every 2 to 3 minutes, until all sides are equally crisp, about 8 to 10 minutes. Remove the pan from the heat and pour the soy sauce mixture over the tofu and mix well. Set aside.

6 - Divide the rice equally between 4 bowls. Top with the edamame, cucumber, mango, and tofu mixture and serve immediately.

Nutrition: Calories: 529 | Fat: 15 g | Carbs: 77 g | Protein: 25 g | Fiber: 8 g

156. Cauliflower Salad

Preparation time: 10 minutes
Cooking time: 35 minutes
Servings: 4

Ingredients:

- Cauliflower – 1 head, florets separated
- Red onion – 1, chopped
- Olive oil – 2 tbsp.
- Balsamic vinegar – 3 tbsp.
- Stevia – 1 ½ tbsp.
- Raisins – 2 tbsp.
- Dills – 1 bunch, chopped
- Almonds – 3 tbsp. toasted and chopped
- Baby spinach – 2 ounces
- Salt and black pepper to taste

Directions:

1 - Spread the onion and cauliflower in a lined baking dish. Season with salt and pepper. Drizzle with oil and roast at 400F for 30 minutes.

2 - Transfer the cauliflower mixture to a bowl. Add the stevia, vinegar, raisins, dill, spinach, and the almonds. Toss and serve.

Nutrition: Calories: 231 Fat: 5g Carb: 15g Protein: 6g

157. Potato And Broccoli Salad
Preparation time: 10 minutes
Cooking time: 20 minutes
Servings: 4

Ingredients:

- Baby potatoes – 1 pound, peeled
- Olive oil – 1 tbsp.
- Zest and juice of 1 lemon
- Broccoli – 1 heard, florets separated and blanched
- Green beans – ¼ pound, trimmed and blanched
- Dill – 1 tbsp. chopped
- Pine nuts – 2 tbsp. toasted

Directions:

1 - Put the baby potatoes in a pot. Add water to cover and boil for 20 minutes.
2 - Drain the potatoes and put them in a bowl. Add oil, broccoli, green beans, dill, pine nuts, lemon zest, and lemon juice. Toss and serve.

Nutrition: Calories: 241 Fat: 6g Carb: 15g Protein: 7g

158. Zucchini Noodles Mix
Preparation time: 10 minutes
Cooking time: 30 minutes
Servings: 4

Ingredients:

- Zucchinis – 2, cut with a spiralizer
- Yellow squashes – 2, cut with a spiralizer
- A pinch of salt and black pepper
- Lemon juice – 1 tbsp.
- Stevia – 1 tsp.
- Basil – 1 cup, chopped
- Olive oil – 4 tbsp.
- Eggplants – 1 ½, sliced

- Garlic – 2 cloves, minced
- Cherry tomatoes – 2 cups, halved
- Black olives – ¼ cup, pitted and sliced

Directions:

1 - In a bowl, mix the basil with the stevia, salt, pepper, lemon juice, and 3 tbsp. oil and whisk well.
2 - Heat a pan with the rest of the oil over medium heat.
3 - Add garlic. Stir-fry for 4 minutes.
4 - Add the tomatoes, eggplant, olives, zucchini, and squash noodles. Stir-fry for 6 minutes.
5 - Add the basil dressing. Toss, divide between plates, and serve.

Nutrition: Calories: 231 Fat: 7g Carb: 15g Protein: 6g

159. Veggie Curry
Preparation time: 10 minutes
Cooking time: 25 minutes
Servings: 4

Ingredients:

- Olive oil – 1 ½ tbsp.
- Sweet potato – 1 cup, cubed
- Cauliflower florets – 1 cup
- Yellow onion – ¼ cup, chopped
- Curry powder – 2 tsp.
- Veggie stock – ½ cup
- A pinch salt and black pepper
- Canned chickpeas – 15 ounces, drained
- Canned tomatoes – 15 ounces, chopped
- Cilantro – 2 tbsp. chopped
- Coconut yogurt - ½ cup

Directions:

1 - In a pot, heat the oil. Add the sweet potato. Stir-fry for 3 minutes.
2 - Add the onion, cauliflower and curry powder, Stir and cook for 1 minute.
3 - Add the salt, stock, pepper, chickpeas, and tomatoes. Stir, and bring to a simmer, then cook for 10 minutes.
4 - Divide the curry into bowls. Sprinkle the cilantro on top. Serve with coconut yogurt.

Nutrition: Calories: 213 Fat: 6g Carb: 16g Protein: 7g

160. Okra And Tomato Mix

Preparation time: 10 minutes
Cooking time: 40 minutes
Servings: 6

Ingredients:

* Green bell pepper – 1, chopped
* Okra – 1 cup
* Yellow onion – 1, chopped
* A drizzle of olive oil
* Garlic – 2 cloves, minced
* Celery ribs – 3, chopped
* Canned tomatoes – 16 ounces, chopped
* Veggie stock - 1 ½ cups
* Sweet paprika - ½ tsp.
* A pinch of salt and pepper

Directions:

1 - Heat oil in a pot. Add onion, garlic, salt, and pepper. Stir-fry for 5 minutes.
2 - Add the bell pepper, celery, tomatoes, paprika, okra, and the stock. Stir and bring to a boil. Cook for 35 minutes.
3 - Divide the mix into bowls and serve.

Nutrition: Calories: 232 Fat: 7g Carb: 15g Protein: 6g

161. Swiss Chard and Tomatoes

Preparation time: 10 minutes
Cooking time: 15 minutes
Servings: 4

Ingredients:
* Swiss chard – 6 cups, chopped
* Yellow onion – ½ cup, chopped
* Cherry tomatoes – ½ pound, halved
* Olive oil – 1 tbsp.
* Garlic – 1 clove, minced
* Salt and black pepper to taste
* A pinch of nutmeg
* Cashew cheese – ¼ cup, grated

Directions:

1 - Heat oil in a pan. Add the onions and garlic. Stir and cook for 3 minutes.
2 - Add Swiss chard, stir and cook for 5 minutes more.
3 - Add the tomatoes, salt, pepper, and nutmeg. Stir and cook for 7 minutes.
4 - Remove from heat and add cheese.

Nutrition: Calories: 272 Fat: 8g Carb: 13g Protein: 7g

162. Catalan Spinach Mix

Preparation time: 10 minutes
Cooking time: 12 minutes
Servings: 4

Ingredients:

* Yellow onion – 1, sliced
* Olive oil – 3 tbsp.
* Raisins – ¼ cup
* Garlic – 6 cloves, chopped
* Pine nuts – ¼ cup, toasted
* Balsamic vinegar - ¼ cup
* Spinach – 5 cups
* Salt and black pepper to taste

Directions:

1 - Heat oil in a pan. Add onion and stir-fry for 6 minutes.
2 - Add raisins, garlic, vinegar, and spinach. Stir-fry for 5 minutes more.
3 - Add salt, nutmeg, and pepper. Stir and cook for a few seconds more.

Nutrition: Calories: 220 Fat: 4g Carb: 14g Protein: 6g

163. Mediterranean Eggplant Mix

Preparation time: 10 minutes
Cooking time: 20 minutes
Servings: 4

Ingredients:

* Red onion – 1, chopped
* Garlic – 2 cloves, chopped

- Cilantro – 1 bunch, chopped
- Salt and black pepper to taste
- Oregano – 1 tsp. dried
- Eggplants – 2, chopped
- Olive oil – 2 tbsp.
- Capers – 2 tbsp., chopped
- Black olives – 1 handful, pitted and sliced
- Tomatoes – 5, chopped
- Balsamic vinegar – 3 tbsp.

Directions:

1 - Heat oil in a pot. Add eggplant, oregano, salt, and pepper. Stir and cook for 5 minutes.
2 - Add garlic, onion, and cilantro. Stir and cook for 4 minutes.
3 - Add olives, capers, vinegar, and tomatoes. Stir and cook for 15 minutes.
4 - Serve.

Nutrition: Calories: 230 Fat: 13g Carb: 15g Protein: 6g

Chapter 18.   Salads

164.   Zucchini & Tomato Salad
Preparation Time: 15 minutes
Cooking Time: 0 minutes
Servings: 4

Ingredients:
- 2 medium zucchinis, sliced thinly
- 2 cups plum tomatoes, sliced
- 2 tablespoons olive oil
- 2 tablespoons fresh key lime juice
- Pinch of Salt

Directions:
1 - In a salad bowl, place all ingredients and gently toss to combine.
2 - Serve immediately.

Nutrition: Calories: 93 Fat: 7.4g Carbohydrates: 6.9g Dietary Fiber: 2.2g Sugar: 4.1g Protein: 2g

165.   Quinoa, Bean, & Mango Salad
Preparation Time: 20 minutes
Cooking Time: 20 minutes
Servings: 6
Ingredients:
- 1¾ cups vegetable broth
- 1 cup quinoa, rinsed
- Salt, as required
- 1½ cups canned black beans, rinsed and drained
- 2 medium bell peppers, seeded and chopped
- 2 cucumbers, chopped
- ½ cup scallion (green part), chopped
- 1 tablespoon olive oil
- 2 tablespoons fresh cilantro leaves, chopped

Directions:
1 - In a saucepan, add the broth over high heat and bring to a boil.
2 - Add the quinoa and salt and cook until boiling.
3 - Now, lower the heat to low and simmer, covered for about 15-20 minutes or until all the liquid is absorbed.
4 - Remove from the heat and set aside, covered for about 5-10 minutes.
5 - Uncover and with a fork, fluff the quinoa.

6 - In a large serving bowl, place the quinoa with the remaining ingredients and gently, toss to coat.
7 - Serve immediately.

Nutrition: Calories: 218 Fat: 4.9g Carbohydrates: 34.8g Dietary Fiber: 7.1g Sugar: 3g Protein: 10.4g

166.   Quinoa & Veggie Salad
Preparation Time: 15 minutes
Cooking Time: 20 minutes
Servings: 6
Ingredients:
For Quinoa:
- 1 cup quinoa, rinsed
- 1 (15-ounce) can unsweetened coconut milk
- ½ cup water

For Dressing:
- 2 tablespoons balsamic vinegar
- 2 tablespoons extra-virgin olive oil
- 2 tablespoons fresh lime juice
- 1 tablespoon maple syrup
- ½ teaspoon Dijon mustard
- Salt and ground black pepper, as required

For Salad:
- 1½ cups frozen shelled edamame, thawed
- 1½ cups tomato, chopped
- 1½ cups cucumber, chopped
- 1 cup fresh baby spinach leaves, chopped
- 2 tablespoons fresh mint leaves, chopped
- 2 tablespoons fresh cilantro, chopped

Directions:
1 - For quinoa: in a medium saucepan, add all ingredients over medium-high heat and bring to a boil.
2 - Now, lower the heat to low and simmer, covered for about 20 minutes or until all the liquid is absorbed.
3 - Remove the saucepan of quinoa from heat and set aside, covered for about 5 minutes.
4 - With a fork, fluff the quinoa and let it cool completely.
5 - For dressing: in a bowl, add all ingredients and beat until well combined.
6 - In a large salad bowl, add the quinoa, salad ingredients and dressing and toss to coat well.

Nutrition: Calories: 276 Fat: 15.1g Carbohydrates: 32.2g Dietary Fiber: 6g Sugar: 3.6g Protein: 14.1g

167.   Red Beans & Corn Salad

Preparation Time: 15 minutes
Cooking Time: 0 minutes
Servings: 6
Ingredients:
For Dressing:
- 5 tablespoons olive oil
- 4 tablespoons fresh lime juice
- 1 tablespoon apple cider vinegar
- 3 tablespoons agave nectar
- Salt and ground black pepper, as required

For Salad:
- 3 (15-ounce) cans red kidney beans, drained and rinsed
- 1 (15¼-ounce) can corn, drained and rinsed
- 2 cups cherry tomatoes, halved
- 1¼ cups onion, sliced
- 1/3 cup fresh cilantro, minced
- 8 cups lettuce, torn

Directions:
1 - For the dressing: add all ingredients in a small bowl and beat until well combined.
2 - In a large serving bowl, add beans, corn, cilantro and lettuce and mix.
3 - Add dressing and toss to coat well.
4 - Serve immediately.

Nutrition: Calories: 396 Fat: 12.6g Carbohydrates: 59.9g Dietary Fiber: 21g Sugar: 13g Protein: 17.1g

168.   Potato   in   Creamy   Avocado Salad

Preparation time: 10 minutes
Cooking time: 1 hour
Servings: 4
Ingredients:

- 5 large potatoes, cut into 1-inch cubes
- 1 large avocado, chopped
- 1/4 cup chopped fresh chives
- 1/2 tablespoon freshly squeezed lemon juice
- 2 tablespoons Dijon mustard
- 1/2 teaspoon onion powder
- 1/2 teaspoon garlic powder
- 1/2 teaspoon dried dill

- 1/4 teaspoon freshly ground black pepper

Directions:
1 - Place potatoes in a pot, then pour in enough water to cover. Bring to a boil for 10 more minutes or until the potatoes are soft.
2 - Let the potatoes to cool for 10 minutes, then put the potatoes in a colander and rinse under running water.
3 - Dry potatoes with paper towels and transfer to a large bowl. Refrigerate for at least 20 minutes.
4 - Meanwhile, combine the avocado with chives, lemon juice, and mustard in a food processor. Sprinkle with onion powder, garlic powder, dill, and pepper. Pulse to mash the avocado until creamy and well combined.
5 - Pour the creamy avocado into the bowl of potatoes, then toss to coat the potato cubes well. Refrigerate for 30 minutes before serving.

Nutrition: Calories: 242 Fat: 9g Carbohydrates: 35g Protein: 7g

169.   Citrus and Grapefruit Salad

Preparation time: 10 minutes
Cooking time: 10 minutes
Servings: 2
Ingredients:
- 2 large oranges, peeled, pith removed, and segmented
- 1 large grapefruit, peeled, pith removed and segmented
- Zest and juice of 1 lime
- 1 teaspoon pure maple syrup (optional)
- 1 tablespoon minced fresh mint

Directions:
1 - Combine all ingredients except for the fresh mint in a mixing bowl, mix until well coated.
2 - Transfer the salad to the serving dishes and top with the fresh mint.
3 - Serve immediately.

Nutrition: Calories: 154 Fat: 0.4g Carbohydrates: 39.2g Protein: 2.9g

170.   Rice and Bean Salad

Preparation time: 10 minutes

Cooking time: 2 hours
Servings: 6 to 8
Ingredients:
- 3 cups cooked brown rice
- 1 (15-ounce / 425-g) can pinto beans, rinsed and drained
- 1 (15-ounce / 425-g) can black beans, rinsed and drained
- 1 (10-ounce / 284-g) package frozen green peas, thawed
- 1 cup sliced celery
- 1 medium red onion, chopped
- 1 (7-ounce / 198-g) can chopped green chilies
- 1/4 cup chopped fresh cilantro
- 1 (8-ounce / 227-g) jar oil-free Italian dressing

Directions:
1 - Prepare all ingredients in a large bowl and mix until well blended.
2 - Wrap the bowl in plastic and set it in the refrigerator for more than 2 hours before serving.

Nutrition: Calories: 224 Fat: 3.1g Carbohydrates: 40.4g Protein: 9.6g

171. Brown Basmati and Currant Salad

Preparation time: 10 minutes
Cooking time: 55 minutes
Servings: 4

Ingredients:
- 2 cups cooked brown basmati
- 1/4 cup maple syrup
- 1/4 cup chopped cilantro
- 1/4 cup brown rice vinegar
- 1/2 cup dried currants
- 1/2 small red onion
- 1 tablespoon curry powder
- 1 jalapeño pepper, minced
- 6 green onions, finely chopped
- Zest and juice of 2 limes
- Salt, to taste (optional)
- Ground black pepper, to taste

Directions:

1 - Add the basmati to a pot, then pour in 4 cups of the water. Bring to a boil over high heat.
2 - Reduce the heat to medium, then put the lid on and simmer for 45 to 50 minutes or until the water is absorbed.
3 - Peel and mince the red onion.
4 - Mix all ingredients in a large bowl. Toss to combine well, then serve immediately.

Nutrition: Calories: 437 Fat: 3.5g Carbohydrates: 93.9g Protein: 9.1g

172. Basmati, Navy, and Spinach Bean Salad

Preparation time: 15 minutes
Cooking time: 1 hour and 20 minutes
Servings: 4

Ingredients:
- 2 cups navy beans
- 1 1/2 cups cooked basmati
- 4 cups baby spinach
- 1/4 cup maple syrup
- 1/4 cup minced basil
- 1/4 cup balsamic vinegar, additional 2 tablespoons
- 1 cup green onion, cut thinly
- 2 tablespoons minced tarragon
- Zest and juice of 1 lemon
- Salt, to taste (optional)
- Ground black pepper, to taste

Directions:

1 - Put the basmati in a pot, then pour in the water to cover the basmati by about 1 inch.
2 - Bring to a boil over medium heat. Simmer in low heat for 40 minutes. Allow to cool before using.
3 - Put the navy beans in a pot, then pour in the water to cover the beans by about 1 inch.
4 - Bring to a boil over medium heat. Simmer for 40 minutes or until the water is absorbed over low heat.
5 - Meanwhile, toast the brown basmati in a nonstick skillet over low heat for 2 to 3 minutes.
6 - Combine the navy beans, toasted basmati, and remaining ingredients in a large serving bowl. Toss to combine well, then serve immediately.

Nutrition: Calories: 269 Fat: 1.5g Carbohydrates: 54.5g Protein: 10.7g

173. Rice, Chickpea, Fennel, and Orange Salad

Preparation time: 15 minutes
Cooking time: 1 hour and 50 minutes
Servings: 4

Ingredients:
- 1 1/2 cups brown basmati, rinsed
- 3 cups water
- 2 cups chickpeas, soaked in water overnight, cooked
- 1 fennel bulb, trimmed and diced
- Zest and segments of 1 orange
- 1/4 cup parsley, finely chopped
- 1/4 cup white wine vinegar, additional 2 tablespoons
- 1/2 teaspoon red pepper flakes

Directions:

1 - Put the soaked chickpeas in a saucepan, then pour in the water to cover by about 1 inch.

2 - Bring to a boil over medium-high heat. Adjust heat to low and simmer for 60 minutes or until soft. Allow to cool before using.

3 - Put the brown basmati in a pot, then pour in the water.

4 - Bring to a boil over high heat. Change heat to medium, then simmer for 45 to 50 minutes or until the water is absorbed.

5 - Combine the cooked basmati with the remaining ingredients in a large serving bowl. Toss to combine well, then serve immediately.

Nutrition: Calories: 438 Fat: 4.4g Carbohydrates: 86.3g Protein: 14.1g

174. Lemony Quinoa and Arugula Salad

Preparation time: 10 minutes
Cooking time: 20 minutes
Servings: 4

Ingredients:
- 1 1/2 cups cooked quinoa
- 4 cups arugula
- 1/4 cup brown rice vinegar
- 1 small red onion
- 1 red bell pepper
- 2 tablespoons toasted pine nuts
- Zest and juice of 1 lime
- Zest and juice of 2 oranges
- Salt, to taste (optional)
- Ground black pepper, to taste

Directions:

1 - Put the quinoa in a saucepan, then pour the water in the pan to cover the quinoa.

2 - Bring to a boil over medium-high heat. Adjust heat to medium, then simmer for 15 minutes or until the water is absorbed. Allow to cool before using.

3 - Peel the red onion and slice thinly. Then, remove the seed of bell pepper and cut it into 1/2-inch cubes.

4 - Prepare all ingredients in a large serving bowl. Toss to combine well, then serve immediately.

Nutrition: Calories: 282 Fat: 4.3g Carbohydrates: 50.6g Protein: 10.4g

175. Ritzy Summer Salad

Preparation time: 10 minutes
Cooking time: 10 minutes
Servings: 2

Ingredients:
Dressing:
- 1 medium avocado, halved, diced, use half for the salad
- 1 teaspoon lemon juice
- 1/4 cup water
- 1/4 cup chopped basil
- Salt, to taste (optional)

Salad:
- 1/4 cup dried chickpeas
- 1/4 cup dried red kidney beans
- 2 radishes, thinly sliced
- 2 cups shredded Brussels sprouts
- 4 cups shredded raw kale
- 1 tablespoon chopped walnuts
- 1 teaspoon flaxseeds
- Salt, to taste (optional)
- Ground black pepper, to taste

Directions:

1 - Combine half of the diced avocado with the remaining ingredients for dressing in a food processor. Pulse until smooth and creamy.

2 - Put a small amount of water during the pulsing. Pour the dressing in a bowl and set aside until ready to serve.

3 - Combine the remaining half of the avocado with all the ingredients for the salad in a large serving bowl.
4 - Top the salad with dressing and serve.

Nutrition: Calories: 371 Fat: 20.8g Carbohydrates: 33.3g Protein: 12.3g

176. Lemony Millet and Fruit Salad

Preparation time: 10 minutes
Cooking time: 15 minutes
Servings: 4
Ingredients:
Dressing:
• 3 tablespoons maple syrup
• Juice of 1 lemon
• Zest and juice of 1 orange
Salad:
• 1 cup cooked millet
• 1/2 cup golden raisins
• 1/2 cup dried currants
• 1/2 cup dried unsulfured apricots, chopped
• 1 Gala apple, cored and diced
• 2 tablespoons finely chopped mint
• Salt, to taste (optional)
Directions:
1 - Put the rinsed millet in a pot, then pour in the water to cover by about 1 inch. Bring to a boil over high heat.
2 - Change the heat to medium and keep boiling for 12 to 14 minutes or until tender. Allow to cool before using.
3 - For the dressing: Prepare and combine all the ingredients in a large bowl. Stir to mix well.
4 - Add the ingredients for the salad to the dressing and toss to combine well.
5 - Refrigerate for half an hour and serve.
Nutrition: Calories: 328 Fat: 2.4g Carbohydrates: 72.6g Protein: 6.8g

177. Endive and Green Lentil Salad

Preparation time: 10 minutes
Cooking time: 10 minutes
Servings: 2
Ingredients:
• 1/2 cup chopped fresh endive, rinsed
• 2 cups cooked green lentils
• 1/4 cup lemon juice
• 2 tablespoons dried oregano

• 1 tablespoon ground black pepper
Directions:
1 - Prepare a larger serving bowl, then combine all the ingredients.
2 - Toss to combine well, then serve immediately.

Nutrition: Calories: 261 Fat: 1.2g Carbohydrates: 48.3g Protein: 19.0g

178. Pinto Bean and Avocado Salad

Preparation time: 10 minutes
Cooking time: 20 minutes
Servings: 2
Ingredients:
• 2 cups cooked pinto beans
• 1 small Hass avocado, peeled, cored, and cubed
• 10 cherry tomatoes, halved
• 1/4 cup corn kernels
• 1/4 cup lime juice
• 1/4 cup fresh cilantro, chopped
• 1 jalapeño, sliced
• 1/2 of 1 red onion
Directions:
1 - Put the soaked pinto beans in a saucepan, then pour in the water to cover by about 1 inch.
2 - Sprinkle with salt, if desired. Bring to a boil over medium-high heat. Simmer over low heat until tender. Allow to cool before using.
3 - Prepare all ingredients in a large serving bowl. Toss to combine well, then serve immediately.

Nutrition: Calories: 399 Fat: 10.3g Carbohydrates: 56.7g Protein: 19.8g

179. White Bean and Carrot Salad

Preparation time: 10 minutes
Cooking time: 10 minutes
Servings: 2
Ingredients:
Dressing:
• 2 tablespoons balsamic vinegar
• 1 tablespoon olive oil (optional)
• 1 tablespoon fresh rosemary, chopped
• 1 tablespoon fresh oregano, chopped
• 1 teaspoon minced fresh chives
• 1 garlic clove, minced
• Pinch sea salt (optional)

Salad:
- 1 (14-ounce / 397-g) can cannellini beans, drained and rinsed
- 2 carrots, diced
- 6 mushrooms, thinly sliced
- 1 zucchini, diced
- 2 tablespoons fresh basil, chopped

Directions:

1 - Prepare all ingredients in a large bowl to make the dressing, then mix well.

2 - Add all the ingredients for the salad to the bowl and toss to combine well.

3 - Divide the salad between 2 bowls and serve immediately.

Nutrition: Calories: 359 Fat: 17.9g Carbohydrates: 7.8g Protein: 18.1g

180. Citrus Kale and Carrot Salad

Preparation time: 15 minutes
Cooking time: 10 minutes
Servings: 3

Ingredients:

Dressing:
- 1/4 cup orange juice
- 1/2 tablespoon maple syrup (optional)
- 1/2 tablespoon sesame oil (optional)
- 1 teaspoon lime juice
- 1/2 teaspoon ginger, finely minced

Salad:
- 4 cups fresh kale, chopped
- 2 cups carrots, shredded
- 1 cup edamame, shelled
- 1/2 cup cooked green lentils
- 1 tablespoon roasted sesame seeds
- 2 teaspoons mint, chopped
- 1 small avocado, peeled, pitted, and diced

Directions:

1 - Stir the orange juice, maple syrup (if desired), sesame oil (if desired), lime juices and ginger in a mixing bowl for the dressing.

2 - Prepare together the fresh kale, carrots, edamame, cooked lentils, sesame seeds and mint in separate bowl then mix until well combined.

3 - Add the dressing over the salad and toss to coat well.

4 - Divide the salad among 3 bowls. Top with avocado and serve immediately.

Nutrition: Calories: 315 Fat: 11.3g Carbohydrates: 38.8g Protein: 14.5g

181. Cucumber Salad with Chili and Lime

Preparation time: 5 minutes
Cooking time: 5 minutes
Servings: 4

Ingredients:
- 1 jalapeno, deseeded, diced
- 2 large cucumbers, sliced
- 1/4 of a medium sliced red onion
- 1/2 bunch cilantro
- 1/2 teaspoon red chili flakes
- 1/2 teaspoon salt
- 1/2 teaspoon coriander
- 3 tablespoons lime juice
- 2 tablespoons olive oil

Directions:

1 - Take a large bowl, place all the ingredients in it, and toss until well coated.

2 - Serve straight away

Nutrition: Calories: 91 Fat: 7.2 g Carbohydrates: 7.6 g Protein: 1.2 g

182. Carrot Salad with Cashews

Preparation time: 15 minutes
Cooking time: 20 minutes
Servings: 4

Ingredients:
- 4 cups grated carrots
- 3 scallions, chopped
- 1/2 cup cilantro, chopped
- 1/2 teaspoon minced garlic
- 1 teaspoon minced ginger
- 1/2 teaspoon salt
- 1/4 teaspoon cayenne pepper
- 1/4 teaspoon ground black pepper
- 1 teaspoon curry powder
- 2 tablespoons maple syrup
- 1/2 teaspoon ground turmeric
- 1/3 cup raisins
- 1/2 cup toasted cashews
- 1 tablespoon orange zest
- 3 tablespoon lime juice
- 1/4 cup olive oil

Directions:

1 - Take a large bowl, place all the ingredients in it, and toss until well coated.

2 - Let the salad refrigerate for 15 minutes and then serve.

Nutrition: Calories: 251 Fat: 16 g Carbohydrates: 29 g Protein: 3 g

183. Penne With Veggies

Preparation time: 5 minutes
Cooking time: 25 minutes
Servings: 6
Ingredients:
- 2 tsps. olive oil
- 2 cloves garlic, crushed and minced
- ½ cup shallots, chopped
- 2 tbsps. dry white wine
- 1 cup Brussels sprouts, trimmed and chopped
- 6 cups bok choy, chopped
- 6 cups cooked penne pasta
- 1 tbsp. vegetable oil spread
- Salt and pepper to taste
- 2 tsps. dried Italian seasoning
- 3 tbsps. Parmesan cheese, grated

Directions:
1. Pour the oil into a pan over medium heat.
2. Cook the garlic and shallots for 3 minutes.
3. Pour in the wine.
4. Scrape the browned bits using a wooden spoon.
5. Stir in the Brussels sprouts.
6. Cook for 3 minutes.
7. Stir in the bok choy and cook for 2 to 3 minutes.
8. Toss the pasta in the veggies.
9. Add the vegetable oil to the mix.
10. Season with the salt, pepper, and Italian seasoning.
11. Sprinkle the Parmesan cheese on top.

Nutrition: Calories: 127; Fat: 4g; Saturated Fat: 1g; Carbs: 17g; Fiber 3g; Protein: 6g.

184. Marinated Veggie Salad

Preparation time: 4 hours and 30 minutes
Cooking time:
Servings: 6
Ingredients:
- 1 zucchini, sliced
- 4 tomatoes, sliced into wedges
- ¼ cup red onion, sliced thinly
- 1 green bell pepper, sliced
- 2 tbsps. fresh parsley, chopped
- 2 tbsps. red-wine vinegar
- 2 tbsps. olive oil
- 1 clove garlic, minced
- 1 tsp. dried basil
- 2 tbsps. water
- Pine nuts, toasted and chopped

Directions:
1 - In a bowl, combine the zucchini, tomatoes, red onion, green bell pepper, and parsley.
2 - Pour the vinegar and oil into a glass jar with a lid.
3 - Add the garlic, basil, and water.
4 - Seal the jar and shake well to combine.
5 - Pour the dressing into the vegetable mixture.
6 - Cover the bowl.
7 - Marinate in the refrigerator for 4 hours.
8 - Garnish with the pine nuts before serving.

Nutrition: Calories: 65; Fat: 4.7g; Saturated Fat: 0.7g; Carbs: 5.3g; Fiber 1.2g; Protein: 0.9g;

185. Mediterranean Salad

Preparation time: 20 minutes
Cooking time: 5 minutes
Servings: 2
Ingredients:
- 2 tsps. balsamic vinegar
- 1 tbsp. basil pesto
- 1 cup lettuce
- ¼ cup broccoli florets, chopped
- ½ cup zucchini, chopped
- ¼ cup tomato, chopped
- ¼ cup yellow bell pepper, chopped
- 2 tbsps. feta cheese, crumbled

Directions:
1 - Arrange the lettuce on a serving platter.
2 - Top with the broccoli, zucchini, tomato, and bell pepper.
3 - In a bowl, mix the vinegar and pesto.
4 - Drizzle the dressing on top.
5 - Sprinkle the feta cheese and serve.

Nutrition: Calories: 100; Fat: 6g; Saturated Fat: 1g; Carbs: 7g; Protein: 4g.

186. Potato Salad

Preparation time: 4 hours and 20 minutes
Cooking time: 10 minutes
Servings: 6

Ingredients:
- Water
- 3 potatoes, peeled and sliced into cubes
- ½ cup plain yogurt
- ½ cup mayonnaise
- 1 clove garlic, crushed and minced
- 1 tbsp. almond milk
- 1 tbsp. fresh dill, chopped
- ½ tsp. lemon zest
- Salt to taste
- 2 hard-boiled eggs, chopped
- 6 cups lettuce, chopped

Directions:
1 - Fill your pot with water.
2 - Add the potatoes and boil.
3 - Cook for 10 minutes or until slightly tender.
4 - Drain and let cool.
5 - In a bowl, mix the yogurt, mayo, garlic, almond milk, fresh dill, lemon zest, and salt.
6 - Stir in the potatoes, flakes, and eggs.
7 - Mix well.
8 - Chill in the refrigerator for 4 hours.
9 - Stir in the shredded lettuce before serving.

Nutrition: Calories: 243; Fat: 9.9g; Saturated Fat: 2g; Carbs: 22.2g; Fiber 4.6g; Protein: 17.5g.

187. Veggie Pasta Salad

Preparation time: 50 minutes
Cooking time: 10 minutes
Servings: 6

Ingredients:
- 8 oz. asparagus, sliced
- Salt and pepper to taste
- 12 oz. farfalle, penne or macaroni pasta, cooked
- 2 tbsps. parsley, chopped
- ½ cup shallots, sliced thinly
- ¼ cup Parmesan cheese, grated
- 2 tbsps. freshly squeezed lemon juice
- ½ cup mayonnaise
- 2 tsps. garlic, minced
- 1 tsp. Worcestershire sauce
- 1 tsp. Dijon mustard
- 1 lemon, sliced into wedges

Directions:
1. Preheat your oven to 400°F.
2. Arrange the asparagus in a baking pan.
3. Season with the salt and pepper.
4. Roast in the oven for 10 minutes.
5. Let cool. Transfer to a bowl.
6. Stir in the cooked pasta, parsley, and shallots.
7. Sprinkle the Parmesan cheese on top.
8. In another bowl, combine the lemon juice, mayonnaise, garlic, Worcestershire sauce, and Dijon mustard.
9. Add this mixture to the pasta salad.
1. Toss to coat evenly.
2. Refrigerate for at least 30 minutes before serving.
3. Garnish with the lemon wedges.

Nutrition: Calories: 429; Fat: 17.1g; Saturated Fat: 2.8g; Carbs: 45.6g; Fiber 7.2g; Protein: 25g.

188. Sautéed Cabbage

Preparation time: 8 minutes
Cooking time: 12 minutes
Servings: 8

Ingredients:
- ¼ cup butter
- 1 onion, sliced thinly
- 1 head cabbage, sliced into wedges
- Salt and pepper to taste
- Crumbled crispy bacon bits

Directions:
1 - Add the butter to a pan over medium-high heat.
2 - Cook the onion for 1 minute, stirring frequently.
3 - Season with the salt and pepper.
4 - Add the cabbage and cook while stirring for 12 minutes.
5 - Sprinkle with the crispy bacon bits.

Nutrition: Calories: 77; Fat: 5.9g; Saturated Fat: 3.6g; Carbs: 6.1g; Fiber 2.4g; Protein: 1.3g.

189. Southwest Style Salad

Preparation time: 10 minutes
Cooking time: 0 minutes
Servings: 3

Ingredients:
- ½ cup dry black beans
- ½ cup dry chickpeas

- 1/3 cup purple onion, diced
- 1 red bell pepper, pitted, sliced
- 4 cups mixed greens, fresh or frozen, chopped
- 1 cup cherry tomatoes, halved or quartered
- 1 medium avocado, peeled, pitted, and cubed
- 1 cup sweet kernel corn, canned, drained
- ½ tsp. chili powder
- ¼ tsp. cumin
- ¼ tsp. Salt
- ¼ tsp. pepper
- 2 tsp. olive oil
- 1 tbsp. vinegar

Directions:

1 - Prepare the black beans and chickpeas according to the method.

2 - Put all of the ingredients into a large bowl.

3 - Toss the mix of veggies and spices until combined thoroughly.

4 - Store, or serve chilled with some olive oil and vinegar on top!

Nutrition: Calories: 635; Fat: 19.9g; Saturated Fat: 3.6g; Sodium: 302mg; Carbs: 95.4g; Dietary Fiber: 28.1g; Protein: 24.3g.

190.   Chickpeas & Veggie Salad

Preparation Time: 15 minutes

Cooking Time: 0 minutes

Servings: 4

Ingredients:

For Salad:
- 3 cups cooked chickpeas
- 2 cups, cucumber, chopped
- 1 cup cherry tomatoes, halved
- 1 cup radishes, trimmed and sliced
- 6 cups fresh baby arugula
- 4 tablespoons scallion greens, chopped
- 4 tablespoons fresh parsley leaves, chopped

For Dressing:
- 1 garlic clove, minced
- 3 tablespoons extra-virgin olive oil
- 1 tablespoon balsamic vinegar
- 1 tablespoon fresh lemon juice
- Salt and ground black pepper, as required

Directions:

1 - For salad: in a large serving bowl, add all the ingredients and mix.

2 - For dressing: in another bowl, add all the ingredients and beat until well combined.

3 - Pour dressing over salad and gently toss to coat well.

Nutrition: Calories: 338 Fat: 13g Carbohydrates: 46.7g Dietary Fiber: 10.1g Sugar: 3.2g Protein: 11.7g

191.   Mango & Avocado Salad

Preparation Time: 15 minutes

Cooking Time: 0 minutes

Servings: 6

Ingredients:
- 2½ cups mango, peeled, pitted and cubed
- 2½ cups avocado, peeled, pitted and cubed
- 1 red onion, sliced
- 6 cups fresh lettuce, torn
- ¼ cup fresh mint leaves, chopped
- 2 tablespoon fresh orange juice
- Salt, as required

Directions:

1 - Place all the ingredients in a salad bowl and gently toss to combine.

2 - Cover and refrigerate to chill before serving.

Nutrition: Calories: 182 Fat: 12.3g Carbohydrates: 18.8g Dietary Fiber: 6.2g Sugar: 11.3g Protein: 2.6g

192.   Apple & Spinach Salad

Preparation Time: 10 minutes

Cooking Time: 0 minutes

Servings: 4

Ingredients:
- 4 large apples, cored and sliced
- 6 cups fresh baby spinach
- 3 tablespoons extra-virgin olive oil
- 2 tablespoons apple cider vinegar

Directions:

1 - In a salad bowl, add all the ingredients and toss to coat well.

2 - Serve immediately.

Nutrition: Calories: 218 Fat: 11.1g Carbohydrates: 32.5g Dietary Fiber: 6.4g Sugar: 23.4g Protein: 1.9g

193.   Cucumber Tomato Chopped Salad

Preparation time: 15 minutes

Cooking time: 0 minute
Servings: 6
Ingredients:
- ½ cup light mayonnaise
- 1 tbsp. lemon juice
- 1 tbsp. fresh dill, chopped
- 1 tbsp. chives, chopped
- ½ cup feta cheese, crumbled
- Salt and pepper to taste
- 1 red onion, chopped
- 1 cucumber, diced
- 1 radish, diced
- 3 tomatoes, diced
- Chives, chopped

Directions:
1 - Combine the mayo, lemon juice, fresh dill, chives, feta cheese, salt, and pepper in a bowl.
2 - Mix well.
3 - Stir in the onion, cucumber, radish, and tomatoes.
4 - Coat evenly.
5 - Garnish with the chopped chives.

Nutrition: Calories: 187; Fat: 16.7g; Saturated Fat: 4.1g; Carbs: 6.7g; Fiber 2g; Protein: 3.3g.

194. Zucchini Pasta Salad

Preparation time: 4 minutes
Cooking time: 0 minute
Servings: 15
Ingredients:
- 5 tbsps. olive oil
- 2 tsps. Dijon mustard
- 3 tbsps. red-wine vinegar
- 1 clove garlic, grated
- 2 tbsps. fresh oregano, chopped
- 1 shallot, chopped
- ¼ tsp. red pepper flakes
- 16 oz. zucchini noodles
- ¼ cup Kalamata olives, pitted
- 3 cups cherry tomatoes, sliced in half
- ¾ cup Parmesan cheese, shaved

Directions:
1 - Mix the olive oil, Dijon mustard, red-wine vinegar, garlic, oregano, shallot, and red pepper flakes in a bowl.
2 - Stir in the zucchini noodles.
3 - Sprinkle on top the olives, tomatoes, and Parmesan cheese.

Nutrition: Calories: 299; Fat: 24.7g; Saturated Fat: 5.1g; Carbs: 11.6g; Fiber 2.8g; Protein: 7g.

195. Avocado Salad

Preparation time: 10 minutes
Cooking time: 0 minute
Servings: 4
Ingredients:
- 1 avocado
- 6 hard-boiled eggs, peeled and chopped
- 1 tbsp. mayonnaise
- 2 tbsps. freshly squeezed lemon juice
- ¼ cup celery, chopped
- 2 tbsps. chives, chopped
- Salt and pepper to taste

Directions:
1 - Add the avocado to a large bowl.
2 - Mash the avocado using a fork.
4 - Add the mayo, lemon juice, celery, chives, salt, and pepper.
5 - Chill in the refrigerator for at least 30 minutes before serving.

Nutrition: Calories: 224; Fat: 18g; Saturated Fat: 3.9g; Carbs: 6.1g; Fiber 3.6g; Protein: 10.6g.

196. Pepper Tomato Salad

Preparation time: 1 hour and 25 minutes
Cooking time: 0 minute
Servings: 8
Ingredients:
- 2 tbsps. balsamic vinegar
- 2 tbsps. olive oil
- ½ tsp. Dijon mustard
- 2 tsps. fresh basil leaves, chopped
- 1 tbsp. fresh chives, chopped
- 1 tsp. sugar
- Pepper to taste
- 2 cups yellow bell peppers, sliced into rings
- 1 cup orange bell pepper, sliced into rings
- 4 tomatoes, sliced into rounds
- ¼ cup blue cheese, crumbled

Directions:
1 - Mix the vinegar, olive oil, mustard, basil, chives, sugar, and pepper in a bowl.
2 - Arrange the tomatoes and pepper rings on a serving plate.
3 - Sprinkle the crumbled blue cheese on top.

4 - Drizzle with the dressing.
5 - Chill in the refrigerator for 1 hour before serving.

Nutrition: Calories: 116; Fat 7g; Saturated Fat: 2g; Carbs: 11g; Fiber 2g; Protein: 3g.

197. Three Grain Salad

Preparation time: 20 minutes
Cooking time: 50 minutes
Servings: 6
Ingredients:
• 1/4 cup dry wheat berries
• 1/4 cup dry barley
• 1/4 cup dry brown rice
• 1/4 cup Boozy Brown Mustard
• 1 tablespoon balsamic vinegar
• 2 garlic cloves, minced
• 6 cups finely shredded Swiss chard leaves
• 1/4 cup chopped unsalted pistachios
Directions:
1 - Pour 2 1/2 cups water in a large saucepan and bring to a boil over high heat.
2 - In a colander, combine the wheat berries, barley, and rice and rinse well.
3 - Add the mixed grains to the boiling water, stir, and return the water to a boil.
4 - Change the heat to medium-low, cover tightly, and cook until the grains are fork-tender and slightly chewy, 45 to 50 minutes. Take it from the heat and let it sit, covered, for 10 minutes.
5 - Using a fork, fluff the grains, lifting and separating them. Transfer the grains to a medium bowl and refrigerate for at least 30 minutes or up to 3 days.
6 - Get a small bowl, whisk together the mustard, vinegar, and garlic.
7 - To assemble the salad, place the chard in a large bowl. Add the cold cooked grains and the mustard dressing and gently toss. Toss in the pistachios before serving.
Store leftovers in a container and keep them in the refrigerator for up to 5 days.
Nutrition: Calories: 125 Fat: 3g Protein: 4g Carbohydrates: 22g

198. Massaged Kale Salad

Preparation time: 5 minutes
Cooking time: 5 minutes

Servings: 4
Ingredients:
• 2 bunches kale, leaves stemmed and torn into bite-size pieces
• 1/4 cup tahini
• 1/4 cup lemon juice
• 2 garlic cloves, minced
• 1/4 cup hemp seeds
• 1 teaspoon salt or Spicy Umami Blend
Directions:
1 - Put kale in a large bowl. Add the tahini, lemon juice, and garlic.
2 - With clean or gloved hands, massage the kale until it brightens and glistens, and the leaves are coated for about 3 minutes.
3 - Dust the hemp seeds and salt over the salad and toss gently, then serve.
Nutrition: Calories: 162 Fats: 13g Protein: 6g Carbohydrates: 9g

199. Artichoke Salad

Preparation time: 10 minutes
Cooking time: 35 minutes
Servings: 4
Ingredients:
• 2 (14-ounce) cans quartered artichoke hearts, drained
• 1/2 cup Tofu Sour Cream
• 1/2 cup diced sweet onion
• 1/2 cup diced celery
• 1 teaspoon dulse flakes, or 1 teaspoon Spicy Umami Blend
Directions:
1 - Coarsely chop the artichoke hearts and transfer them to a medium bowl.
2 - Add the sour cream, onion, celery, and dulse and stir to combine.
3 - Move the mixture to a sealed container and refrigerate for at least 30 minutes before serving.
Nutrition: Calories: 157 Fats: 3g Protein: 10g Carbohydrates: 27g

200. Chickpea Pecan Salad

Preparation time: 10 minutes
Cooking time: 5 minutes
Servings: 4
Ingredients:

- 1 (15-ounce) can chickpeas, drained and rinsed
- 1 (4-ounce) jar hearts of palm, drained
- 1/2 teaspoon ground thyme
- 1/2 teaspoon ground sage
- 1 large celery stalk, chopped
- 1/4 cup dried cranberries
- 2 tablespoons rice vinegar
- 1/4 cup chopped pecans

Directions:

1 - Add in chickpeas and hearts of palm in a food processor and pulse in 1-second bursts until the mixture has a flaky texture. Be careful not to over process.

2 - Transfer the mixture to a medium bowl.

3 - Add the thyme, sage, celery, cranberries, vinegar, and pecans and stir to combine.

4 - Serve immediately.

Nutrition: Calories: 225 Fats: 7g Protein: 8g Carbohydrates: 35g

201.　Loaded Potato with Tofu "Egg" Salad

Preparation time: 10 minutes
Cooking time: 30 minutes + 1-hour chill
Servings: 4

Ingredients:

- 2 large russet potatoes, unpeeled, scrubbed
- 1 (14-ounce) package extra-firm tofu, pressed, and drained
- 1/2 cup chopped celery
- 1/2 cup chopped red onion
- 1/2 cup Tofu Sour Cream
- 1 teaspoon ground mustard
- 1/2 teaspoon black salt, or 1 teaspoon Spicy Umami Blend
- 1/4 teaspoon freshly ground black pepper
- 1/2 teaspoon smoked paprika

Directions:

1 - Fill up a deep saucepan with 1 to 2 inches of water, insert a steamer basket, and bring to a boil.

2 - Once boiling, lower the heat and place the potatoes in the steamer. Cover and steam for 30 minutes until the potatoes are tender.

3 - Transfer the potatoes to a bowl and refrigerate for at least 1 hour.

4 - Prepare tofu in a large bowl and gently mash it with a fork or potato masher until crumbled.

5 - Add the celery, onion, sour cream, ground mustard, black salt, and pepper and stir until combined.

6 - Put the mixture in a safe container and refrigerate for at least 1 hour.

7 - Cut the chilled potatoes in half. Slowly scoop out the flesh using a spoon, leaving about 1/2 inch attached to the skins; reserve the flesh for another use.

8 - Put 1/4 cup of the tofu mixture into each potato skin and sprinkle with paprika, then serve.

Nutrition: Calories: 287 Fats: 8g Protein: 18g Carbohydrates: 38g

202.　The Waldorf salad

Preparation time: 15 minutes
Cooking time: 10 minutes
Servings: 4

Ingredients:

- 1/2 cup Tofu Sour Cream
- 3 tablespoons lemon juice
- 2 tablespoons nutritional yeast
- 2 garlic cloves, minced
- 1 Medjool date, pitted (optional)
- 1/2 cup chopped walnuts
- Zest of 1 lemon (optional)
- 2 large Gala apples, cored and cut into 1/4-inch pieces
- 2 celery stalks, chop into 1/2-inch pieces
- 1 cup grapes (any kind), halved
- 1 head red-leaf lettuce, chopped or torn into bite-size pieces
- 1 head Bibb or Boston lettuce, chopped or torn into bite-size pieces

Directions:

1 - With a food processor or blender, mix in the sour cream, lemon juice, nutritional yeast, garlic, and date. Purée until creamy and pourable.

2 - If needed, put in 2 tablespoons of water to make it thinner. Set aside.

3 - In a small bowl, combine the walnuts and lemon zest (if using).

4 - Get a large bowl, combine the apples, celery, and grapes. Add the lettuces and toss to combine. Put dressing over the salad and toss until evenly coated.

5 - Portion the salad into four bowls. Sprinkle 2 tablespoons of the walnut–lemon zest mixture over each salad and serve.

Nutrition: Calories: 255 Fats: 12g Protein: 9g Carbohydrates: 34g

203. Classic Wedge Salad

Preparation time: 15 minutes
Cooking time: 15 minutes
Servings: 4

Ingredients:

- 2 carrots, finely diced
- 2 tablespoons low-sodium soy sauce or tamari
- 2 teaspoons pure maple syrup
- 1/2 teaspoon smoked paprika
- 2 ripe avocados
- 1/4 cup cashews
- 2 tablespoons apple cider vinegar
- 1 tablespoon nutritional yeast
- 1 teaspoon spirulina powder (optional)
- 1 small red onion, sliced
- 1 cup cherry or grape tomatoes, halved
- 1 head iceberg lettuce, cut into 4 wedges
- Freshly ground black pepper

Directions:

1 - Prepare carrots in a small bowl and let sit for 10 minutes.

2 - Whisk the soy sauce, maple syrup, and paprika, then pour it over the carrots. Set aside.

3 - Remove the avocado pits by slicing them in half. Dice the flesh of one of the avocado halves in the peel, then gently scoop it out into a small bowl. Set aside.

4 - Scoop the flesh from the 3 remaining avocado halves into a blender.

5 - Add the cashews, vinegar, nutritional yeast, spirulina (if using), and purée until smooth, creamy, and pourable.

6 - Put more water if needed to reach the right consistency. Pour the dressing into a medium bowl.

7 - Add the onion, tomatoes, and carrots (along with the liquid in the bowl) to the bowl.

8 - Pour the dressing and stir to combine. Gently fold the diced avocado into the dressing.

9 - Place a wedge of lettuce on each of the four salad plates. Dress the lettuce by spooning about 1/2 cup of dressing over each wedge, then repeat until the dressing is used up.

10 - Sprinkle with black pepper over each salad and serve.

Nutrition: Calories: 298 Fats: 20g Protein: 8g Carbohydrates: 29g

204. Caper Caesar Salad

Preparation time: 10 minutes
Cooking time: 35 minutes
Servings: 4

Ingredients:

- 1/2 cup plus 1 tablespoon raw cashews, divided
- 2 heads romaine lettuce, chopped
- 2 tablespoons Boozy Brown Mustard or Dijon mustard
- 3 tablespoons lemon juice
- 1 tablespoon capers, drained
- 2 garlic cloves, minced
- 1 Medjool date, pitted
- 1 teaspoon Spicy Umami Blend, or 1/2 teaspoon kosher salt
- 1/2 teaspoon ground white pepper
- 1/4 cup hemp seeds

Directions:

1 - Place 1/2 cup of cashews in a measuring cup and add hot water to cover. Set aside to soak for 30 minutes.

2 - Prepare lettuce in a large bowl. Set aside.

3 - Put the drained cashews in a blender. Add the mustard, lemon juice, capers, garlic, date, umami blend, and white pepper and purée until creamy and pourable. Add additional water or lemon juice, if needed, to make it thinner.

4 - Pour the dressing over the lettuce and toss until evenly coated.

5 - Chop the remaining 1 tablespoon of cashews and combine with the hemp seeds in a small bowl. Sprinkle the cashew mixture over the lettuce and gently stir to combine.

6 - Portion the salad into four bowls and serve.

Nutrition: Calories: 235 Fats: 14g Protein: 9g Carbohydrates: 24g

205. Jackfruit Louie Avocado Salad

Preparation time: 10 minutes
Cooking time: 10 minutes
Servings: 4

Ingredients:

- 1/2 cup Tofu Sour Cream
- 2 teaspoons apple cider vinegar

- 1 garlic clove, minced
- 1/4 teaspoon ground ginger
- 1/4 teaspoon ground mustard
- 1/4 teaspoon onion powder
- 1 (14-ounce) can jackfruit, drained
- 1 teaspoon chili powder
- 8 cups chopped lettuce
- 2 ripe avocados, halved and pitted

Directions:

1 - Get a small bowl, then mix together the sour cream, vinegar, garlic, ginger, ground mustard, and onion powder. Set aside.

2 - Place the jackfruit in a medium bowl. Dust with the chili powder and stir until evenly coated. Add the sour cream mixture and stir to combine. Set aside.

3 - Plate 2 cups of the chopped lettuce on each of the four salad plates. Scoop the flesh from 1 avocado half over the lettuce on each plate.

4 - Spoon 1/2 cup of the jackfruit mixture into each avocado half. Spoon the remaining jackfruit mixture equally over each plate and serve.

Nutrition: Calories: 337 Fats: 18g Protein: 11g Carbohydrates: 39g

206. Corn Cobb Salad

Preparation time: 15 minutes

Cooking time: 20 minutes

Servings: 4

Ingredients:

- 6 fingerling potatoes, unpeeled, cut in half
- 2 ears corn, shucked and halved crosswise
- 1/2 cup red wine vinegar
- 1/4 cup raw hulled pumpkin seeds
- 3 green onions, chopped
- 1 head Bibb lettuce, chopped
- 1 head romaine lettuce, chopped
- 1/2 teaspoon ground turmeric
- 1/2 teaspoon freshly ground black pepper
- 1/4 teaspoon black salt
- 4 pieces Tempeh Bacon chopped

Directions:

1 - Add a few waters to a large saucepan, insert a steamer basket, and boil over medium heat.

2 - Adjust heat to medium-high and place the potatoes in the steamer—cover and steam for 10 minutes.

3 - Place corn to the steamer, cover, and steam for 5 minutes more.

4 - While the potatoes and corn are steaming, in a small bowl, mix together the vinegar, pumpkin seeds, and green onions to make a dressing. Set aside.

5 - In a large bowl, toss together the chopped lettuce. Set aside.

6 - Transfer the corn to a wire rack and let cool. Transfer the potatoes to a medium bowl, and add the turmeric, pepper, and black salt. Stir until the potatoes are evenly coated. Set aside.

7 - Add dressing over the lettuce and gently toss.

8 - Portion the lettuce into four large bowls. Place one piece of corn in the middle of each bowl. Line three pieces of potato along one side of each bowl and sprinkle the tempeh bacon along the other side. Serve.

Nutrition: Calories: 357 Fat: 8g Protein: 16g Carbohydrates: 59g

207. Mixed Berries Salad

Preparation Time: 15 minutes

Cooking Time: 0 minutes

Servings: 4

Ingredients:

- 1 cup fresh strawberries, hulled and sliced
- ½ cup fresh blackberries
- ½ cup fresh blueberries
- ½ cup fresh raspberries
- 6 cups fresh arugula
- 2 tablespoons olive oil
- Salt, as required

Directions:

1 - In a salad bowl, place all ingredients and toss to coat well.

2 - Serve immediately.

Nutrition: Calories: 105 Fat: 7.6g Carbohydrates: 10.1g Dietary Fiber: 3.6g Sugar: 5.7g Protein: 1.6g

208. Beet & Spinach Salad

Preparation Time: 15 minutes

Cooking Time: 1 hour

Servings: 2

Ingredients:

- 3 medium beets, trimmed
- 1 tablespoon extra-virgin olive oil
- 1 tablespoon balsamic vinegar
- 1 teaspoon maple syrup
- Salt and ground black pepper, as required
- 4 cups fresh spinach, torn
- ¼ cup walnuts, chopped

Directions:

1 - Preheat your oven to 400 °F.

2 - With a piece foil, wrap each beet completely.

3 - Arrange the foil packets onto a baking sheet and roast for about 1 hour.

4 - Remove from the oven and carefully, open the foil packets.

5 - Set aside to cool slightly.

6 - With a paper towel, remove the peel of beets and then cut into chunks.

7 - In a serving bowl, add the oil, vinegar, maple syrup, salt and black pepper and beat well.

8 - Add beet chunks, spinach and walnuts and toss to coat well.

10. Serve immediately.

Nutrition: Calories: 247 Fat: 16.7g Carbohydrates: 21g Dietary Fiber: 5.4g Sugar: 14.4g Protein: 8g

209. Cucumber & Tomato Salad

Preparation Time: 15 minutes

Cooking Time: 0 minutes

Servings: 4

Ingredients:

• 2 cups plum tomatoes, chopped
• 2 cups cucumbers, chopped
• 2 cups mixed fresh lettuce, torn
• 2 cups fresh baby spinach
• 2 tablespoons extra virgin olive oil
• 2 tablespoons fresh lime juice
• Salt, as required

Directions:

1.Place all the ingredients in a salad bowl and gently, toss to combine.

2. Serve immediately.

Nutrition: Calories: 96 Fat: 7.4g Carbohydrates: 7.9g Dietary Fiber: 1.8g Sugar: 4.8g Protein: 2g

Chapter 19.   Rice & Grains

210.   Almond Crackers

Preparation Time: 15 minutes
Cooking Time: 15 minutes
Servings: 8

Ingredients:

- 1 tablespoon sesame seeds
- 4 tablespoons water
- 1 cup almond flour
- ½ teaspoon sea salt
- 2 tablespoons flaxseed meal

Directions:

1 - Set the oven to 350 degrees Fahrenheit.
2 - Prepare a baking sheet with parchment paper.
3 - Mix flaxseed meal and water in a small bowl.
4 - Leave for 10 minutes, stirring occasionally.
5 - After 10 minutes, the mixture should be gooey. It acts as binding agent for the mixture.
6 - Combine almond flour, flax mixture, salt, and sesame seeds in a medium bowl.
7 - Roll the dough into a ball and place it on a parchment-lined surface.
8 - Then, cover again with a piece of parchment paper, press with your hand to flatten.
9 - Roll with a pin until it is about 1/8 inch thick.
10 - The thinner the crackers, the crispier they will be.
11 - Remove cover paper.
12 - Using a pizza cutter or knife, cut any shape to your desired size.
13 - Poke the center with a toothpick to prevent puffing.
14 - Add a little salt if desired.
15 - Put the leftover parchment paper on the baking sheet. Put each cracker on the sheet carefully.
16 - Bake for 15 minutes or until the edges are slightly golden brown.
17 - Allow it to cool and serve.
Nutrition: Calories: 87 Fat: 2.5g Saturated Fat: 0g Cholesterol: 0mg Sodium: 72.7mg Carbohydrates: 2.5g Fiber: 1g Sugars: 0.5g Protein: 2.4g

211.   Cauliflower Black Bean Rice

Preparation Time: 10 minutes
Cooking Time: 20 minutes
Servings: 4

Ingredients:

- 15.5 oz. cooked black beans
- 3 cups cauliflower rice
- ½ cup chopped onion
- 1 ½ teaspoon minced garlic
- ¼ teaspoon ground cayenne pepper
- ½ cup diced red bell pepper
- 3 tablespoons chopped pickled jalapeno
- ¼ teaspoon ground black pepper
- 1/3 teaspoon sea salt
- 2 tablespoons extra-virgin olive oil
- ½ cup diced parsley

Directions:

1 - Add oil and garlic in a large skillet over medium heat and cook for 2 minutes.
2 - Sauté onion and red bell pepper, seasoning with all spices.
3 - Cook it for 5 minutes, and sauté in cauliflower rice and jalapeno.
4 - Add salt and black pepper, cook for 7 minutes while stirring.
5 - Add beans and cook them for 2 minutes until hot.
6 - Serve topped with parsley
Nutrition: Calories: 270.3 Fat: 1.6 g Carbohydrates: 52.7 g Protein: 13.5 Fiber: 13.1 g

212.   Skillet Quinoa

Preparation Time: 20 minutes
Cooking Time: 25 minutes
Servings: 4

Ingredients:

- 1 cup sweet potato, cubed
- ½ cup water
- 1 tablespoon olive oil
- 1 onion, chopped
- 3 cloves garlic, minced
- 1 teaspoon ground cumin
- 1 teaspoon ground coriander
- ½ teaspoon chili powder
- ½ teaspoon dried oregano
- 15 oz. black beans, rinsed and drained
- 15 oz. roasted tomatoes
- 1 ¼ cup vegetable broth
- 1 cup frozen corn
- 1 cup quinoa (uncooked)

- Salt to taste
- ½ cup light sour cream
- ½ cup fresh cilantro leaves

Directions:

1 - Add the water and sweet potato to a pan over medium heat.

2 - Bring to a boil.

3 - Decrease heat and cook sweet potatoes.

4 - Add the oil and onion.

5 - Cook for 3 minutes.

6 - Cook garlic and spices for 1 minute.

7 - Add the rest of the ingredients, except the sour cream and cilantro.

8 - Cook for 20 minutes.

9 - Serve with sour cream and top with the cilantro before serving.

Nutrition: Calories: 421; Fiber: 11 g; Proteins: 16 g.

213. Green Beans with Balsamic Sauce

Preparation Time: 10 minutes
Cooking Time: 15 minutes
Servings: 6

Ingredients:

- 2 shallots, sliced
- 8 cups green beans, trimmed
- 2 tablespoons olive oil
- Salt and pepper to taste
- 2 tablespoons balsamic vinegar
- ¼ cup parmesan cheese, grated

Directions:

1 - Preheat your oven to 425° F.

2 - Line you're baking with foil.

3 - In the pan, toss the shallots and beans in oil, salt, and pepper.

4 - Roast in the oven for 15 minutes.

5 - Drizzle with vinegar and top with cheese.

Nutrition: Calories: 78; Fiber: 0.6 g; Proteins: 1.9 g.

214. Grain Dishes Cranberry and Walnut Brown Rice

Preparation Time: 10 minutes
Cooking Time: 15 minutes
Servings: 5

Ingredients:

- 1/4 cup water
- 1/4 cup dried cranberries
- 14 oz. vegetable broth
- 3/4 cup brown rice
- 1/4 cup chopped walnuts
- 1/8 teaspoon ground cinnamon
- Salt to taste

Directions:

1 - To begin this recipe, you should first cook your brown rice in the vegetable broth according to the directions on the package.

2 - Once this is done, allow the rice to cool slightly before adding it to a mixing bowl.

3 - With the rice in place, add the walnuts and cranberries. Begin to season with the salt and ground cinnamon.

4 - Once everything is in place, toss the flavors together, and your dish is set.

Nutrition: Calories: 150; Carbs: 25 g; Fat: 5 g; Proteins: 5 g.

215. Curried Rice

Preparation Time: 5 minutes
Cooking Time: 25 minutes
Servings: 4

Ingredients:

- 1 tablespoon olive oil
- 1 broccoli, chopped
- 2 teaspoons ginger
- 1 cup spinach, chopped
- 1 tablespoon water
- 1 teaspoon curry powder
- 1 cup brown rice
- 2 garlic cloves, minced
- Salt to taste
- 2 carrots, chopped
- Pepper to taste

Directions:

1 - Whether you are using this recipe as a base or a side, it is sure to offer a kick to any dish it is served with! To save yourself some time, you should prepare all the vegetables ahead of time.

2 - When you are set to cook the dish, bring a skillet above moderate temperature and toss the oil, ginger, and garlic together. Once you can smell these ingredients, you can add the broccoli and carrot pieces. At this point, you should stir the ingredients and season to your fancy.

3 - Next, flash steam the vegetables.

4 - You can complete this task by placing one tablespoon of water into the bottom of the skillet and place a lid over the top for one minute.

5 - When that is set, add your cooked brown rice along with the curry powder. Be sure to toss everything and coat the ingredients well.

6 - If the rice is seasoned to your fancy, allow to cool off slightly and then serve.

Nutrition: Calories: 250; Carbs: 45 g; Fat: 5 g; Proteins: 10 g.

216. Cilantro and Avocado Lime Rice

Preparation Time: 5 minutes
Cooking Time: 20 minutes
Servings: 4

Ingredients:
- 2 avocados, sliced
- 5 cups brown rice, cooked
- 1/2 teaspoon cumin
- 1/4 cup cilantro, chopped
- 2 tablespoon lime juice
- 1 garlic clove, minced
- Salt to taste

Directions:

1 - For a rice recipe with a twist, you need to try this recipe! Begin by taking out a mixing bowl and mashing down the avocado pieces until they are perfectly smooth.

2 - Once the avocado is set, add in your seasonings, cilantro, and squeeze in the lime juice.

3 - Finally, stir in your brown rice that has already been cooked and blend together well before serving.

Nutrition: Calories: 450; Carbs: 60 g; Fat: 15 g; Proteins: 5 g.

217. Fried Veggie Brown Rice

Preparation Time: 10 minutes
Cooking Time: 35 minutes
Servings: 4

Ingredients:
- 4 garlic cloves, chopped
- 1/2 teaspoon sesame oil
- 3 1/2 cups water
- 2 cups brown rice
- 4 green onions
- 1 cup green peas
- 1 carrot, diced

- 1/2 red bell pepper, diced
- 1 tablespoon rice vinegar
- 1 1/2 tablespoon soy sauce

Directions:

1 - Fried rice is a classic dish; now you can make the healthy version of it! You should start this recipe cooking your rice in some water according to the directions on the package.

2 - As the rice cooks, take out a skillet and bring it over high heat.

3 - Once warm, add in the olive oil, scallions, ginger, and chopped garlic. When everything is in place, cook the ingredients for two or three minutes.

4 - Next, toss in the peas, carrots, and the diced peppers. You will only be cooking these for another three minutes. Be sure to stir everything consistently to help avoid anything burning to the bottom.

5 - With the vegetables all cooked, it is time to add in the rice vinegar, soy sauce, and the rice you just cooked. At this point, feel free to season the dish however you desire.

6 - Finally, portion out your meal, and enjoy your rice.

Nutrition: Calories: 410; Carbs: 80 g; Fat: 4 g; Proteins: 10 g.

218. Vegetable Stir-fry

Preparation Time: 10 minutes
Cooking Time: 40 minutes
Servings: 3

Ingredients:
- 2 tablespoon olive oil
- 1/2 zucchini
- 1/2 red bell pepper
- 4 garlic cloves
- 1/2 broccoli
- 1 cup cabbage
- 1/2 cup brown rice
- 2 tablespoons tamari sauce
- 1 red chili pepper
- 1 teaspoon cayenne powder
- 1 parsley
- Optional: sesame seeds

Directions:

1 - First things first, go ahead and cook your brown rice according to the directions provided on the package.

2 - As the rice cooks, get out your frying pan and place some water at the bottom. Once it is boiling, add in

all of the diced vegetables from the list above. Once in place, be sure the ingredients are covered by the water, and then cook everything for two minutes under high heat. Once done, drain the vegetables and place them to the side.

3 - Next, put some olive oil in the pan and add garlic, cayenne, and parsley. After this has cooked for a minute or so, add the vegetables back in along with the tamari sauce and your rice.

4 - Cook everything here for an additional two minutes before removing it from heat.

5 - When it is ready, add some sesame seeds as garnish.

Nutrition: Calories: 280; Carbs: 35 g; Fat: 10 g; Proteins: 10 g.

219. Sweet Coconut Pilaf

Preparation Time: 5 minutes
Cooking Time: 30 minutes
Servings: 4
Ingredients:
- 2 tablespoons coconut oil
- 1 cinnamon stick
- 1 teaspoon ground cumin
- 1 cauliflower
- 1 onion, diced
- 3 garlic cloves
- 2 bay leaves
- 1 teaspoon ground coriander
- 1 cup coconut milk
- 1 1/2 teaspoon ground ginger
- 1 teaspoon ground cardamom
- 1 1/2 teaspoon ground turmeric
- 1 tablespoon ginger, grated

Directions:
1 - If you are looking to switch up your grains, this is the perfect dish for you. Begin by heating your oven to 400° F.

2 - As the oven begins to warm up, it is now time to prepare the cauliflower. Start by cutting the cauliflower into bite-sized pieces and then carefully place them onto your baking pan. Once in place, drizzle some coconut oil over the cauliflower and dash with salt, coriander, and cumin. When the cauliflower is set, pop the dish into the oven for about twenty-five minutes.

3 - As the cauliflower cooks, take out a saucepan and begin heating up another tablespoon of coconut oil over medium heat. Once warm, you can also add in the ginger, garlic, onion, coriander, and a bit of salt. Cook these ingredients together for about five minutes.

4 - With the garlic and onion cooked, add the rest of the spices before also throwing in the quinoa, a half cup of water, cinnamon, coconut milk, and the bay leaves. Throw a lid on top and simmer the ingredients for fifteen minutes.

5 - When the quinoa is done, mix together the cauliflower and quinoa together, and your meal is set!

Nutrition: Calories: 150; Carbs: 20 g; Fat: 7 g; Proteins: 5 g.

220. Vegetable Quinoa Tots

Preparation Time: 5 minutes
Cooking Time: 1 hour
Servings: 4
Ingredients:
- 1 broccoli, cut
- 1/2 cup peas
- 2 carrots, chopped
- 1 cup quinoa, cooked
- 1 garlic powder
- 1/4 cup nutritional yeast
- Salt to taste
- 1/2 cup water
- 3/4 cup garbanzo bean flour

Directions:
1 - These tots are easy to make and even easier to enjoy! You should start this recipe by prepping the oven to 400°F and getting out your sheet pan.

2 - Before you begin creating the tots, cook the quinoa according to the directions provided on the package. In the meantime, take a small bowl and mix the flour and water. Once complete, set the bowl to the side.

3 - Now, it is time to get your food processor out. Once you have this set, place the peas, carrot, and broccoli in. Blend these ingredients until the vegetables are broken down into tiny bits. When this step is complete, add it into the flour mixture along with the quinoa, salt, garlic powder, and nutritional yeast. Be sure to mix everything as well as possible.

4 - When you are set, use your hands to create tots from the mixture. Once created, place them onto your baking sheet and pop the dish into the oven for twenty minutes.

5 - After twenty minutes, take away the dish from the cooker and flip the tots over. Once they are all flipped, place the dish back into the oven for another twenty minutes, and by the end, you will have crispy and healthy tots.

Nutrition: Calories: 260; Carbs: 50 g; Fat: 3 g; Proteins: 15 g.

221. Easy Millet Nuggets

Preparation Time: 5 minutes
Cooking Time: 10 minutes
Servings: 4
Ingredients:
- 1/2 cup millet
- 3 scallions, sliced
- 1 lemon zest
- 1/4 cup mint
- 1 can chickpeas
- 2 tablespoons olive oil
- Pepper to taste

Directions:
1 - Begin this recipe by first cooking the millet. You can do this by following the instructions provided on the packet.
2 - As the millet cooks, place your chickpeas into a mixing dish and smash them down using a fork. When this is done, incorporate the remainder of the ingredients along with the cooked millet.
3 - Next, use your hands to create nugget shapes from the mixture.
4 - With this set, heat a skillet over intermediate heat and bake the nuggets for about five minutes on every side.
5 - Finally, remove from the pan and dip in your favorite plant-friendly dipping sauce!

Nutrition: Calories: 250; Carbs: 35 g; Fat: 10 g; Proteins: 5 g.

222. Millet Fritters

Preparation Time: 5 minutes
Cooking Time: 20 minutes
Servings: 4
Ingredients:
- 2 tablespoons coconut oil
- 1/3 cup psyllium husk
- 1/2 cup chickpea flour
- 1 cup millet
- 1/8 teaspoon mustard powder
- Pepper to taste
- 1/2 teaspoon onion powder
- 1/2 teaspoon paprika
- 1 teaspoon dried parsley
- 1/8 teaspoon coriander
- Salt to taste

Directions:
1 - To start this recipe, first cook your millet according to the directions on the package. Once this is cooked through, place the millet into a mixing bowl.
2 - Next, add the flour, psyllium husk, and all of the seasonings into your bowl and mix everything well.
3 - Once you have a "dough" formed, use your hands to create patties from the ingredients and set on a plate to the side.
4 - When you bake the fritters, take a medium skillet and put it over a medium heat. As it warms up, add some coconut oil and your first batch of fritters into the pan.
5 - You should grill the fritters for nearly five minutes on either side or up until the fritter is a nice, golden color and crunchy on the outer surface.
6 - Finally, remove the dish from the stove and enjoy your creation!

Nutrition: Calories: 410; Carbs: 50 g; Fat: 15 g; Proteins: 10 g.

223. Classic Garlicky Rice

Preparation Time: 4 minutes
Cooking Time: 16 minutes
Servings: 4
Ingredients:
- 4 tablespoons olive oil
- 4 cloves garlic, chopped
- 1 ½ cups white rice
- 2 ½ cups vegetable broth

Directions:
1 - In a saucepan, heat the olive oil over a moderately high flame. Add in the garlic and sauté for about 1 minute or until aromatic.
2 - Add in the rice and broth. Bring to a boil; immediately turn the heat to a medium flame.
3 - Cook for about 15 minutes or until all the liquid has been absorbed. Fluff the rice with a fork; season with salt and pepper, and serve hot!

Nutrition: Calories: 422; Fat: 15.1 g; Carbs: 61.1 g; Proteins: 9.3 g.

224. Brown Rice with Vegetables and Tofu

Preparation Time: 12 minutes
Cooking Time: 33 minutes
Servings: 4

Ingredients:

- 4 teaspoons sesame seeds
- 2 spring garlic stalks, minced
- 1 cup spring onions, chopped
- 1 carrot, trimmed and sliced
- 1 celery rib, sliced
- 1/4 cup dry white wine
- 10 ounces tofu, cubed
- 1 ½ cups long-grain brown rice, rinsed thoroughly
- 2 tablespoons soy sauce
- 2 tablespoons tahini
- 1 tablespoon lemon juice

Directions:

1 - In a wok or large saucepan, heat 2 teaspoons of the sesame oil over medium-high fire. Now, cook the garlic, onion, carrot, and celery for about 3 minutes, stirring periodically to ensure even cooking.

2 - Add the wine to deglaze the pan and push the vegetables to one side of the wok. Add in the remaining sesame oil and fry the tofu for 8 minutes, stirring occasionally.

3 - Bring 2 ½ cups of water to a boil over medium-high heat. Bring to a simmer and cook the rice for about 30 minutes or until it is tender; fluff the rice and stir it with the soy sauce and tahini.

4 - Stir the vegetables and tofu into the hot rice; add a few drizzles of the fresh lemon juice and serve warm. Bon appétit!

Nutrition: Calories: 410; Fat: 13.2 g; Carbs: 60 g; Proteins: 14.3 g.

225. Basic Amaranth Porridge

Preparation Time: 30 minutes
Cooking Time: 5 minutes
Servings: 4

Ingredients:

- 3 cups water
- 1 cup amaranth
- 1/2 cup coconut milk
- 4 tablespoons agave syrup
- A pinch of kosher salt
- A pinch of grated nutmeg

Directions:

1 - Bring the water to a boil over medium-high heat; add in the amaranth and turn the heat to a simmer.

2 - Let it cook for about 30 minutes, stirring periodically to prevent the amaranth from sticking to the bottom of the pan.

3 - Stir in the remaining ingredients and continue to cook for 1 to 2 minutes more until cooked through. Bon appétit!

Nutrition: Calories: 261; Fat: 4.4 g; Carbs: 49 g; Proteins: 7.3 g.

226. Country Cornbread with Spinach

Preparation Time: 25 minutes
Cooking Time: 25 minutes
Servings: 8

Ingredients:

- 1 tablespoon flaxseed meal
- 1 cup all-purpose flour
- 1 cup yellow cornmeal
- 1/2 teaspoons baking soda
- 1/2 teaspoons baking powder
- 1 teaspoon kosher salt
- 1 teaspoon brown sugar
- A pinch of grated nutmeg
- 1 ¼ cups oat milk, unsweetened
- 1 teaspoon white vinegar
- 1/2 cup olive oil
- 2 cups spinach, torn into pieces

Directions:

1 - Start by preheating your oven to 420° F. Now, coat a baking pan with a nonstick cooking spray.

2 - To make the flax eggs, mix the flaxseed meal with 3 tablespoons of water. Stir and let it sit for about 15 minutes.

3 - In a mixing bowl, thoroughly combine the flour, cornmeal, baking soda, baking powder, salt, sugar, and grated nutmeg.

4 - Gradually add in the flax egg, oat milk, vinegar, and olive oil, whisking constantly to avoid lumps. Afterward, fold in the spinach.

5 - Scrape the batter into the prepared baking pan. Bake your cornbread for about 25 minutes or until a tester inserted in the middle comes out dry and clean.

6 - Let it stand for about 10 minutes before slicing and serving. Bon appétit!

Nutrition: Calories: 282; Fat: 15.4 g; Carbs: 30 g; Proteins: 4.6 g.

227. Rice Pudding with Currants

Preparation Time: 5 minutes
Cooking Time: 40 minutes
Servings: 4
Ingredients:
- 1 ½ cups water
- 1 cup white rice
- 2 ½ cups oat milk, divided
- 1/2 cup white sugar
- A pinch of salt
- A pinch of grated nutmeg
- 1 teaspoon ground cinnamon
- 1/2 teaspoons vanilla extract
- 1/2 cup dried currants

Directions:
1 - In a saucepan, bring the water to a boil over medium-high heat. Immediately turn the heat to a simmer; add in the rice and let it cook for about 20 minutes.
2 - Add the milk, sugar, and spices and continue to cook for 20 minutes more, stirring constantly to prevent the rice from sticking to the pan.
3 - Top with dried currants and serve at room temperature. Bon appétit!
Nutrition: Calories: 423; Fat: 5.3 g; Carbs: 85 g; Proteins: 8.8 g.

228. Chard Wraps with Millet

Preparation Time: 5 minutes
Cooking Time: 10 minutes
Servings: 4
Ingredients:
- 1 cut into thin strips carrot
- ½ cut into thin strips cucumber
- ½ cup cooked chickpeas
- ½ cooked millet
- 1 cup sliced cabbage
- Hemp seeds as needed
- 1 bunch Swiss rainbow chard
- Mint leaves as needed
- 1/3 cup hummus

Directions:
1 - Apply hummus on one side of chard, put some millet, veggies, and chickpeas.

2 - Add mint leaves and hemp seeds as a topping and turn it into a burrito.
Nutrition: Calories: 152 Fat: 4.5 g Carbohydrates: 25 g Protein: 3.5 g Fiber: 2.4 g

229. Corn Kernel Black Bean Rice

Preparation Time: 10 minutes
Cooking Time: 25 minutes
Servings: 8
Ingredients:
- 15.25 oz. cooked kernel corn
- 8 oz. yellow rice mix
- 2 tablespoons extra-virgin olive oil
- 1 teaspoon ground cumin
- 1 1/4 cups water
- 15 oz. cooked black beans
- 2 teaspoons lemon juice

Directions:
1 - Heat a saucepan over high heat by adding oil, water and rice.
2 - Bring it to a boil and reduce heat to medium.
3 - Let it simmer until rice is tender and the liquid has vanished.
4 - Place the rice in a large bowl.
5 - Add the rest of the ingredients to the rice.
6 - Mix to combine and serve immediately!
Nutrition: Calories: 100 Fat: 4.4 g Carbohydrates: 15.1 g Protein: 2 g Fiber: 1.4 g

230. Rice & Cuban Beans

Preparation Time: 20 minutes
Cooking Time: 55 Minutes
Servings: 6
Ingredients:
- 2 ½ cups vegetable broth
- 1 cup uncooked rice
- 1 cup chopped onion
- 1 teaspoon sea salt
- 1 teaspoon minced garlic
- 4 tablespoons tomato paste
- 1 cored & chopped green bell pepper
- 15.25 oz. cooked kidney beans
- 1 tablespoon extra-virgin olive oil

Directions:
1 - Heat oil in a saucepan over medium heat.

2 - Add onion, garlic, bell pepper and sauté for 5 minutes until tender.

3 - Sauté in tomato and salt and cook for a minute.

4 - Mix in the rice and beans, pour in the stock and stir.

5 - Cook for 45 minutes or until the liquid has absorbed.

6 - Serve hot!

Nutrition: Calories: 258 Fat: 3.2g Carbohydrates: 49.3g Protein: 7.3g Fiber: 5g

231. Potato & Corn Chowder

Preparation Time: 10 minutes
Cooking Time: 16 minutes
Servings: 6

Ingredients:
- 2 medium peeled & chopped carrots
- 1 rib chopped celery
- 1 medium peeled onion
- 1 tablespoon extra-virgin olive oil
- ¼ cup all-purpose flour
- 1 teaspoon dried thyme
- 1 ½ teaspoon minced garlic
- 2 cups vegetable broth
- 4 cups chopped white potatoes
- 2 cups vegetable broth
- 3 tablespoons nutritional yeast
- 1 cup frozen corn kernels
- 2 cups unsweetened almond milk
- 1 teaspoon sea salt
- ¼ teaspoon ground black pepper

Directions:
1 - Heat oil in a large pot over medium heat.

2 - Add onion, garlic, carrots, celery and cook for 5 minutes until golden-brown.

3 - Sprinkle thyme and flour and stir to coat for a minute or until the flour turns brown.

4 - Next, add yeast, milk, potatoes, vegetable stock and stir until combined.

5 - Cook for 8 minutes or until tender.

6 - Lastly, add corn and sprinkle sea salt and black pepper.

Nutrition: Calories: 126 Fat: 3 g Carbohydrates: 18 g Protein: 6 g Fiber: 3 g

232. Tomato Pesto Quinoa

Preparation Time: 10 minutes

Cooking Time: 25 minutes
Servings: 1

Ingredients:
- 2 tablespoons sun dried chopped tomatoes
- 1 cup chopped onion
- 1 minced garlic clove
- A pinch of sea salt
- 1 cup chopped zucchini
- 1 chopped tomato
- 3 tablespoons Basil Pesto
- 2 cups cooked Quinoa
- 1 cup chopped spinach
- 1 tablespoon nutritional yeast

Directions:
1 - Heat oil in a skillet over medium heat.

2 - Add onion and garlic and cook for 5 minutes until translucent.

3 - Add in zucchini and sea salt, and cook for 5 minutes.

4 - Next, put in sun dried tomatoes and combine well.

5 - Stir in the pesto and combine well.

6 - Put spinach, quinoa and zucchini mixture in a bowl or plate, and serve with nutritional yeast.

Nutrition: Calories: 535 Protein: 20g Fat: 23g Carbohydrates: 69g

233. Oatmeal Cookies

Preparation Time: 10 minutes
Cooking Time: 25 minutes
Servings: 12

Ingredients:
- 2 cups oatmeal
- ½ teaspoon cinnamon
- 1/3 cup raisins
- ¼ cup applesauce
- 1/3 teaspoon pure vanilla extract
- 1 cup mashed ripe banana

Directions:
1 - Preheat oven to 350 degrees Fahrenheit.

2 - Combine everything to a gooey consistency.

3 - Spoon it on an ungreased baking sheet and then apply pressure to flatten.

4 - Bake for fifteen minutes or until done.

5 - Allow it to cool on a baking wire and serve!

Nutrition: Calories: 79.1 Protein: 2g Fat: 1g Carbohydrates: 16.4g

234. No-Bake Peanut Butter Oat Bars

Preparation Time: 10 minutes
Cooking Time: 10 minutes
Servings: 20

Ingredients:

- ½ cup maple syrup
- 2 cups gluten free oats
- ¾ cup creamy peanut butter
- ¼ cup pepitas
- 2 tablespoons cacao nibs
- 4oz. vegan chopped dark chocolate bar
- 1 tablespoon coconut oil
- 3 tablespoons hemp hearts
- ¼ cup shredded & unsweetened coconut flakes
- A pinch of sea salt

Directions:

1 - Use parchment paper to line an 8inchx8inch baking sheet.
2 - Place a saucepan on low heat with peanut butter and maple syrup
3 - Cook and stir until well combined.
4 - Remove from stove when done.
5 - In a skillet, add oats and pepitas and toast on low heat for 5 minutes
6 - Put the oats and peanut butter mixture in a mixing bowl with hemp hearts and cacao nibs stirred well.
7 - Pour the mixture onto the lined baking sheet and use a glass to press down the mixture firmly into the dish until no cracks.
8 - Let chill in the fridge.
9 - Melt chocolate and coconut oil in a double boiler, or use the microwave.
10 - Toast coconut flakes in the pan in which the oats were toasted.
11 - Take out the peanut butter mixture from the fridge and pour chocolate over it.
12 - Refrigerate for half an hour or until firm.
13 - Season with salt before cutting the bars.
14 - Store them in the fridge and serve however you like.
Nutrition: Calories: 170 Sugar: 8 g Sodium: 158 mg Fat: 7.5 g Saturated Fat: 3 g Carbohydrates: 21 g Fiber: 3 g Protein: 4.5 g Cholesterol: 0 mg

235. Peanut Butter Rice Crispy Treats

Preparation Time: 5 minutes
Cooking Time: 35 minutes
Servings: 6

Ingredients:

- 1 cup brown rice syrup
- 1/3 cup cacao nibs
- 5 cups rice crispy cereal
- 1 cup natural peanut butter
- 1 teaspoon coconut oil

Directions:

1 - Prepare a 9 x 9 square pan with parchment paper.
2 - You may also grease with coconut oil
3 - Place a large pan on low heat and carefully heat up brown rice syrup and peanut butter while stirring.
4 - Take off from stove and mix in the rice crispy cereal until combined. Stir in the cacao nibs well.
5 - Put the mixture in the lined square pan and carefully put pressure until evenly distributed.
6 - Cut into squares and serve. Or chill for 30 minutes in the fridge before serving.
Nutrition: Calories: 359 Fat: 17.6g Saturated Fat: 4.6g Cholesterol: 0.2mg Sodium: 259.8mg Carbohydrates: 46.1g Fiber: 2.2g Sugars: 27g Protein: 7.9g

236. Easy Chickpea Tacos

Preparation Time: 20 minutes
Cooking Time: 20 minutes
Servings: 2

Ingredients:

- 1 tablespoon tamari
- 2 teaspoons garlic powder
- 1 ½ cups drained & rinsed cooked chickpeas
- ½ teaspoon cumin
- ½ teaspoon onion powder
- ½ teaspoon paprika
- 1/1 cup cilantro
- 2 thinly sliced green onions
- ½ sliced avocado
- 1 tablespoon Sriracha hot sauce
- ¼ shredded head cabbage
- 2 thinly sliced green onions
- Vegan sour cream
- Lime wedges

Directions:

1 - Add chickpeas, garlic, onion powder, cumin, paprika, tamari, and hot sauce in a small pan.

2 - Heat the mixture over medium heat and remove once done.

3 - Warm the tortillas on the stove until slightly charring on the edges. Keep warm in the pot!

4 - Top each tortilla with the chickpea mixture, cabbage, green onions, avocado, cilantro and some vegan cream

5 - Serve warm with lime wedges!

Nutrition: Calories: 362 Total Fat: 14.1g Saturated Fat: 1.9g Cholesterol: 0 mg Sodium: 1207.1mg Carbohydrates: 52.6g Fiber: 14.5g Sugars 0.8g Protein 12g

237. Instant & Yummy Steel Cut Oats

Preparation Time: 1 minute
Cooking Time: 20 minutes
Ingredients:

- 2 ½ cups water
- A pinch of salt
- 1 cup steel cut oats
- 1 teaspoon vanilla
- 2 tablespoons maple syrup
- A handful of berries
- 2 tablespoons of any favorite nuts
- ¼ unsweetened almond milk

Directions:

1 - In the Instant Pot insert, combine the steel cut oats, spices, vanilla, and water.

2 - Lock the lid by twisting it. Put the valve in the sealed position. Adjust the pressure manually too high for 4 minutes. Then let natural release for 15 minutes.

3 - Serve this with nuts and berries, pure maple syrup and almond milk in individual bowls.

Nutrition: Calories: 150 Protein 5g Carbohydrates 27g Fiber: 4g Sugars: 2g Fat: 2.5g Saturated fat: 5g

238. Simple Gluten-Free Bread

Preparation Time: 1 hour 30 minutes
Cooking Time: 1 hour 15 minutes
Servings: 12
Ingredients:

- 2 cups warm water
- 1 packet active dry yeast
- 2 tablespoons organic cane sugar

- Avocado oil
- ¼ ground chia seeds
- ¾ cup gluten-free oat flour
- 1 cup brown rice flour
- ¾ cup sorghum flour
- 1 cup potato starch
- 2 teaspoons sea salt

Directions:

1 - Grease and flour an 8 x 4-inch loaf pan with oil and brown rice flour.

2 - Whisk the sugar and warm water together in a medium mixing bowl until the sugar dissolves.

3 - Stir in the yeast and let it rise on the counter for 10 minutes. In case it doesn't, try again - it could be too hot water or an expired yeast packet.

4 - Whisk in the ground chia seeds once the yeast has risen and set it aside for 10 minutes.

5 - Take a large bowl and whisk all the flours, potato starch and sea salt.

6 - Add the wet ingredients in the middle and mix together with a wooden spatula.

7 - The batter should be thick and sticky.

8 - Transfer the batter to your greased pan and cover with a kitchen towel.

9 - Put it in a warm and enclosed space for an hour to rise even more.

10 - Pre-heat the oven to 425 F once the batter has doubled in size.

11 - Bake for 45 minutes, then switch the temperature 375 F for 30 minutes.

12 - Take the bread out of the oven and let it cool for 10 minutes in the pan.

13 - Let cool completely before slicing and serving.

Nutrition: Calories: 167 Carbohydrates: 35.6 g Protein: 2.8 g Fat: 1.7 g Saturated Fat: 0.3 g Cholesterol: 0 mg Sodium: 392 mg Potassium: 102 mg Fiber: 2.4 g Sugar: 2.3 g

239. Millet Porridge with Sultanas

Preparation Time: 5 minutes
Cooking Time: 20 minutes
Servings: 3
Ingredients:

- 1 cup water
- 1 cup coconut milk
- 1 cup millet, rinsed
- 1/4 teaspoon grated nutmeg

- 1/4 teaspoon ground cinnamon
- 1 teaspoon vanilla paste
- 1/4 teaspoon kosher salt
- 2 tablespoons agave syrup
- 4 tablespoons sultana raisins

Directions:

1 - Place the water, milk, millet, nutmeg, cinnamon, vanilla, and salt in a saucepan; bring to a boil.

2 - Turn the heat to a simmer and let it cook for about 20 minutes; fluff the millet with a fork and spoon into individual bowls.

3 - Serve with agave syrup and sultanas. Bon appétit!

Nutrition: Calories: 353; Fat: 5.5 g; Carbs: 65.2 g; Proteins: 9.8 g

240. Quinoa Porridge with Dried Figs

Preparation Time: 5 minutes
Cooking Time: 20 minutes
Servings: 3

Ingredients:

- 1 cup white quinoa, rinsed
- 2 cups almond milk
- 4 tablespoons brown sugar
- A pinch of salt
- 1/4 teaspoon grated nutmeg
- 1/2 teaspoons ground cinnamon
- 1/2 teaspoons vanilla extract
- 1/2 cup dried figs, chopped

Directions:

1 - Place the quinoa, almond milk, sugar, salt, nutmeg, cinnamon, and vanilla extract in a saucepan.

2 - Bring it to a boil over medium-high heat. Turn the heat to a simmer and let it cook for about 20 minutes; fluff with a fork.

3 - Divide between three serving bowls and garnish with dried figs. Bon appétit!

Nutrition: Calories: 414; Fat: 9 g; Carbs: 71.2 g; Proteins: 13.8 g.

241. Bread Pudding with Raisins

Preparation Time: 15 minutes
Cooking Time: 45 minutes
Servings: 4

Ingredients:

- 4 cups day-old bread, cubed
- 1 cup brown sugar
- 4 cups coconut milk

- 1/2 teaspoons vanilla extract
- 1 teaspoon ground cinnamon
- 2 tablespoons rum
- 1/2 cup raisins

Directions:

1 - Start by preheating your oven to 360° F. Lightly oil a casserole dish with a nonstick cooking spray.

2 - Place the cubed bread in the prepared casserole dish.

3 - In a mixing bowl, thoroughly combine the sugar, milk, vanilla, cinnamon, rum, and raisins. Pour the custard evenly over the bread cubes.

4 - Let it soak for about 15 minutes.

5 - Bake in the preheated oven for about 45 minutes or until the top is golden and set. Bon appétit!

Nutrition: Calories: 474; Fat: 12.2 g; Carbs: 72 g; Proteins: 14.4 g.

242. Bulgur Wheat Salad

Preparation Time: 12 minutes
Cooking Time: 13 minutes
Servings: 4

Ingredients:

- 1 cup bulgur wheat
- 1 ½ cups vegetable broth
- 1 teaspoon sea salt
- 1 teaspoon fresh ginger, minced
- 4 tablespoons olive oil
- 1 onion, chopped
- 8 ounces canned garbanzo beans, drained
- 2 large roasted peppers, sliced
- 2 tablespoons fresh parsley, roughly chopped

Directions:

1 - In a deep saucepan, bring the bulgur wheat and vegetable broth to a simmer; let it cook, covered, for 12 to 13 minutes.

2 - Let it stand for about 10 minutes and fluff with a fork.

3 - Add the remaining ingredients to the cooked bulgur wheat; serve at room temperature or well-chilled. Bon appétit!

Nutrition: Calories: 359; Fat: 15.5 g; Carbs: 48.1 g; Proteins: 10.1 g.

243. Rye Porridge with Blueberry Topping

Preparation Time: 9 minutes
Cooking Time: 6 minutes
Servings: 3

Ingredients:
- 1 cup rye flakes
- 1 cup water
- 1 cup coconut milk
- 1 cup fresh blueberries
- 1 tablespoon coconut oil
- 6 dates, pitted

Directions:

1 - Add the rye flakes, water, and coconut milk to a deep saucepan; bring to a boil over medium-high. Turn the heat to a simmer and let it cook for 5 to 6 minutes.

2 - In a blender or food processor, puree the blueberries with coconut oil and dates.

3 - Ladle into three bowls and garnish with the blueberry topping. Bon appétit!

Nutrition: Calories: 359; Fat: 11 g; Carbs: 56.1 g; Proteins: 12.1 g.

244.   Coconut Sorghum Porridge

Preparation Time: 10 minutes
Cooking Time: 15 minutes
Servings: 2

Ingredients:
- 1/2 cup sorghum
- 1 cup water
- 1/2 cup coconut milk
- 1/4 teaspoon grated nutmeg
- 1/4 teaspoon ground cloves
- 1/2 teaspoons ground cinnamon
- Kosher salt, to taste
- 2 tablespoons agave syrup
- 2 tablespoons coconut flakes

Directions:

1 - Place the sorghum, water, milk, nutmeg, cloves, cinnamon, and kosher salt in a saucepan; simmer gently for about 15 minutes.

2 - Spoon the porridge into serving bowls. Top with agave syrup and coconut flakes. Bon appétit!

Nutrition: Calories: 289; Fat: 5.1 g; Carbs: 57.8 g; Proteins: 7.3 g.

245.   Dad's Aromatic Rice

Preparation Time: 5 minutes
Cooking Time: 15 minutes
Servings: 4

Ingredients:
- 3 tablespoons olive oil

- 1 teaspoon garlic, minced
- 1 teaspoon dried oregano
- 1 teaspoon dried rosemary
- 1 bay leaf
- 1 ½ cups white rice
- 2 ½ cups vegetable broth
- Sea salt and cayenne pepper, to taste

Directions:

1 - In a saucepan, heat the olive oil over a moderately high flame. Add garlic, oregano, rosemary, and bay leaf; sauté for about 1 minute or until aromatic.

2 - Add in the rice and broth. Bring to a boil; immediately turn the heat to a gentle simmer.

3 - Cook for about 15 minutes or until all the liquid has been absorbed. Fluff the rice with a fork; season with salt and pepper, and serve immediately. Bon appétit!

Nutrition: Calories: 384; Fat: 11.4 g; Carbs: 60.4 g; Proteins: 8.3 g.

246.   Every Day Savory Grits

Preparation Time: 5 minutes
Cooking Time: 30 minutes
Servings: 4

Ingredients:
- 2 tablespoons vegan butter
- 1 sweet onion, chopped
- 1 teaspoon garlic, minced
- 4 cups water
- 1 cup stone-ground grits
- Sea salt and cayenne pepper, to taste

Directions:

1 - In a saucepan, melt the vegan butter over medium-high heat. Once hot, cook the onion for about 3 minutes or until tender.

2 - Add in the garlic and continue to sauté for 30 seconds more or until aromatic; reserve.

3 - Bring the water to a boil over moderately high heat. Stir in the grits, salt, and pepper.

4 - Turn the heat to a simmer; cover, and cook for about 30 minutes or until cooked through.

5 - Stir in the sautéed mixture and serve warm. Bon appétit!

Nutrition: Calories: 238; Fat: 6.5 g; Carbs: 38.7 g; Proteins: 3.7 g.

247.   Greek-Style Barley Salad

Preparation Time: 5 minutes

Cooking Time: 30 minutes
Servings: 4
Ingredients:
- 1 cup pearl barley
- 2 ¾ cups vegetable broth
- 2 tablespoons apple cider vinegar
- 4 tablespoons extra-virgin olive oil
- 2 bell peppers, seeded and diced
- 1 shallot, chopped
- 2 ounces sun-dried tomatoes in oil, chopped
- 1/2 green olives, pitted and sliced
- 2 tablespoons fresh cilantro, roughly chopped

Directions:
1 - Bring the barley and broth to a boil over medium-high heat; now, turn the heat to a simmer. Continue to simmer for about 30 minutes until all the liquid has absorbed; fluff with a fork.
2 - Toss the barley with vinegar, olive oil, peppers, shallots, sun-dried tomatoes, and olives; toss to combine well.
3 - Garnish with fresh cilantro and serve at room temperature or well-chilled. Enjoy!
Nutrition: Calories: 378; Fat: 15.6 g; Carbs: 50 g; Proteins: 10.7 g.

248. Easy Sweet Maize Meal Porridge
Preparation Time: 5 minutes
Cooking Time: 10 minutes
Servings: 2
Ingredients:
- 2 cups water
- 1/2 cup maize meal
- 1/4 teaspoon ground allspice
- 1/4 teaspoon salt
- 2 tablespoons brown sugar
- 2 tablespoons almond butter

Directions:
1 - In a saucepan, bring the water to a boil; then gradually add in the maize meal and turn the heat to a simmer.
2 - Add in the ground allspice and salt. Let it cook for 10 minutes.
3 - Add in the brown sugar and almond butter and gently stir to combine. Bon appétit!
Nutrition: Calories: 278; Fat: 12.7 g; Carbs: 37.2 g; Proteins: 3 g.

249. Mom's Millet Muffins
Preparation Time: 10 minutes
Cooking Time: 25 minutes
Servings: 8
Ingredients:
- 2 cup whole-wheat flour
- 1/2 cup millet
- 2 teaspoons baking powder
- 1/2 teaspoons salt
- 1 cup coconut milk
- 1/2 cup coconut oil, melted
- 1/2 cup agave nectar
- 1/2 teaspoons ground cinnamon
- 1/4 teaspoon ground cloves
- A pinch of grated nutmeg
- 1/2 cup dried apricots, chopped

Directions:
1 - Begin by preheating your oven to 400° F. Lightly oil a muffin tin with nonstick oil.
2 - In a mixing bowl, mix all dry ingredients. In a separate bowl, mix the wet ingredients. Stir the milk mixture into the flour mixture; combine just until evenly moist and do not overmix your batter. Fold in the apricots and scrape the batter into the prepared muffin cups.
3 - Bake the muffins in the preheated oven for about 15 minutes or until a tester inserted in the center of your muffin comes out dry and clean. Let it stand for 10 minutes on a wire rack before unmolding and serving. Enjoy!
Nutrition: Calories: 367; Fat: 15.9 g; Carbs: 53.7 g; Proteins: 6.5 g.

250. Vegan Bean Quesadilla
Preparation Time: 10 minutes
Cooking Time: 15 minutes
Servings: 4
Ingredients:
- 1 avocado
- 4 tortillas
- ¼ cup vegetable broth
- ¼ teaspoon cumin
- ¼ teaspoon chili powder
- ¼ teaspoon garlic powder
- ¼ teaspoon onion powder
- 1 adobo chipotle pepper
- 15oz. rinsed & drained pinto beans

Directions
1 - Add all the ingredients in a food processor or blender.
2 - Process until creamy and use more broth if needed for desired consistency.
3 - Layer the mixture on the side of the tortilla, fold it, and put it on a non-stick pan.
4 - Cook both sides until brown.
5 - Take off from heat, cut and serve!
Nutrition: Calories: 179 Carbohydrates: 21g Protein: 4g Fat: 10g Saturated Fat: 2g Sodium: 272 mg Potassium: 299mg Fiber: 5g Sugar: 3g

251. Easy Quinoa Sweet Potato Chili

Preparation Time: 10 minutes
Cooking Time: 35 minutes
Servings: 4
Ingredients:
- 3 medium cubed sweet potatoes
- 2 teaspoons ground cumin
- 1 tablespoon extra-virgin olive oil
- 1 diced yellow or white onion
- ½ teaspoon chipotle powder
- 3 teaspoons hot sauce
- ½ teaspoon ground cinnamon
- 1 tablespoon chili powder
- 16 ounces salsa
- 15 ounces black beans
- 2 cups cooked quinoa
- 2 cups vegetable broth
- 2 cups water
- 1 avocado
- Sea salt as needed
- Black pepper as needed

Directions:
1 - Heat the oil in a large pot over medium heat. Combine the onions and a pinch of salt and pepper.
2 - Then stir in the cumin, cinnamon, sweet potatoes, chipotle powder, hot sauce, chili powder.
3 - After 3 to 4 minutes, add the salsa, vegetable stock, and water.
4 - On medium heat, bring the pot to a low boil and then let it simmer.
5 - Add black beans let it cook with a lid on for 20 minutes or until the sweet potatoes are fork-tender and the liquid has thickened.

6 - Stir in the quinoa at the end.
7 - Serve with avocado and enjoy!
Nutrition: Calories: 525 Carbohydrates: 89g Protein: 17g Fat: 14g Saturated Fat: 2g Sodium: 1853 mg Potassium: 1729 mg Fiber: 22g Sugar: 15g

252. Easy Tomato Basil Pasta

Preparation Time: 10 minutes
Cooking Time: 45 minutes
Servings: 6
Ingredients:
- ¾ teaspoon sea salt
- ½ cup extra-virgin olive oil
- 1 small chopped cherry tomato basket
- 2 finely chopped garlic cloves
- 1 oz. vegan pasta
- ½ cup chopped fresh basil
- Salt & pepper as needed

Directions:
1 - Mix garlic, olive oil and salt in a bowl.
2 - Add 1 cup of chopped cherry tomatoes to the olive oil bowl.
3 - Allow it to rest for half an hour while stirring often.
4 - Cook the pasta according to the guidelines.
5 - Drain and reserve ½ pasta water.
6 - Mix pasta and tomato mixture. Serve with basil, a little pasta water for consistency, and salt & pepper.
Nutrition: Calories: 448 Carbohydrates: 58g Protein: 10g Fat: 19g Saturated Fat: 3g Sodium: 300mg Potassium: 261mg Fiber: 3g Sugar: 3g

253. Simple & Vegan Mexican Style Rice

Preparation Time: 10 minutes
Cooking Time: 20 minutes
Servings: 4
Ingredients:
- 1 teaspoon sea salt
- ½ teaspoon black pepper
- 8oz.can tomato sauce
- 1 ½ cups water
- ¼ of a diced yellow onion
- 2 minced garlic cloves
- ½ tablespoon extra-virgin olive oil
- 1 cup brown rice

Directions:

1 - Warm the vegetable oil in a medium saucepan.
2 - Add the uncooked rice and sauté until golden.
3 - Add the onion and garlic and cook until translucent.
4 - Add the tomato sauce and water, as well as salt and pepper.
5 - Bring water to a boil, cover the pan, and lower the heat.
6 - Cook for 20 minutes.
7 - Serve when done with extra seasoning.

Nutrition: Calories: 203 Carbohydrates: 41g Protein: 4g Fat: 2g Saturated Fat: 2g Sodium: 886 mg Potassium: 260mg Fiber: 2g Sugar:3g

254. Parsley Lemon Pasta

Preparation Time: 5 minutes
Cooking Time: 10 minutes
Servings: 3
Ingredients:

- 3 tablespoons extra-virgin olive oil
- 8 oz long pasta
- ½ cup lemon juice
- 1 teaspoon lemon zest
- 3 minced garlic cloves
- ¼ teaspoon red chili flakes
- Sea salt as needed
- ¼ cup chopped parsley
- Black pepper as needed

Directions:
1 - As directed on the package, cook the pasta al dente.
2 - Drain the pasta water and save 1/2 cup of pasta water.
3 - Run the pasta under cool running water for a moment before setting aside.
4 - Heat oil in the pot in which the pasta was cooked.
5 - Add the garlic and red pepper flakes, and cook for about a minute.
6 - Then, add the pasta and ¼ cup of pasta water, and heat until the pasta is warm.

7 - Put the heat on low and add the lemon juice, lemon zest, and parsley.
8 - Stir and season with pepper and salt to taste.
9 - Serve Immediately!

Nutrition: Calories: 366 Fat: 9.9g Saturated Fat: 1.4g Cholesterol: 0 mg Sodium: 33.2mg Carbohydrates: 59.2g Fiber: 3.4g Sugars: 0.8g Protein: 10.1g

255. Fried Pineapple Rice

Preparation Time: 10 minutes
Cooking Time: 30 minutes
Servings: 6
Ingredients:

- 1 tablespoon sesame oil
- 2 tablespoons fresh & chopped cilantro
- ½ cup chopped pineapple
- ½ teaspoon turmeric
- 1 chopped tomato
- 1 teaspoon curry powder
- 1 tablespoon chopped pineapple
- 1 small chopped onion
- 3 cups cooked & cooled brown rice
- 1 tablespoon soy sauce
- Sea salt as needed
- Black pepper as needed

Directions:
1 - Add the sesame oil to a saucepan and heat
2 - Sauté onions until translucent.
3 - Stir in your cooked rice, soy sauce, pineapple, curry powder, and turmeric.
4 - Cook for ten minutes while mixing well.
5 - Season with salt and pepper and serve with cilantro.

Nutrition: Calories: 179 Protein: 3g Fat: 4.4g Carbohydrates: 32.6g

Chapter 20.　　Soup & Stews

256.　Sweet Potato Soup

Preparation Time: 20 minutes
Cooking Time: 25 minutes
Servings: 4

Ingredients:

- 400 grams of sweet potatoes
- 100 grams of corn kernels
- 1 shallot
- 1 clove of garlic
- 80 ml of soy cream
- 2 liters of vegetable broth
- 1 teaspoon of thyme leaves
- 1 tablespoon Olive oil
- Salt and pepper to taste

Directions:

1 - Peel and wash the shallots and garlic and then chop them.
2 - Peel the sweet potatoes, wash them, and then dry them. Cut them into cubes.
3 - Put some oil in a saucepan. As soon as it is hot, brown the garlic and shallot.
4 - After 2 minutes, add the sweet potatoes and vegetable broth. Cook for 15 minutes.
5 - Now add the corn and season with salt and pepper.
6 - Cook for another 5 minutes and then add the cream. Stir and then turn off.
7 - Put the soup on the plates, sprinkle them with the thyme leaves, and serve.

Nutrition: Calories: 110 Fat: 1g Carbohydrates: 23g Protein: 2g

257.　Bean and Cabbage Soup

Preparation Time: 20 minutes
Cooking Time: 2 hours
Servings: 4
Calories: 240

Ingredients:

- 200 grams of cabbage leaves
- 150 grams of beans already soaked
- 1 carrot
- 1 shallot
- 100 grams of tomato pulp
- 4 bay leaves
- 1 1/2 liters of vegetable broth
- Olive oil to taste
- Salt and pepper to taste

Directions:

1 - Add broth to the saucepan and add the beans.
2 - Bring to a boil and continue cooking for another 20 minutes.
3 - Meanwhile, wash the cabbage leaves, dry them, and cut them into strips.
4 - Peel off the carrot, wash it, and then cut it into cubes.
5 - Peel and wash the shallot and then chop it.
6 - Wash and dry the bay leaves.
7 - Add the cabbage to the beans after 20 minutes.
8 - Stir and, after 5 minutes, add the carrot, shallot, bay leaves, and tomato pulp.
9 - Put salt and pepper, stir, and continue cooking for another 30 minutes.
10 - After 30 minutes, turn off and remove the bay leaves.
11 - Put the soup on plates, season with oil and pepper, and serve.

Nutrition: Calories: 164 Fat: 4g Carbohydrates: 30g Protein: 11g

258.　Soup with Red Onion

Preparation Time: 20 minutes
Cooking Time: 40 minutes
Servings: 4

Ingredients:

- 200 grams of cabbage
- 2 carrots
- 1 potato
- 2 sticks of celery
- 1 red onion
- 100 grams of beans already boiled
- 100 grams of tomato pulp
- 2 liters of vegetable broth
- Salt and pepper to taste
- Olive oil to taste

Directions:

1 - Wash and dry the cabbage leaves. Keep only the tenderest leaves and then cut them into strips.
2 - Clean and peel the carrot and then cut it into cubes.
3 - Peel the potato, wash it well under running water, and then cut it into cubes.
4 - Remove the celery stalk and the side filaments. Wash it and chop it.
5 - Peel the onion, wash it, and then slice it.

6 - Add vegetable broth in a saucepan, and as soon as it starts to boil, add the potato, cabbage, carrots, and celery.

7 - Stir, cook for more minutes, and then add the tomato pulp.

8 - Season with salt, pepper, and cook for 30 minutes.

9 - Now add the beans, stir, and continue cooking for another 10 minutes.

10 - Turn off once cooked and put the soup on serving plates.

11 - Season with a drizzle of oil, sprinkle with onion, and serve.

Nutrition: Calories: 80 Fat: 3g Carbohydrates: 12g Protein: 2g

259.   Basil Soup

Preparation Time: 15 minutes
Cooking Time: 40 minutes
Servings: 4

Ingredients:
- 2 carrots
- 1 onion
- 1 potato
- 2 liters of hot vegetable broth
- 8 basil leaves
- Olive oil to taste
- Salt and pepper to taste

Directions:
1 -Wash and peel off the carrots, then cut them into slices.

2 - Peel and wash the potato and then cut it into cubes.

3 - Peel and wash the onion and then cut it into thin slices.

4 - Pour two tablespoons of olive oil into a saucepan and as soon as it is hot, add the onion.

5 - Sauté for 2 minutes and then add the carrots and potato.

6 - Season with salt and pepper, stir and then add the broth.

7 - Put a cover and cook for 30 minutes over medium heat.

8 - Meanwhile, wash and dry the basil leaves and then cut them into small pieces.

9 - After the cooking time, turn off and put the soup on the plates.

10 - Season with a drizzle of oil, sprinkle with basil, and serve.

Nutrition: Calories: 210 Fat: 10g Carbohydrates: 14g Protein: 2g

260.   Potato and Carrot Soup

Preparation Time: 20 minutes
Cooking Time: 20 minutes
Servings: 4

Ingredients:
400 grams of potatoes
- 300 grams of carrots
- 1 onion
- 1 1 /2 liters of vegetable broth
- 40 grams of soy butter
- 2 sprigs of chopped parsley
- Salt and pepper to taste

Directions:
1 - Peel off and wash the potatoes. Then cut them into cubes.

2 - Peel off and wash the carrots. Then cut them into slices.

3 - Peel and wash the onion and then chop it.

4 - Put the vegetable broth in a saucepan and bring to a boil.

5 - Put the carrots, potatoes, onion, and season with salt and pepper.

6 - Cook for 20 minutes over medium heat.

7 - After 20 minutes, turn off and blend everything with an immersion blender.

8 - Put the butter cut into chunks and stir until melted.

9 - Also, add the parsley and mix.

10 - Now put the soup on the serving plates and serve.

Nutrition: Calories: 147 Fat: 4g Carbohydrates: 16g Protein: 0g

261.   Spinach and Kale Soup

Preparation Time: 5 minutes
Cooking Time: 5 minutes
Servings: 2

Ingredients:
- 3 oz. Plant-based butter
- 1 cup fresh spinach, chopped coarsely
- 1 cup fresh kale, chopped coarsely
- 1 large avocado
- 3 tbsp. chopped fresh mint leaves
- 3 1/2 cups coconut cream
- 1 cup vegetable broth
- Salt and black pepper to taste
- 1 lime, juiced

Directions:
1 - Liquefy butter in a pot over medium heat and sauté the kale and spinach until wilted, 3 minutes. Turn the heat off.

2 - Stir in the remaining ingredients, and using an immersion blender, puree the soup until smooth.

3 - Dish the soup and serve warm.

Nutrition: Calories: 743 Proteins: 27g Carbohydrates: 28g Fat: 62g

262. Coconut and Grilled Vegetable Soup

Preparation Time: 10 minutes
Cooking Time: 45 minutes
Servings: 4

Ingredients:
- 2 small red onions cut into wedges
- 2 garlic cloves
- 10 oz. butternut squash, peeled and chopped
- 10 oz. pumpkins, peeled and chopped
- 4 tbsp. melted butter
- Salt and black pepper to taste
- 1 cup of water
- 1 cup unsweetened coconut milk
- 1 lime juiced
- 3/4 cup plant-based mayonnaise
- Toasted pumpkin seeds for garnishing

Directions:
1 - Preheat the oven to 400 F.
2 - On a baking sheet, spread the onions, garlic, butternut squash, and pumpkins and drizzle half of the butter on top. Season with salt, black pepper, and rub the seasoning well onto the vegetables. Roast in the oven for 45 minutes or until the vegetables are golden brown and softened.
3 - Transfer the vegetables to a pot; add the remaining ingredients except for the pumpkin seeds.
4 - Use a blender to puree the ingredients until smooth.
5 - Dish the soup, garnish with the pumpkin seeds, and serve warm.

Nutrition: Calories: 672 Proteins: 15g Carbohydrates: 12g Fat: 182g

263. Celery Dill Soup

Preparation Time: 5 minutes
Cooking Time: 25 minutes
Servings: 4

Ingredients:
- 2 tbsp. coconut oil
- 1/2 lb. celery root, trimmed
- 1 garlic clove
- 1 medium white onion
- 1/4 cup fresh dill, roughly chopped
- 1 tsp cumin powder
- 1/4 tsp nutmeg powder

- 1 small head cauliflower, cut into florets
- 3 1/2 cups seasoned vegetable stock
- 5 oz. Plant-based butter
- Juice from 1 lemon
- 1/4 cup coconut cream
- Salt and black pepper to taste

Directions:
1 - Get a large pot and melt coconut oil. Sauté the celery root, garlic, and onion until softened and fragrant, 5 minutes.
2 - Stir in the dill, cumin, and nutmeg, and stir-fry for 1 minute.
3 - Mix in the cauliflower and vegetable stock.
4 - Let it boil for 15 minutes and turn the heat off.
5 - Add the butter and lemon juice, and puree the soup using an immersion blender.
6 - Stir in the coconut cream, salt, black pepper, and dish the soup. Serve warm.

Nutrition: Calories: 205 Proteins: 3g Carbohydrates: 12g Fat: 232g

264. Quick Jackfruit and Bean Stew

Preparation Time: 10 minutes
Cooking Time: 10 minutes
Servings: 2

Ingredients:
- ½ cup jackfruit cut into 1-inch pieces
- ½ cup kidney bean rinsed and drained
- ½ cup pinto beans rinsed and drained
- 1 tomato
- ½ onion chopped
- 2 cup vegetable broth or water
- ½ orange juiced
- ½ teaspoon salt and pepper
- ½ teaspoon cumin
- 1 bay leaf
- Fresh basil

Directions:
1. Combine kidney beans, jackfruit, pinto beans, tomato, onion, broth, orange juice, pepper, salt, cumin, and bay leaf in Instant Pot; mix them well.
2. Lock lid in place and turn the valve to Sealing. Press Manual or Pressure Cooker; cook at High Pressure 6 minutes.
3. When cooking is complete, use Natural-release for 5 minutes, then release remaining pressure.

4. Press Sauté, cook for 3 to 5 minutes or until the stew thickens slightly, stirring frequently. Remove and discard bay leaf. Garnish with basil.

Nutrition: Calories 222, Total Fat 2. 3g, Saturated Fat 0. 6g, Cholesterol 0mg, Sodium 1617mg, Total Carbohydrate 38. 5g, Dietary Fiber 9. 2g, Total Sugars 5. 9g, Protein 13. 6g

265. Pasta Tofu Soup

Preparation Time:10 minutes
Cooking Time: 10 minutes
Servings: 2
Ingredients:
- ½ tablespoon butter
- ½ teaspoon garlic ginger, crushed
- ¼ onion chopped
- ½ green chilies, finely chopped (or adjust to taste)
- ½ big tomato, chopped
- Salt to taste
- ¼ cup pasta
- ½ cup of tofu cubes
- 2 cups water or broth as needed
- Cilantro to garnish

Directions:
1. Put Instant Pot on Sauté mode High and add butter. Once butter is hot, add garlic ginger and fry until aromatic.
2. Add onions and green chili, fry till edges of onions brown, then add tomatoes and fry for 2 to 3 minutes.
3. Add the pasta and tofu. Mix gently.
4. Add salt, and the water about 1/2 inch to 1 inch covering the pasta and mix well. Turn off the Sauté mode. Lock lid in place and turn the valve to Sealing.
5. Do Manual (Pressure Cooker) High 5 to 6 minutes. Let it naturally release or quick release after 10 minutes in Warm mode.
6. Garnish with cilantro if desired and serve hot.

Nutrition: Calories 196, Total Fat 9. 2g, Saturated Fat 2. 7g, Cholesterol 19mg, Sodium 161mg, Total Carbohydrate 18g, Dietary Fiber 4g, Total Sugars 3. 3g, Protein 13. 3g

266. Creamy Garlic Onion Soup

Preparation Time: 45 minutes
Cooking Time: 15-60 minutes

Servings: 4
Ingredients:
- 1 onion, sliced
- 4 cups vegetable stock
- 1 1/2 tbsp olive oil
- 1 shallot, sliced
- 2 garlic cloves, chopped
- 1 leek, sliced
- Salt to taste

Directions:
1. Add stock and olive oil in a saucepan and bring to boil.
2. Add remaining ingredients and stir well.
3. Cover and simmer for 25 minutes.
4. Puree the soup using an immersion blender until smooth.
5. Stir well and serve warm.

Nutrition: Calories 90; Fat 7.4 g; Carbohydrates 10.1 g; Sugar 4.1 g; Protein 1 g; Cholesterol 0 mg

267. Avocado Broccoli Soup

Preparation Time: 25 minutes
Cooking Time: 15-60 minutes
Servings: 4
Ingredients:
- 2 cups broccoli florets, chopped
- 5 cups vegetable broth
- 2 avocados, chopped
- Pepper to taste
- Salt to taste

Directions:
1. Cook broccoli in boiling water for 5 minutes. Drain well.
2. Add broccoli, vegetable broth, avocados, pepper, and salt to the blender and blend until smooth.
3. Stir well and serve warm.

Nutrition: Calories 269; Fat 21.5 g; Carbohydrates 12.8 g; Sugar 2.1 g; Protein 9.2 g; Cholesterol 0 mg

268. Green Spinach Kale Soup

Preparation Time: 15 minutes
Cooking Time: 15-60 minutes
Servings: 6
Ingredients:
- 2 avocados
- 8 oz spinach

- 8 oz kale
- 1 fresh lime juice
- 1 cup of water
- 3 1/3 cup coconut milk
- 3 oz olive oil
- 1/4 tsp pepper
- 1 tsp salt

Directions:
1. Heat olive oil in a saucepan over medium heat.
2. Add kale and spinach to the saucepan and sauté for 2-3 minutes. Remove saucepan from heat. Add coconut milk, spices, avocado, and water. Stir well.
3. Puree the soup using an immersion blender until smooth and creamy. Add fresh lime juice and stir well.
4. Serve and enjoy.

Nutrition: Calories 233; Fat 20 g; Carbohydrates 12 g; Sugar 0.5 g; Protein 4.2 g; Cholesterol 0 mg

269. Cauliflower Asparagus Soup

Preparation Time: 30 minutes
Cooking Time: 15-60 minutes
Servings: 4
Ingredients:
- 20 asparagus spears, chopped
- 4 cups vegetable stock
- ½ cauliflower head, chopped
- 2 garlic cloves, chopped
- 1 tbsp coconut oil
- Pepper to taste
- Salt to taste

Directions:
1. Heat coconut oil in a large saucepan over medium heat.
2. Add garlic and sauté until softened.
3. Add cauliflower, vegetable stock, pepper, and salt. Stir well and bring to boil.
4. Reduce heat to low and simmer for 20 minutes.
5. Add chopped asparagus and cook until softened.
6. Puree the soup using an immersion blender until smooth and creamy.
7. Stir well and serve warm.

Nutrition: Calories 74; Fat 5.6 g; Carbohydrates 8.9 g; Sugar 5.1 g; Protein 3.4 g; Cholesterol 2 mg

270. African Pineapple Peanut Stew

Preparation Time: 30 minutes
Cooking Time: 15-60 minutes
Servings: 4
Ingredients:
- 4 cups sliced kale
- 1 cup chopped onion
- 1/2 cup peanut butter
- 1 tbsp. hot pepper sauce or 1 tbsp. Tabasco sauce
- 2 minced garlic cloves
- 1/2 cup chopped cilantro
- 2 cups pineapple, undrained, canned & crushed
- 1 tbsp. vegetable oil

Directions:
1. In a saucepan (preferably covered), sauté the garlic and onions in the oil until the onions are lightly browned, approximately 10 minutes, stirring often.
2. Wash the kale. Get rid of the stems. Mound the leaves on a cutting surface & slice crosswise into slices (preferably 1" thick).
3. Now put the pineapple and juice to the onions & bring to a simmer. Stir the kale in, cover, and simmer until just tender, stirring frequently for approximately 5 minutes.
4. Mix in the hot pepper sauce, peanut butter & simmer for another 5 minutes.
5. Add salt according to your taste.

Nutrition: 382 Calories, 20.3 g Total Fat, 0 mg Cholesterol, 27.6 g Total Carbohydrate, 5 g Dietary Fiber, 11.4 g Protein

271. Fuss-Free Cabbage and Tomatoes Stew

Preparation Time: 15-30 minutes
Cooking Time: 3 hours and 10 minutes
Servings: 6
Ingredients:
- 1 medium-sized cabbage head, chopped
- 1 medium-sized white onion, peeled and sliced
- 28-ounce of stewed tomatoes
- 3/4 teaspoon of salt
- 1/4 teaspoon of ground black pepper
- 10-ounce of tomato soup

Directions:

1. Using a 6 quarts slow cooker, place all the ingredients, and stir properly.
2. Cover it with the lid, plug in the slow cooker and let it cook at the high heat setting for 3 hours or until the vegetables get soft.
3. Serve right away.

Nutrition: Calories:103 Cal, Carbohydrates:17g, Protein:4g, Fats:2g, Fiber:4g.

272. Awesome Spinach Artichoke Soup

Preparation Time: 15-30 minutes
Cooking Time: 4 hours and 45 minutes
Servings: 6

Ingredients:

- 15 ounces of cooked white beans
- 2 cups of frozen artichoke hearts, thawed
- 2 cups of spinach leaves
- 1 small red onion, peeled and chopped
- 1 teaspoon of minced garlic
- 1 teaspoon of salt
- 1/2 teaspoon of ground black pepper
- 2 teaspoons of dried basil
- 1 teaspoon of dried oregano
- 1/2 teaspoon of whole-grain mustard paste
- 2 1/2 tablespoons of nutritional yeast
- 1 1/2 teaspoons of white miso
- 4 tablespoons of lemon juice
- 16 fluid ounces of almond milk, unsweetened
- 3 cups of vegetable broth
- 1 cups of water

Directions:

1. Grease a 6-quarts slow cooker with a non-stick cooking spray, add the artichokes, spinach, onion, garlic, salt, black pepper, basil, and oregano.
2. Pour in the vegetable broth and water, stir properly and cover it with the lid.
3. Then plug in the slow cooker and let it cook at the high heat setting for 4 hours or until the vegetables get soft.
4. While waiting for that, place the white beans in a food processor, add the yeast, miso, mustard, lemon juice, and almond milk.
5. Mash until it gets smooth, and set it aside.

6. When the vegetables are cooked thoroughly, add the prepared bean mixture and continue cooking for 30 minutes at the high heat setting or until the soup gets slightly thick.
7. Garnish it with cheese and serve.

Nutrition: Calories:200 Cal, Carbohydrates:13g, Protein:4g, Fats:12g, Fiber:2g.

273. Brazilian Black Bean Stew

Preparation Time: 15 minutes
Cooking Time: 30 minutes
Servings: 2

Ingredients:

- ½ tablespoon olive oil
- 1 medium onion, chopped
- 1 teaspoon garlic powder
- ½ cup sweet potatoes, peeled and diced
- ½ large red bell pepper, diced
- 1 cup diced tomatoes with juice
- ½ cup of corn
- ½ cup broccoli
- 1 small hot green chili pepper, diced
- 1 1/2 cups water
- ½ cup black beans
- 1 mango - peeled, seeded, and diced
- ¼ cup chopped fresh cilantro
- ¼ teaspoon salt

Directions:

1. Select the Sauté setting on the Instant Pot. Add olive oil and onions to the Instant Pot. Stir in garlic powder, and cook until tender, then mix in the sweet potatoes, bell pepper, tomatoes with juice, chili pepper, corn, broccoli, and water.
2. Stir the beans into the Instant Pot. Select Pressure Cook or Manual, and adjust the pressure to High and the time to 12 minutes. After cooking, let the pressure release naturally for 10 minutes, then quickly release any remaining pressure.
3. Open the lid and mix in the mango and cilantro, and season with salt.

Nutrition: Calories 434, Total Fat 5. 8g, Saturated Fat 1g, Cholesterol 0mg, Sodium 325mg, Total Carbohydrate 86. 6g, Dietary Fiber 16. 1g, Total Sugars 32. 4g, Protein 16. 3g

274.   Split Pea and Carrot Stew

Preparation Time: 10 minutes
Cooking Time:20 minutes
Servings: 2
Ingredients:

- 1 tablespoon avocado oil
- 1 small onion, diced
- ½ carrot, diced into small cubes
- ½ leek stick, diced into cubes
- 4–5 cloves garlic, diced finely
- 1 bay leaf
- 1 teaspoon paprika powder
- 1 1/2 teaspoons cumin powder
- ½ teaspoon salt
- ¼ teaspoon cinnamon powder
- ¼ teaspoon chili powder or cayenne pepper
- 2 cups green split peas (rinsed well
- ½ cup chopped tinned tomatoes
- Juice of ½ lemon
- 2 cups vegetable stock

Directions:

1. Press the Sauté key to the Instant Pot. Add the avocado oil, onions, carrots, and leeks and cook for 4 minutes, stirring a few times.
2. Add the rest of the ingredients and stir. Cancel the Sauté function by pressing the Keep Warm/Cancel button.
3. Place and lock the lid, make sure the steam releasing handle is pointing to Sealing. Press Manual and adjust to 10 minutes.
4. Once the timer goes off, allow the pressure to release for 4-5 minutes and then use the Quick-release method before opening the lid.
5. Serve.

Nutrition: Calories 337, Total Fat 20. 5g, Saturated Fat 4. 2g, Cholesterol 0mg, Sodium 661mg, Total Carbohydrate 32. 6g, Dietary Fiber 16. 3g, Total Sugars 7. 9g, Protein 10g

275.   Broccoli Fennel Soup

Preparation Time: 15 minutes
Cooking Time: 10 minutes
Servings: 4
Ingredients:

- 1 fennel bulb, white and green parts coarsely chopped

- 10 oz. broccoli, cut into florets
- 3 cups vegetable stock
- Salt and freshly ground black pepper
- 1 garlic clove
- 1 cup dairy-free cream cheese
- 3 oz. Plant-based butter
- 1/2 cup chopped fresh oregano

Directions:

1 - In a medium pot, combine the fennel, broccoli, vegetable stock, salt, and black pepper.
2 - Bring to a boil until the vegetables soften, 10 to 15 minutes.
3 - Stir in the remaining ingredients and simmer the soup for 3 to 5 minutes.
4 - Taste, then adjust the season with salt and black pepper.
5 - Serve warm.

Nutrition: Calories: 690 Proteins: 2g Carbohydrates: 15g Fat: 188g

276.   Tofu Goulash Soup

Preparation Time: 35 minutes
Cooking Time: 20 minutes
Servings: 4
Ingredients:

- 4 1/4 oz. Plant-based butter
- 1 white onion, chopped
- 2 garlic cloves, minced
- 1 1/2 cups butternut squash
- 1 red bell pepper, deseeded and chopped
- 1 tbsp. paprika powder
- 1/4 tsp red chili flakes
- 1 tbsp. dried basil
- 1/2 tbsp. crushed cardamom seeds
- Salt and black pepper to taste
- 1 1/2 cups crushed tomatoes
- 3 cups vegetable broth
- 1 1/2 tsp red wine vinegar
- Chopped parsley to serve

Directions:

1 - Put tofu between two paper towels and allow draining of water for 30 minutes. After, crumble the tofu and set it aside.
2 - Dissolve butter in a large pot over medium heat and sauté the onion and garlic until the veggies are fragrant and soft, 3 minutes.
3 - Stir in the tofu and cook until golden brown, 3 minutes.

4 - Add the butternut squash, bell pepper, paprika, red chili flakes, basil, cardamom seeds, salt, and black pepper.

5 - Cook for 2 minutes to release some flavor and mix in the tomatoes and 2 cups of vegetable broth.

6 - Close the lid, bring the soup to a boil, and then simmer for 10 minutes.

7 - Stir in the remaining vegetable broth, the red wine vinegar, and adjust the taste with salt and black pepper.

8 - Garnish with the parsley and serve warm.

Nutrition: Calories: 358 Proteins: 4g Carbohydrates: 8g Fat: 36g

277.   Vegetable Broth

Preparation Time: 10 minutes
Cooking Time: 60 minutes
Servings: 2

Ingredients:
- 8 cups Water
- 1 Onion, chopped
- 4 Garlic cloves, crushed
- 2 Celery Stalks, chopped
- Pinch of Salt
- 1 Carrot, chopped
- Dash of Pepper
- 1 Potato, medium and chopped
- 1 tbsp. Soy Sauce
- 3 Bay Leaves

Directions:
1 - To make the vegetable broth, you need to place all of the ingredients in a deep saucepan.

2 - Heat the pan over medium-high heat. Bring the vegetable mixture to a boil.

3 - Lower the heat to medium-low once it starts boiling. Allow it to simmer for at least an hour or so. Then, cover it with a lid.

4 - When the time is up, pass it through a filter and strain the vegetables, garlic, and bay leaves.

5 - Allow the stock to cool completely and store in an air-tight container.

Nutrition: Calories: 40 Protein: 1 g Carbohydrates: 9g Fat: 0g

278.   Cucumber Dill Gazpacho

Preparation Time: 10 minutes
Cooking Time: 2 hours
Servings: 4

Ingredients:

- 4 large cucumbers, peeled, deseeded, and chopped
- 1/8 tsp salt
- 1 tsp chopped fresh dill + more for garnishing
- 2 tbsp. freshly squeezed lemon juice
- 1 1/2 cups green grape, seeds removed
- 3 tbsp. extra virgin olive oil
- 1 garlic clove, minced

Directions:
1 - Prepare food processor and put all ingredients. Blend until smooth.

2 - Pour the soup into serving bowls and chill for 1 to 2 hours.

3 - Garnish with dill and serve chilled.

Nutrition: Calories: 118cal   Proteins: 2g Carbohydrates: 17g Fat: 5g

279.   Red Lentil Soup

Preparation Time: 5 minutes
Cooking Time: 25 minutes
Servings: 6

Ingredients:
- 2 tbsp. Nutritional Yeast
- 1 cup Red Lentil, washed
- 1/2 tbsp. Garlic, minced
- 4 cups Vegetable Stock
- 1 tsp. Salt
- 2 cups kale, shredded
- 3 cups Mixed Vegetables

Directions:
1 - To start with, place all ingredients needed to make the soup in a large pot.

2 - Heat the pot over medium-high heat and bring the mixture to a boil.

3 - Once it starts boiling, lower the heat to low. Allow the soup to simmer.

4 - Simmer it for 1o to 15 minutes or until cooked.

5 - Serve and enjoy.

Nutrition: Calories: 406   Proteins: 11.8g Carbohydrates: 77.3g Fat: 0.6g

280.   Pesto Pea Soup

Preparation Time: 10 minutes
Cooking Time: 20 minutes
Servings: 4

Ingredients:
- 2 cups Water

- 8 oz. Tortellini
- 1/4 cup Pesto
- 1 Onion, small and finely chopped
- 1 lb. Peas, frozen
- 1 Carrot, medium and finely chopped
- 1 3/4 cup Vegetable Broth, less sodium
- 1 Celery Rib, medium and finely chopped

Directions:

1 - To start with, boil the water in a large pot over medium-high heat.

2 - Stir in the tortellini to the pot and cook it following the Directions given in the packet.

3 - In the meantime, cook the onion, celery, and carrot in a deep saucepan along with the water and broth.

4 - Cook the celery-onion mixture for 6 minutes or until softened.

5 - Now, spoon in the peas and allow it to simmer while keeping it uncovered.

6 - Cook the peas for few minutes or until they are bright green and soft.

7 - Then, spoon in the pesto to the pea's mixture. Combine well.

8 - Place mixture into a high-speed blender and blend for 2 to 3 minutes or until you get a rich, smooth soup.

9 - Return the soup to the pan. Spoon in the cooked tortellini.

10 - Finally, pour into a serving bowl and top with more cooked peas if desired.

Nutrition: Calories: 396 Protein: 16.7g Carbohydrates: 51g Fat: 14.3g

281. Tofu and Mushroom Soup

Preparation Time: 15 minutes
Cooking Time: 10 minutes
Servings: 4

Ingredients:

- 2 tbsp. olive oil
- 1 garlic clove, minced
- 1 large yellow onion, finely chopped
- 1 tsp freshly grated ginger
- 1 cup vegetable stock
- 2 small potatoes, peeled and chopped
- 1/4 tsp salt
- 1/4 tsp black pepper
- 2 (14 oz.) silken tofu, drained and rinsed
- 2/3 cup baby Bella mushrooms, sliced
- 1 tbsp. chopped fresh oregano
- 2 tbsp. chopped fresh parsley to garnish

Directions:

1 - Heat olive oil in a medium pot. Sauté the garlic, onion, and ginger until soft and fragrant.

2 - Pour in the vegetable stock, potatoes, salt, and black pepper. Cook until the potatoes soften, 12 minutes.

3 - Stir in the tofu, and using an immersion blender, puree the ingredients until smooth.

4 - Mix in the mushrooms and simmer with the pot covered until the mushrooms warm up while occasionally stirring to ensure that the tofu doesn't curdle 7 minutes.

5 - Stir oregano and dish the soup.

6 - Garnish with the parsley and serve warm.

Nutrition: Calories: 325cal Proteins: 33g Carbohydrates: 41g Fat: 27g

282. Avocado Green Soup

Preparation Time: 5 minutes
Cooking Time: 5 minutes
Servings: 4

Ingredients:

- 2 tbsp. olive oil
- 1 1/2 cup fresh kale, chopped coarsely
- 1 1/2 cup fresh spinach, chopped coarsely
- 3 large avocados, halved, pitted, and pulp extracted
- 2 cups of soy milk
- 2 cups no-sodium vegetable broth
- 3 tbsp. chopped fresh mint leaves
- 1/4 tsp salt
- 1/4 tsp black pepper
- 2 limes, juiced

Directions:

1 - Put and heat olive oil in a saucepan over medium flame. Mix in the kale and spinach. Cook until wilted, 3 minutes, and turn off the heat.

2 - Add the remaining ingredients, and using an immersion blender, puree the soup until smooth.

3 - Dish the soup and serve immediately.

Nutrition: Calories: 625cal Proteins: 27g Carbohydrates: 29g Fat: 48g

283. Potato Leek Soup

Preparation Time: 5 minutes
Cooking Time: 20 minutes
Servings: 4

Ingredients:

- 1 cup fresh cilantro leaves

- 6 garlic cloves, peeled
- 3 tbsp. vegetable oil
- 3 leeks, white and green parts chopped
- 2 lb. russet potatoes, peeled and chopped
- 1 tsp cumin powder
- 1/4 tsp salt
- 1/4 tsp black pepper
- 2 bay leaves
- 6 cups no-sodium vegetable broth

Directions:

1 - In a spice blender, process the cilantro and garlic until smooth paste forms.

2 - Prepare vegetable oil in a large pot. Once hot, sauté the garlic mixture and leeks until the leeks are tender, 5 minutes.

3 - Mix in the remaining ingredients and allow boiling until the potatoes soften 15 minutes.

4 - Turn the heat off, open the lid, remove, and discard the bay leaves.

5 - Blend the soup using a blender until smooth.

6 - Serve warm.

Nutrition: Calories: 128 Proteins: 4g Carbohydrates: 19g Fat: 5g

284. Spicy Corn Chowder

Preparation Time: 5 minutes
Cooking Time: 20 minutes
Servings: 8

Ingredients:

- 2 medium yellow potatoes
- 2 cups low-sodium vegetable broth
- 1 (13.5-ounce) can coconut milk
- 1 (16-ounce) bag frozen corn
- 2 tablespoons nutritional yeast
- 1 teaspoon chipotle powder
- 1 teaspoon canned diced green chiles, drained
- 1/2 teaspoon ground mustard
- 1/2 teaspoon paprika

Directions:

1 - Peeled and cut potatoes into 1-inch cubes

2 - In a large pot, combine the potatoes, vegetable broth, coconut milk, corn, nutritional yeast, chipotle powder, green chiles, mustard, and paprika, and stir to combine.

3 - Bring to a soft boil and reduce the heat to medium-low.

4 - Place cover and let it simmer for 25 minutes until the potatoes are tender.

5 - Remove the soup from the heat, partially blend with a blender, leaving some of the soup chunky.

6 - Return to the pot and serve.

Nutrition: Calories: 176 Fat: 9g Carbohydrates: 24g Protein: 5g

285. Vegetable Pho

Preparation Time: 10 minutes
Cooking Time: 20 minutes
Servings: 6

Ingredients:

For the broth

- 8 cups low-sodium vegetable broth
- 3 cups water
- 1 large onion, quartered
- 1 cinnamon stick
- 3 whole star anise
- 3 whole cloves
- 2-inch piece fresh ginger, peeled
- 2 garlic cloves, halved
- 2 tablespoons tamari
- 8 ounces wide rice noodles
- 3 baby bok choy heads, separated into individual leaves
- 2 cups broccoli florets
- 2 carrots, thinly sliced
- 2 scallions, cut both green and white parts

For serving:

- 1 (15-ounce) can corn, drained
- 1 cup bean sprouts
- 1 jalapeño or Thai chile pepper, sliced into rings
- 1 bunch of fresh basil leaves (Thai or Italian)
- Sriracha
- Hoisin sauce

Directions:

1 - In a large pot, combine the broth, water, onion, cinnamon, anise, cloves, ginger, garlic, and tamari and bring almost to a boil.

2 - Lower heat slightly and simmer, covered, for 20 minutes.

3 - While the soup is cooking, bring a medium pot of water to a boil and cook the rice noodles according to package directions. Drain.

4 - During the last 5 minutes of the broth's cooking time, add the bok choy, broccoli, carrots, and scallions.

5 - Put soup into bowls and add the noodles. Top with corn, bean sprouts, jalapeño, and basil leaves.

6 - Season with sriracha and hoisin sauce to taste.

Nutrition: Calories: 230 Fat: 1g Carbohydrates: 49g Protein: 7g

286.   Tortilla Soup

Preparation Time: 10 minutes

Cooking Time: 20 minutes

Servings: 4

Ingredients:

- 6 corn or flour tortillas, cut into strips
- 2 tablespoons grapeseed or extra-virgin olive oil, divided
- 3/4 teaspoon salt, divided
- 1 medium onion, diced
- 1 jalapeño pepper, sliced into rings or 2 tablespoons canned chopped jalapeños
- 1 teaspoon minced garlic
- 1 teaspoon ground cumin
- 1 teaspoon chili powder
- 1/2 teaspoon ground black pepper
- 1/2 teaspoon ground cayenne pepper
- 4 cups low-sodium vegetable broth
- 1 (28-ounce) can crushed tomatoes
- 2 cups frozen mixed vegetables
- 1 can black beans (15-ounce), drained and rinsed

Directions:

1 - Prepare oven to 475 F and line a rimmed baking sheet with parchment paper.

2 - Put together the tortillas, cut them in half, and cut them into strips about 1/2 inch wide.

3 - Toss with 1 tablespoon of oil and spread in a single layer on the prepared sheet.

4 - Bake for 6 - 7 minutes, or until lightly golden. Remove from the pan, sprinkle with 1/4 teaspoon of salt, and set aside.

5 - Get a large pot, heat the remaining 1 tablespoon of oil on medium-high heat.

6 - Add the onion and cook for 3 to 4 minutes, or until just translucent. Add the jalapeño, garlic, cumin, chili powder, black pepper, cayenne pepper and remaining 1/2 teaspoon of salt. Cook for 30 seconds, until fragrant.

7 - Pour in the broth and tomatoes. When boiling, adjust the heat to medium and simmer for 5 minutes.

8 - Add the frozen vegetables and black beans and cook for another 3 to 4 minutes, or until the vegetables are warmed through.

9 - Prepare in bowls topped with tortilla strips and your choice of toppings.

Nutrition: Calories: 363 Fat: 9g Carbohydrates: 59g Protein: 13g

287.   Chickpea, Leek, and Rosemary Soup

Preparation Time: 15 minutes+2 hours to rest

Cooking Time: 1 hour and 15 minutes

Servings: 4

Ingredients:

- 200 grams of chickpeas
- 3 leeks
- 2 sprigs of rosemary
- The grated rind of one lemon
- 2 tablespoon Olive oil
- Salt and pepper to taste

Directions:

1 - Start by putting the chickpeas in a bowl with cold water. Let it sit for 2 hours.

2 - Remove the root and the green part of the leeks, wash them, and cut them into thin slices.

3 - Put oil in a saucepan, and as soon as it is hot, put the leeks to dry.

4 - Cook them for about 10 minutes and then add the chickpeas. Mix and season with salt and pepper.

5 - Now add 1 liter of water and bring to a boil.

6 - Wash the rosemary, put it in the pot with the chickpeas, and continue cooking for another 60 minutes.

7 - When cooked, remove the rosemary, and take half of the soup.

8 - Put it in the blender glass and blend until thick and creamy.

9 - Put it back in the pot with the rest of the chickpeas and add the grated lemon zest.

10-Stir to flavor well. Put the soup on the plates and serve.

Nutrition: Calories: 225 Fat: 7g Carbohydrates: 53g Protein: 11g

288.   Zucchini and Spinach Soup

Preparation Time: 10 minutes

Cooking Time: 30 minutes

Servings: 4

Ingredients:

- 600 grams of zucchini
- 500 grams of spinach
- 2 tomatoes
- 1 carrot
- 1 onion
- 8 basil leaves
- Olive oil to taste
- Salt and pepper to taste

Directions:

1 - Wash the zucchinis and then cut them into thin slices.

2 - Wash and dry the spinach and then cut them into thin strips.

3 - Peel and wash the onion and carrot and then chop them.

4 - Wash and dry the basil leaves.

5 - Clean the tomatoes and then cut into cubes.

6 - Pour a liter of water into a saucepan and put onion, carrots, tomatoes, spinach, and zucchini inside.

7 - Let it boil and season with salt and pepper. Continue cooking for another 25 minutes.

8 - After 25 minutes, drain some of the vegetables and put them in the glass of the blender together with the basil leaves. Blend well to get a smooth and homogeneous mixture.

9 - Put the vegetable smoothie in the pot and bring it to a boil again.

10 - At this point, turn off, put the soup on the plates, season with a drizzle of oil, and serve.

Nutrition: Calories: 133 Fat: 4g Carbohydrates: 21g Protein: 6g

289. Seitan Stew with Barley

Preparation Time:10 minutes
Cooking Time: 20 minutes
Servings: 2

Ingredients:

- 1 teaspoon coconut oil
- ½ onion chopped
- 1 parsnip cut into thin half-circles
- 1 leek stalks diced
- 1 teaspoon garlic minced
- 1 teaspoon dried basil
- ½ teaspoons dried parsley
- 1 1/2 tablespoons tomato paste
- 2 cups vegetable broth
- 1 cup seitan
- 1 cup dry barley

- ½ teaspoon salt
- ½ teaspoon ground pepper

Directions:

1. Set the Instant Pot to Sauté mode. Heat the coconut oil, then add the onion, parsnips, and leek. Sauté the vegetables, stirring occasionally, until starting to soften, 3 to 4 minutes.

2. Add the garlic, basil, parsley, and tomato paste. Cook, stirring constantly, for 1 minute.

3. Pour in the vegetable broth and stir to combine.

4. Add the seitan, barley, and salt and pepper to the Instant Pot.

5. Put the lid on the Instant Pot, close the steam vent, and set it to High Pressure using the Manual setting. Set the time to 20 minutes.

6. Once the time is expired, use Natural-release for 10 minutes, then quickly release.

7. Serve soup with salt and pepper to taste.

Nutrition: Calories 376, Total Fat 5. 8g, Saturated Fat 2. 9g, Cholesterol 0mg, Sodium 1600mg, Total Carbohydrate 57. 9g, Dietary Fiber 13. 7g, Total Sugars 8. 2g, Protein 23. 5g

290. Cottage Cheese Soup

Preparation Time:10 minutes
Cooking Time: 35 minutes
Servings: 2

Ingredients:

- 1 stalks leek, diced
- 1 tablespoon bell pepper, diced
- ¼ cup Swiss chard, sliced into strips
- 1/8 cup fresh kale
- 1 eggplant
- ½ tablespoon avocado oil
- 1/8 cup button mushrooms, diced
- 1 small onion, diced
- ½ cup cottage cheese
- 2 cups vegetable broth
- 1 bay leaf
- ½ teaspoon salt
- ¼ teaspoon garlic, minced
- 1/8 teaspoon paprika

Directions:

1. Place leek, bell pepper, Swiss chard, eggplant, and kale into a medium bowl, set aside in a separate medium bowl.

2. Press the Sauté button and add the avocado oil to Instant Pot. Once the oil is hot, add mushrooms and onion. Sauté for 4–6 minutes until the onion is translucent and fragrant.
3. Add leek, bell pepper, Swiss chard, and kale to Instant Pot. Cook for an additional 4 minutes. Press the Cancel button.
4. Add diced cottage cheese, broth, bay leaf, and seasonings to Instant Pot. Click the lid closed. Press the Soup button and set the time for 20 minutes.
5. When the timer beeps, allow a 10-minute natural release and quickly release the remaining pressure. Add eggplant on Keep Warm mode and cook for additional 10 minutes or until tender. Serve warm.

Nutrition: Calories 212, Total Fat 3. 6g, Saturated Fat 1. 2g, Cholesterol 5mg, Sodium 1603mg, Total Carbohydrate 30. 7g, Dietary Fiber 11. 9g, Total Sugars 12. 7g, Protein 17g

291. Fresh Corn & Red Pepper Stew

Preparation Time:15 minutes
Cooking Time: 30 minutes
Servings: 2

Ingredients:

- 1 teaspoon coconut oil
- ¼ cup sweet onion, chopped,
- 1 1/2 cups fresh corn kernels
- 1 teaspoon garlic, minced
- 2 cups vegetable broth,
- ¼ teaspoon salt
- 1/8 cup coconut cream
- ½ tablespoon cornmeal
- ½ small red bell pepper, diced
- Enough water

Directions:

1. Select the Sauté setting on the Instant Pot and heat the coconut oil. Add the onion, garlic, and salt and sauté for about 5 minutes, until the onion has softened and is translucent.
2. Add the fresh corn, broth, water, bell pepper, and stir well.
3. Lock lid and set the Pressure Release to Sealing. Press the Cancel button to reset the cooking program, then select the Soup/Broth setting and

set the cooking time for 15 minutes at High Pressure.
4. Meanwhile add water, coconut cream, and cornmeal.
5. Let the pressure release naturally for at least 10 minutes, then move the Steam Release to Vent to release any remaining steam.
6. Open the pot and stir in the cornmeal mixer into soup, then taste and adjust the seasoning with salt if needed.

Nutrition: Calories 183, Total Fat 8. 3g, Saturated Fat 5. 7g, Cholesterol 0mg, Sodium 1070mg, Total Carbohydrate 21. 8g, Dietary Fiber 3. 3g, Total Sugars 5. 8g, Protein 8. 4g

292. Zucchini & White Bean Stew

Preparation Time:10 minutes
Cooking Time: 35 minutes
Servings: 2

Ingredients:

- ¼ ounce mushrooms
- 1 cup hot water
- ½ large zucchini
- 1 tablespoon coconut oil, divided
- 1 small onion, thinly sliced
- ½ teaspoon garlic powder
- ¼ teaspoons dried basil, crumbled
- 1 small (1-inch) cinnamon stick
- ¼ teaspoon salt
- 1/8 teaspoon freshly ground pepper
- 1 bay leaf
- 2 cups vegetable broth
- ¼ cup dried white beans, rinsed and soaked overnight and drained
- 1 tomato
- ¼ cup finely chopped fresh cilantro

Directions:

1. Select the Sauté setting on the Instant Pot and heat ¼ tablespoon coconut oil. Add zucchini and roast it and keep aside.
2. Add remaining coconut oil, add onion and sauté for about 5 minutes, until the onion has softened and is translucent. Add garlic powder, basil, cinnamon stick, salt, pepper, bay leaf, and the chopped mushrooms cook, stirring, for 1 minute

add vegetable broth and add white beans and roast zucchini.

3. Lock lid and set the Pressure Release to Sealing. Press the Cancel button to reset the cooking program, then select the Soup/Broth setting and set the cooking time for 25 minutes at High Pressure.
4. Let the pressure release naturally for at least 10 minutes, then move the Steam Release to Vent to release any remaining steam.
5. Open the pot and remove the cinnamon stick and bay leaf. Stir in tomatoes and cilantro.

Nutrition: Calories 210, Total Fat 7. 5g, Saturated Fat 6g, Cholesterol 0mg, Sodium 307mg, Total Carbohydrate 30. 9g, Dietary Fiber 11. 1g, Total Sugars 8g, Protein 8. 5g

293. Potato Tofu Soup

Preparation Time:10 minutes
Cooking Time: 35 minutes
Servings: 2
Ingredients:

- ½ tablespoon olive oil
- ½ celery cleaned and sliced
- ½ teaspoon garlic powder
- 1 sweet potato peeled and cut into 2-inch cubes
- ½ large potato peeled and cut into 2-inch cubes
- ½ cup tofu
- 2 cups vegetable broth
- Juice from one lemon
- A handful of chopped parsley
- Salt and pepper to taste

Directions:

1. Hit the Sauté button and when it's hot, heat the olive oil in your Instant Pot and sauté the celery and garlic powder until they soften down, stirring often.
2. Add in the potatoes, sweet potatoes, tofu, broth, salt, and pepper, and stir well.
3. Lock lid, make sure the vent is sealed, and program for 6 minutes on High Pressure. You can do a Quick-release if you like or leave it to release on its own with soup like this it doesn't matter.
4. Once the pressure is released, open the lid and throw in the parsley and add the lemon juice.

Nutrition: Calories 216, Total Fat 7.6g,Saturated 1.5g,Cholesterol 0mg, Sodium 809mg,Total Carbohydrate 27.2g, Dietary Fiber 3.6g,Total Sugars 5.2g, Protein 12.2g

294. Tomato Gazpacho

Preparation Time: 2 Hours 25 minutes
Cooking Time: 15-60 minutes
Servings: 6
Ingredients:

- 2 Tablespoons + 1 Teaspoon Red Wine Vinegar, Divided
- ½ Teaspoon Pepper
- 1 Teaspoon Sea Salt
- 1 Avocado,
- ¼ Cup Basil, Fresh & Chopped
- 3 Tablespoons + 2 Teaspoons Olive Oil, Divided
- 1 Clove Garlic, crushed
- 1 Red Bell Pepper, Sliced & Seeded
- 1 Cucumber, Chunked
- 2 ½ lbs. Large Tomatoes, Cored & Chopped

Directions:

1. Place half of your cucumber, bell pepper, and ¼ cup of each tomato in a bowl, covering. Set it in the fridge.
2. Puree your remaining tomatoes, cucumber, and bell pepper with garlic, three tablespoons oil, two tablespoons of vinegar, sea salt, and black pepper into a blender, blending until smooth. Transfer it to a bowl, and chill for two hours.
3. Chop the avocado, adding it to your chopped vegetables, adding your remaining oil, vinegar, salt, pepper, and basil.
4. Ladle your tomato puree mixture into bowls, and serve with chopped vegetables as a salad.
5. Interesting Facts:
6. Avocados themselves are ranked within the top five of the healthiest foods on the planet, so you know that the oil that is produced from them is too. It is loaded with healthy fats and essential fatty acids. Like race bran oil it is perfect to cook with as well! Bonus: Helps in the prevention of diabetes and lowers cholesterol levels.

Nutrition: Calories 70; Fat 2.7 g; Carbohydrates 13.8 g; Sugar 6.3 g; Protein 1.9 g; Cholesterol 0 mg

295. Tomato Pumpkin Soup

Preparation Time: 25 minutes
Cooking Time: 15-60 minutes

Servings: 4

Ingredients:

- 2 cups pumpkin, diced
- 1/2 cup tomato, chopped
- 1/2 cup onion, chopped
- 1 1/2 tsp curry powder
- 1/2 tsp paprika
- 2 cups vegetable stock
- 1 tsp olive oil
- 1/2 tsp garlic, minced

Directions:

1. In a saucepan, add oil, garlic, and onion and sauté for 3 minutes over medium heat.
2. Add remaining ingredients into the saucepan and bring to boil.
3. Reduce heat and cover and simmer for 10 minutes.
4. Puree the soup using a blender until smooth.
5. Stir well and serve warm.

Nutrition: Calories 70; Fat 2.7 g; Carbohydrates 13.8 g; Sugar 6.3 g; Protein 1.9 g; Cholesterol 0 mg

296. Cauliflower Spinach Soup

Preparation Time: 45 minutes
Cooking Time: 15-60 minutes
Servings: 5

Ingredients:

- 1/2 cup unsweetened coconut milk
- 5 oz fresh spinach, chopped
- 5 watercress, chopped
- 8 cups vegetable stock
- 1 lb. cauliflower, chopped
- Salt to taste

Directions:

1. Add stock and cauliflower in a large saucepan and bring to boil over medium heat for 15 minutes.
2. Add spinach and watercress and cook for another 10 minutes.
3. Remove from heat and puree the soup using a blender until smooth.
4. Add coconut milk and stir well. Season with salt.
5. Stir well and serve hot.

Nutrition: Calories 153; Fat 8.3 g; Carbohydrates 8.7 g; Sugar 4.3 g; Protein 11.9 g; Cholesterol 0 mg

297. Avocado Mint Soup

Preparation Time: 10 minutes
Cooking Time: 15-60 minutes
Servings: 2

Ingredients:

- 1 medium avocado, peeled, pitted, and cut into pieces
- 1 cup of coconut milk
- 2 romaine lettuce leaves
- 20 fresh mint leaves
- 1 tbsp fresh lime juice
- 1/8 tsp salt

Directions:

1. Add all ingredients into the blender and blend until smooth. The soup should be thick not as a puree.
2. Pour into the serving bowls and place in the refrigerator for 10 minutes.
3. Stir well and serve chilled.

Nutrition: Calories 268; Fat 25.6 g; Carbohydrates 10.2 g; Sugar 0.6 g; Protein 2.7 g; Cholesterol 0 mg

298. Creamy Squash Soup

Preparation Time: 35 minutes
Cooking Time: 15-60 minutes
Servings: 8

Ingredients:

- 3 cups butternut squash, chopped
- 1 ½ cups unsweetened coconut milk
- 1 tbsp coconut oil
- 1 tsp dried onion flakes
- 1 tbsp curry powder
- 4 cups of water
- 1 garlic clove
- 1 tsp kosher salt

Directions:

1. Add squash, coconut oil, onion flakes, curry powder, water, garlic, and salt into a large saucepan. Bring to boil over high heat.
2. Turn heat to medium and simmer for 20 minutes.
3. Puree the soup using a blender until smooth. Return soup to the saucepan and stir in coconut milk and cook for 2 minutes.
4. Stir well and serve hot.

Nutrition: Calories 146; Fat 12.6 g; Carbohydrates 9.4 g; Sugar 2.8 g; Protein 1.7 g; Cholesterol 0 mg

299. Zucchini Soup

Preparation Time: 20 minutes
Cooking Time: 15-60 minutes
Servings: 8
Ingredients:
- 2 ½ lbs. zucchini, peeled and sliced
- 1/3 cup basil leaves
- 4 cups vegetable stock
- 4 garlic cloves, chopped
- 2 tbsp olive oil
- 1 medium onion, diced
- Pepper to taste
- Salt to taste

Directions:
1. Heat olive oil in a pan over medium-low heat.
2. Add zucchini and onion and sauté until softened. Add garlic and sauté for a minute.
3. Add vegetable stock and simmer for 15 minutes.
4. Remove from heat. Stir in basil and puree the soup using a blender until smooth and creamy. Season with pepper and salt.
5. Stir well and serve.

Nutrition: Calories 62; Fat 4 g; Carbohydrates 6.8 g; Sugar 3.3 g; Protein 2 g; Cholesterol 0 mg

300. Creamy Celery Soup

Preparation Time: 40 minutes
Cooking Time: 15-60 minutes
Servings: 4
Ingredients:
- 6 cups celery
- ½ tsp dill
- 2 cups of water
- 1 cup of coconut milk
- 1 onion, chopped
- Pinch of salt

Directions:
1. Add all ingredients into the electric pot and stir well.
2. Cover the electric pot with the lid and select the soup setting.
3. Release pressure using a quick-release method than opening the lid.
4. Puree the soup using an immersion blender until smooth and creamy.
5. Stir well and serve warm.

Nutrition: Calories 174; Fat 14.6 g; Carbohydrates 10.5 g; Sugar 5.2 g; Protein 2.8 g; Cholesterol 0 mg

301. Avocado Cucumber Soup

Preparation Time: 40 minutes
Cooking Time: 15-60 minutes
Servings: 3
Ingredients:
- 1 large cucumber, peeled and sliced
- ¾ cup of water
- ¼ cup lemon juice
- 2 garlic cloves
- 6 green onions
- 2 avocados, pitted
- ½ tsp black pepper
- ½ tsp pink salt

Directions:
1. Add all ingredients into the blender and blend until smooth and creamy.
2. Place in the refrigerator for 30 minutes.
3. Stir well and serve chilled.

Nutrition: Calories 73; Fat 3.7 g; Carbohydrates 9.2 g; Sugar 2.8 g; Protein 2.2 g; Cholesterol 0 mg

302. Quinoa and Spinach Soup

Preparation Time: 30 minutes
Cooking Time: 50 minutes
Servings: 4
Ingredients:
- 150 grams of quinoa
- 8 mushrooms
- 1 clove of garlic
- 100 grams of spinach
- 2 liters of vegetable broth
- 2 teaspoons of grated ginger
- 1 onion
- 1 carrot
- 150 grams of tofu
- Salt and pepper to taste
- Olive oil

Directions:
1 - Wash and dry the mushrooms and then cut them into slices.
2 - Bring the vegetable broth to a boil and then add the mushrooms and ginger.
3 - Cook for 20 minutes and then remove the mushrooms and turn them off.

4 - Peel the onion and carrots and then chop them.

5 - Wash the spinach thoroughly and then pat dry.

6 - Warm tablespoon of olive oil in a saucepan. Then put the onion and carrots to fry for 10 minutes.

7 - Now add the vegetable broth, and when it starts to boil, add the quinoa.

8 - Cook over medium heat for 20 minutes.

9 - Once the quinoa is cooked, put in the spinach, season with salt and pepper, then mix well. Let it sit for a minute once done.

10 - Meanwhile, pat the tofu with absorbent paper and then cut it into cubes.

Nutrition: Calories: 110 Fat: 3.5g Carbohydrates: 17g Protein: 2g

303. Board Beans Cream

Preparation Time: 15 minutes

Cooking Time: 30 minutes

Servings: 4

Ingredients:

- 600 grams of fresh broad beans
- 800 ml of vegetable broth
- 1 shallot
- A tablespoon of cumin seeds
- 2 tablespoons Olive oil
- Salt and pepper to taste

Directions:

1 - Shell the beans, remove the skin and then wash them.

2 - Peel and wash the shallot and then chop it.

3 - Heat olive oil in a saucepan.

4 - As soon as it is hot, brown the shallot for a couple of minutes.

5 - Add the broad beans and cumin and sauté them for 10 minutes, stirring often.

6 - Now add the vegetable broth and continue cooking for another 15 minutes.

7 - Lower the heat and blend everything with an immersion blender.

8 - Cook for another 2 minutes, stirring constantly.

9 - Turn off, put the cream on the plates, season with olive oil, and serve.

Nutrition: Calories: 159 Fat: 3.8g Carbohydrates: 23g Protein: 8g

304. Peas Cream

Preparation Time: 15 minutes

Cooking Time: 25 minutes

Servings: 4

Ingredients:

- 300 grams of peas
- 1 onion
- 5 mint leaves
- Salt and pepper to taste
- 1 tablespoon Olive oil

Directions:

1 - Peel and wash the onion, then chop it.

2 - Wash the peas under running water and then let them drain.

3 - Put some olive oil in a saucepan, and once hot, put the onion to fry for a couple of minutes.

4 - Now add the peas, mix, and season with salt and pepper.

5 - Now add 300 ml of water and cook for 20 minutes.

6 - After 20 minutes, take half of the peas and set them aside.

7 - Blend the rest with an immersion blender until you get a smooth and creamy mixture.

8 - Wash and dry the mint leaves and then chop them.

9 - Put the whole peas back into the pot with the mint.

10 - Stir, leave to flavor for 2 minutes, and then turn off.

11 - Put the cream on the plates, season it with a drizzle of olive oil and serve.

Nutrition: Calories: 236 Fat: 18g Carbohydrates: 13g Protein: 7g

Chapter 21.   Snacks & Appetizers

305.   Roasted Cashews

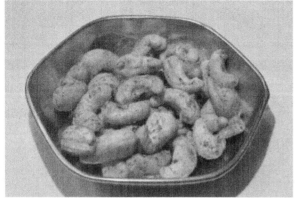

Preparation Time: 5 minutes
Cooking Time: 4 minutes
Servings: 8
Ingredients:
*   2 cups raw cashews
*   1 teaspoon coconut oil, melted
*   Salt and ground black pepper, as required
Directions:
1 - In a bowl, mix together all the ingredients.
2 - Set the temperature of Air Fryer to 355 degrees F to preheat for 5 minutes.
3 - After preheating, place the cashews into the greased Air Fryer Basket in a single layer.
4 - Slide the basket into Air Fryer and set the time for 4 minutes.
5 - While cooking, shake the basket once halfway through.
6 - When cooking time is completed, transfer the cashews into a bowl.
7 - Set aside to cool before serving.
Nutrition: Calories: 202 Fat: 16.4g Carbohydrates: 11.2g Fiber: 1g Sugar: 1.7gProtein: 5.2g

306.   Roasted Mixed Nuts

Preparation Time: 10 minutes
Cooking Time: 20 minutes
Servings: 6
Ingredients:
*   ½ cup walnuts
*   ½ cup pecans
*   ½ cup almonds
*   3-4 tablespoons unsweetened applesauce

*   ½ tablespoon ground cinnamon
*   Pinch of cayenne pepper
Directions:
1 - In a bowl, mix together all the ingredients.
2 - Set the temperature of Air Fryer to 320 degrees F to preheat for 5 minutes.
3 - After preheating, place the nuts into the greased Air Fryer Basket in a single layer.
4 - Slide the basket into Air Fryer and set the time for 20 minutes.
5 - While cooking, stir the nuts once halfway through.
6 - When cooking time is completed, transfer the nuts into a bowl.
7 - Set aside to cool before serving.
Nutrition: Calories: 188 Fat: 17.6g Carbohydrates: 5.6g Fiber: 3.2g Sugar: 1.6g Protein: 5.3g

307.   Tortilla Chips

Preparation Time: 10 minutes
Cooking Time: 6 minutes
Servings: 3
Ingredients:
*   4 corn tortillas, cut into triangles
*   1 tablespoon olive oil
*   Salt, as required
Instructions:
1 - Coat the tortilla chips with oil and then sprinkle each side of with salt.
2 - Set the temperature of Air Fryer to 390 degrees F to preheat for 5 minutes.
3 - After preheating, place them into the greased Air Fryer Basket in a single layer in 2 batches.
4 - Slide the basket into Air Fryer and set the time for 3 minutes.
5 - When cooking time is completed, transfer the tortilla chips into a bowl.
6 - Set aside to cool before serving.
Nutrition: Calories: 110 Fat: 5.6g Carbohydrates: 14.3g Fiber: 2g Sugar: 0.3g Protein: 1.8g

308.   Apple Chips

Preparation Time: 10 minutes
Cooking Time: 8 minutes
Servings: 2
Ingredients:
*   1 apple, peeled, cored and thinly sliced

- 1 tablespoon white sugar
- ½ teaspoon ground cinnamon
- Pinch of ground cardamom
- Pinch of ground ginger
- Pinch of salt

Directions:

1 - In a bowl, add all the ingredients and toss to coat well.

2 - Set the temperature of Air Fryer to 390 degrees F to preheat for 5 minutes.

3 - After preheating, arrange the apple slices into the greased Air Fryer Basket in a single layer.

4 - Slide the basket into Air Fryer and set the time for 7-8 minutes.

5 - While cooking, flip the chips once halfway through.

6 - When cooking time is completed, transfer the apple chips onto a platter.

7 - Set aside to cool before serving.

Nutrition: Calories: 83 Fat: 0.2g Carbohydrates: 22g Fiber: 3.1g Sugar: 17.6g Protein: 0.3g

309.   Banana Chips

Preparation Time: 10 minutes

Cooking Time: 10 minutes

Servings: 4

Ingredients:

- 2 raw bananas, peeled and sliced
- 2 tablespoons olive oil
- Salt and ground black pepper, as required

Directions:

1 - Drizzle the banana slices with oil evenly.

2 - Set the temperature of Air Fryer to 355 degrees F to preheat for 5 minutes.

3 - After preheating, arrange the banana slices into the greased Air Fryer Basket in a single layer.

4 - Slide the basket into Air Fryer and set the time for 10 minutes.

5 - When cooking time is completed, transfer the banana chips onto a platter and sprinkle with salt and black pepper.

6 - Set aside to cool before serving.

Nutrition: Calories: 113 Fat: 7.2g Carbohydrates: 13.5g Fiber: 1.5g Sugar: 7.2g Protein: 0.6g

310.   Sweet Potato Chips

Preparation Time: 10 minutes

Cooking Time: 15 minutes

Servings: 2

Ingredients:

- 1 medium sweet potato, cut into 1/8-inch-thick slices
- 1 tablespoon canola oil
- ¼ teaspoon sea salt
- ¼ teaspoon freshly ground black pepper
- Olive oil cooking spray

Directions:

1 - In a large bowl of cold water, place the sweet potato slices for about 20 minutes.

2 - Drain the sweet potatoes slices and with paper towels, pat dry them.

3 - In a large dry bowl, add the sweet potatoes slices, oil, salt and black pepper and gently toss to coat.

4 - Set the temperature of Air Fryer to 350 degrees F to preheat for 5 minutes.

5 - After preheating, arrange the sweet potato slices into the greased Air Fryer Basket.

6 - Slide the basket into Air Fryer and set the time for 15 minutes.

7 - When cooking time is completed, remove the sweet potato chips and set aside to cool before serving.

Nutrition: Calories: 125 Fat: 7.1g Carbohydrates: 14.5g Fiber: 2.3g Sugar: 4.5g Protein: 1.4g

311.   Beet Chips

Preparation Time: 10 minutes

Cooking Time: 15 minutes

Servings: 3

Ingredients:

- 2 medium beets, peeled and thinly sliced
- 1 tablespoon olive oil
- ¼ teaspoon smoked paprika
- Salt, as required

Directions:

1 - In a large bowl and mix together all the ingredients.

2 - Set the temperature of Air Fryer to 325 degrees F to preheat for 5 minutes.

3 - After preheating, arrange the beet slices into the greased Air Fryer Basket.

4 - Slide the basket into Air Fryer and set the time for 15 minutes.

5 - While cooking, flip the chips once halfway through.

6 - When cooking time is completed, remove the beet chips and set aside to cool before serving.

Nutrition: Calories: 70 Fat: 4.8g Carbohydrates: 6.7g Fiber: 1.4g Sugar: 5.3g Protein: 1.2g

312.   French Fries

Preparation Time: 10 minutes
Cooking Time: 30 minutes
Servings: 4
Ingredients:
- 1-pound potatoes, peeled and cut into strips
- 2 tablespoons olive oil
- 1 teaspoon paprika
- ½ teaspoon garlic powder
- ½ teaspoon onion powder

Directions:
1 - In a large bowl of water, add the potato strips and set aside for about 1 hour.
2 - Drain the potato strips well and pat them dry with paper towels.
3 - In a large bowl, add the potato strips and the remaining ingredients and toss to coat well.
4 - Set the temperature of Air Fryer to 375 degrees F to preheat for 5 minutes.
5 - After preheating, arrange the potato strips into the greased Air Fryer Basket in a single layer.
6 - Slide the basket into Air Fryer and set the time for 30 minutes.
7 - When cooking time is completed, transfer the French fries onto a platter and serve immediately.
Nutrition: Calories: 142 Fat: 7.2g Carbohydrates: 18.6g Fiber: 3g Sugar: 1.6g Protein: 2.1g

313. Avocado Fries

Preparation Time: 15 minutes
Cooking Time: 7 minutes
Servings: 2
Ingredients:
- 2 tablespoons brown rice flour
- ½ teaspoon garlic powder
- Salt and ground black pepper, as required
- 2 tablespoons unsweetened almond milk
- 1/3 cup nutritional yeast
- 1 avocado, peeled, pitted and cut into 6 wedges
- Non-stick cooking spray

Directions:
1 - In a shallow dish, mix together the flour, garlic powder, salt and black pepper.
2 - In a second shallow dish, add the nutritional yeast and almond milk and beat lightly.
3 - Roll the avocado wedges with flour mixture, then coat with yeast mixture.

4 - Spray the avocado wedges with cooking spray generously.
5 - Set the temperature of Air Fryer to 400 degrees F to preheat for 5 minutes.
6 - After preheating, arrange the avocado wedges into the greased Air Fryer Basket in a single layer and spray with cooking spray lightly.
7 - Slide the basket into Air Fryer and set the time for 7 minutes.
8 - Flip the avocado wedges once halfway through.
9 - When cooking time is completed, transfer the avocado fries onto a platter and serve immediately.
Nutrition: Calories: 340 Fat: 21.6g Carbohydrates: 29.1g Fiber: 14g Sugar: 0.8g Protein: 5.1g

314. Banana Bulgur Bars

Preparation Time: 10 minutes
Cooking Time: 30 minutes
Servings: 9
Ingredients:
- 2 ripe large bananas
- 1 tablespoon pure maple syrup
- ½ teaspoon pure vanilla extract
- 1 cup rolled oats
- 1 cup medium-grind or coarse bulgur
- ¼ cup chopped walnuts

Directions:
1 - Preheat the oven to 350°Fahrenheit. Prepare an 8-inch square baking pan lined using parchment paper.
2 - In a medium bowl, mash the bananas with a fork. Add the maple syrup and vanilla and mix well. Add the oats, bulgur, and walnuts and mix until combined.
3 - Transfer the mixture to the prepared baking pan and bake for 25 to 30 minutes, until the top is crispy.
4 - Let cool, then slice into 9 bars and transfer to an airtight container or a large zip-top plastic bag. Store at room temperature for up to 5 days.
Nutrition: Calories: 142 Fat: 3 g Carbohydrates: 26 g Protein: 4 g

315. Italian Tomato Snack

Preparation Time: 10 minutes
Cooking Time: 60 minutes
Servings: 6
Ingredients:
- 50 ounces canned tomatoes, drained
- A pinch salt and black pepper
- ¼ cup extra virgin olive oil

- 15 basil leaves, sliced
- 1 tablespoon burgundy or merlot wine vinegar
- A pinch stevia
- 10 baguette pieces, toasted

Directions:

1 - Spread the tomatoes on the lined baking sheet. Drizzle half of the oil; season with salt and pepper and bake them at 300°Fahrenheit for one hour.

2 - Slice the tomatoes into cubes and put them inside a bowl with the oil, basil, vinegar and stevia and toss. Split the tomatoes on each baguette slice and serve as a snack.

Nutrition: Calories: 191 Fat: 4 g Carbohydrates: 9 g Protein: 7 g

316. Easy Dried Grapes

Preparation Time: 5 minutes

Cooking Time: 4 hours

Servings: 10

Ingredients:

- 3 bunches seedless grapes
- A drizzle vegetable oil

Directions:

1 - Spread the grapes over a lined baking sheet and drizzle the oil. Toss and bake at 225°Fahrenheit for 4 hours.

2 - Separate the grapes into bowls and serve.

Nutrition: Calories: 131 Fat: 1 g Protein: 3 g Carbohydrates: 5 g

317. Banana Nut Bread Bars

Preparation Time: 5 minutes

Cooking Time: 30 minutes

Servings: 9

Ingredients:

- Non-stick cooking spray (optional)
- 2 large ripe bananas
- 2 tablespoons maple syrup
- ½ teaspoon vanilla extract
- 2 cups old-fashioned rolled oats
- ½ teaspoons salt
- ¼ cup chopped walnuts

Directions:

1 - Preheat the oven to 350°Fahrenheit. Lightly coat a 9-by-9-inch baking pan with non-stick cooking spray (if using) or line with parchment paper for oil-free baking.

2 - In a medium bowl, mash the bananas with a fork. Add the maple syrup and vanilla extract and mix well. Add the oats, salt, and walnuts, mixing well.

3 - Move the batter to the baking pan and bake for 25 to 30 minutes, until the top is crispy. Cool completely before slicing into 9 bars. Transfer to an airtight storage container or a large plastic bag.

Nutrition: Calories: 73 Fat: 1 g Carbohydrates: 15 g Protein: 2 g

318. Rosemary and Lemon Zest Popcorn

Preparation Time: 10 minutes

Cooking Time: 0 minutes

Servings: 2

Ingredients:

- 1 cup popcorn kernels
- 2 tablespoons vegan butter, melted
- 1 tablespoon chopped rosemary
- 1 teaspoon lemon zest
- ¼ teaspoon salt

Directions:

1 - Pop the kernels, and when done, transfer them into a large bowl. Drizzle butter over the popcorns, sprinkle with salt, lemon zest, and rosemary, and then toss until combined.

2 - Serve straight away.

Nutrition: Calories: 201 Protein: 3 g Carbohydrates: 25 g Fat: 10 g

319. Strawberry Avocado Toast

Preparation Time: 5 minutes

Cooking Time: 0 minutes

Servings: 4

Ingredients:

- 1 avocado, peeled, pitted, and quartered
- 4 whole-wheat bread slices, toasted
- 4 ripe strawberries, cut into ¼-inch slices
- 1 tablespoon balsamic glaze or reduction

Directions:

1 - Mash one-quarter of your avocado on a slice of toast. Put one-quarter of the strawberry slices over your avocado, then finish with a drizzle of balsamic glaze.

2 - Repeat with the remaining fixings, and serve.

Nutrition: Calories: 150 Fat: 8 g Carbohydrates: 17 g Protein: 5 g

320. Strawberry Watermelon Ice Pops

Preparation Time: 6 hours and 5 minutes
Cooking Time: 0 minutes
Servings: 6
Ingredients:
- 4 cups diced watermelon
- 4 strawberries, tops removed
- 2 tablespoons freshly squeezed lime juice

Directions:
1 - Combine the watermelon, strawberries, and lime juice in a blender. Blend within 1 to 2 minutes, or until well combined.
2 - Pour evenly into 6 ice-pop molds, insert ice-pop sticks, and freeze for at least 6 hours before serving.
Nutrition: Calories: 61 Fat: 0 g Carbohydrates: 15 g Protein: 1 g

321. Carrot Energy Balls

Preparation Time: 10 minutes
Cooking Time: 0 minutes
Servings: 8
Ingredients:
- 1 large carrot, grated carrot
- 1-½ cups old-fashioned oats
- 1 cup raisins
- 1 cup dates, pitied
- 1 cup coconut flakes
- ¼ teaspoon ground cloves
- ½ teaspoon ground cinnamon

Directions:
1 - Pulse all fixings in your food processor until it forms a sticky and uniform mixture. Shape the batter into equal balls.
2 - Place in your refrigerator until ready to serve. Bon Appetit!
Nutrition: Calories: 495 Protein: 22 g Carbohydrates: 58 g Fat: 21 g

322. Zucchini Muffins

Preparation Time: 10 minutes
Cooking Time: 30 minutes
Servings: 12
Ingredients:
- 2 cups almond flour
- 2 teaspoons baking powder
- 2 tablespoons coconut sugar
- A pinch black pepper
- 2 tablespoons flaxseed meal plus 3 tablespoons water, mixed
- ¾ cup almond milk
- 1 cup zucchinis, grated
- ½ cup tofu, shredded

Directions:
1 - In a bowl, combine the flour with baking powder, flaxseed, and the other ingredients. Stir well and divide into a lined muffin tray. Introduce in the oven and bake at 400°Fahrenheit for 30 minutes.
2 - Serve as a snack.
Nutrition: Calories: 149Fat: 4 g Carbohydrates: 14 g Protein: 5 g

323. Nuts and Seeds Squares

Preparation Time: 20 minutes
Cooking Time: 5 minutes
Servings: 8
Ingredients:
- ½ cup hazelnuts, toasted
- ½ cup walnuts, toasted
- ½ cup almonds, toasted
- ½ cup white sesame seeds
- ½ cup pumpkin seeds, shelled
- 1 cup unsweetened dried cherries
- 2 cups unsweetened dried coconut flakes
- ¼ cup coconut oil
- 1 cup maple syrup
- ½ teaspoon ground cinnamon
- ½ teaspoon salt

Directions:
1 - Prepare a 13x9 inch baking dish lined using parchment paper. Set aside. In a large bowl, add the hazelnuts, walnuts, and almonds and mix well.
2 - Transfer 1 cup of the nut mixture into another large bowl and chop them roughly. In the food processor, add the remaining nut mixture and pulse until finely ground.
3 - Now, transfer the ground nut mixture into the bowl of the chopped nuts. Add the seeds and coconut flakes and mix well.
4 - In a small pan, add the oil, maple syrup, and cinnamon over medium-low heat and cook for about 3–5 minutes or until it starts to boil, stirring continuously.

5 - Remove from the heat and immediately pour over the nut mixture, stirring continuously until well combined. Set aside to cool slightly.

6 - Now, place the mixture into the prepared baking dish evenly, and with the back of a spoon, smooth the top surface by pressing slightly.

7 - Refrigerate for about 1 hour or until set completely. Remove from refrigerator and cut into equal-sized squares then serve.

Nutrition: Calories: 496 Protein: 10 g Carbohydrates: 24 g Fat: 42 g

324. Carrot Fries

Preparation Time: 10 minutes
Cooking Time: 12 minutes
Servings: 2

Ingredients:
- 1 large carrot, peeled and cut into sticks
- 1 tablespoon fresh rosemary, chopped finely
- 1 tablespoon olive oil
- ¼ teaspoon cayenne pepper
- Salt and ground black pepper, as required

Directions:
1 - In a bowl, add all the ingredients and mix well.

2 - Set the temperature of Air Fryer to 390 degrees F to preheat for 5 minutes.

3 - After preheating, arrange the carrot sticks into the greased Air Fryer Basket in a single layer.

4 - Slide the basket into Air Fryer and set the time for 12 minutes.

5 - When cooking time is completed, transfer the fries onto a platter and serve immediately.

Nutrition: Calories: 81 Fat: 7.3g Carbohydrates: 4.7g Fiber: 1.7g Sugar: 1.8g Protein: 0.4g

325. Eggplant Fries

Preparation Time: 15 minutes
Cooking Time: 15 minutes
Servings: 4

Ingredients:
- 1 medium eggplant
- 1-1½ tablespoons olive oil
- 2 teaspoons maple syrup
- 1 teaspoon smoked paprika
- Salt and ground black pepper, as required
- 1 cup almond flour

Directions:

1 - Cut the eggplant into ½-inch rounds and then cut each round into ¼-inch sticks.

2 - With paper towels, pat dry the eggplant sticks.

3 - In a shallow bowl, mix together the oil, maple syrup, paprika, salt and black pepper.

4 - In a second shallow bowl, place the flour.

5 - Dip the eggplant sticks into the oil mixture and then coat with flour.

6 - Arrange the coated eggplant sticks onto a platter and set aside for about 5 minutes.

7 - Set the temperature of Air Fryer to 370 degrees F to preheat for 5 minutes.

8 - After preheating, arrange the eggplant sticks into the greased Air Fryer Basket.

9 - Slide the basket into Air Fryer and set the time for 14-16 minutes.

10 - After 10 minutes of cooking, shake the basket once.

11 - When cooking time is completed, transfer the eggplant fries onto a platter and serve immediately.

Nutrition: Calories: 229 Fat: 17.8g/ Carbohydrates: 15.3g/ Fiber: 7.2g / Sugar: 6.5g/ Protein: 7.2g

326. Pumpkin Fries

Preparation Time: 10 minutes
Cooking Time: 10 minutes
Servings: 6

Ingredients:
- 2 pounds pumpkin, peeled and cut into ½-inch thick wedges
- Olive oil cooking spray
- ½ teaspoon ground nutmeg

Directions:

1 - Set the temperature of Air Fryer to 360 degrees F to preheat for 5 minutes.

2 - After preheating, arrange the pumpkin wedges into the Air Fryer Basket and spray with the cooking spray.

3 - Slide the basket into Air Fryer and set the time for 10 minutes.

4 - Shake the basket once halfway through.

5 - When cooking time is completed, transfer the pumpkin wedges onto a platter.

6 - Sprinkle with nutmeg and serve.

Nutrition: Calories: 52/ Fat: 0.5g/ Carbohydrates: 12.3g/ Fiber: 4.4g / Sugar: 5g/ Protein: 1.7g

327. Onion Rings

Preparation Time: 15 minutes

Cooking Time: 10 minutes
Servings: 4

Ingredients:
- 2 large yellow onions
- ½ cup all-purpose flour
- 2/3 cup unsweetened almond milk
- 1 teaspoon paprika, divided
- ½ teaspoon ground turmeric, divided
- Salt, as required
- 1 cup vegan panko breadcrumbs

Directions:
1 - Carefully cut each onion into ½-inch circular slices.
2 - In a shallow bowl, mix together the flour, almond milk, ½ teaspoon of paprika, ¼ teaspoon of turmeric and salt.
3 - In another shallow bowl, mix together the breadcrumbs, ½ teaspoon of paprika, ¼ teaspoon of turmeric and salt.
4 - Coat each onion ring with flour mixture and then roll in breadcrumb mixture.
5 - Set the temperature of Air Fryer to 400 degrees F to preheat for 5 minutes.
6 - After preheating, arrange the onion rings into the greased Air Fryer Basket in a single layer.
7 - Slide the basket into Air Fryer and set the time for 10 minutes.
8 - Serve warm.
Nutrition: Calories: 1944/ Fat: 2.8g/ Carbohydrates: 23.9g/ Fiber: 2.6g / Sugar: 3.3g/ Protein: 3.4g

328. Corn on the Cob

Preparation Time: 10 minutes
Cooking Time: 10 minutes
Servings: 4

Ingredients:
- 4 ears of corn, husked and trimmed
- Non-stick cooking spray
- Salt and ground black pepper, as required
- 2 tablespoon olive oil

Directions:
1 - Set the temperature of Air Fryer to 400 degrees F to preheat for 5 minutes.
2 - Spray ears of corn with cooking spray evenly and then sprinkle with salt and black pepper.
3 - After preheating, arrange the ears of corn into the greased Air Fryer Basket.

4 - Slide the basket into Air Fryer and set the time for 8-10 minutes.
5 - Flip the ears of corn once halfway through.
6 - When cooking time is completed, transfer the ears of corn onto a platter.
7 - Drizzle with oil and serve.
Nutrition: Calories: 192 Fat: 8.8g Carbohydrates: 29g Fiber: 4.2g Sugar: 5g Protein: 5g

329. Mushroom Bites

Preparation Time: 10 minutes
Cooking Time: 6 minutes
Servings: 2

Ingredients:
- 2 Portobello mushroom caps, stemmed
- 2 tablespoons olive oil
- 1/8 teaspoon dried Italian seasoning
- Salt, as required
- 2 tablespoons canned tomatoes, chopped
- 2 Kalamata olives, pitted and sliced
- 2 tablespoons nutritional yeast
- Pinch of red pepper flakes, crushed

Directions:
1 - With a spoon, scoop out the center of each mushroom cap.
2 - Coat each mushroom cap with oil from both sides.
3 - Sprinkle the inside of caps with Italian seasoning and salt.
4 - Place the tomato pieces over both caps, followed by the olives and nutritional yeast.
5 - Set the temperature of Air Fryer to 320 degrees F to preheat for 5 minutes.
6 - After preheating, arrange the mushroom caps into the greased Air Fryer Basket.
7 - Slide the basket into Air Fryer and set the time for 6 minutes.
8 - When cooking time is completed, transfer the mushroom caps onto a platter.
9 - Sprinkle with the red pepper flakes and serve immediately.
Nutrition: Calories: 190/ Fat: 15.4g/ Carbohydrates: 10.4g/ Fiber: 4.3g / Sugar: 2.1g/ Protein: 7.2g

330. Seed Bars

Preparation Time: 15 minutes
Cooking Time: 15 minutes
Servings: 10

Ingredients:

- 1-¼ cups creamy salted peanut butter
- 5 Medjool dates, pitted
- ½ cup unsweetened vegan protein powder
- 1 cup hemp seeds
- 1 cup chia seeds

Directions:

1 - Line a loaf pan with parchment paper. Set aside. In a food processor, add the peanut butter and dates and pulse until well combined.

2 - Add the protein powder, hemp seeds, and chia seeds and pulse until well combined. Now, place the mixture into the prepared loaf pan, and with the back of a spoon, smooth the top surface.

3 - Freeze for at least 10–15 minutes, or until set. Cut into 10 equal-sized bars and serve.

Nutrition: Calories: 308 Fat: 21 g Carbohydrates: 17 g Protein: 16 g

331. Zucchini Fritters

Preparation Time: 10 minutes
Cooking Time: 6 minutes
Servings: 12

Ingredients:

- 1/2 cup quinoa flour
- 3 1/2 cups shredded zucchini
- 1/2 cup chopped scallions
- 1/3 teaspoon ground black pepper
- 1 teaspoon salt
- 2 tablespoons coconut oil
- 2 flax eggs

Directions:

1. Squeeze moisture from the zucchini by wrapping it in a cheesecloth and then transfer it to a bowl.
2. Add remaining ingredients, except for oil, stir until combined, and then shape the mixture into twelve patties.
3. Take a skillet pan, place it over medium-high heat, add oil and when hot, add patties and cook for 3 minutes per side until brown.
4. Serve the patties with your favorite vegan sauce.

Nutrition: Calories: 37 Cal Fat: 1 g Carbs: 4 g Protein: 2 g Fiber: 1 g

332. Zucchini Chips

Preparation Time: 10 minutes
Cooking Time: 120 minutes
Servings: 4

Ingredients:

- 1 large zucchini, thinly sliced
- 1 teaspoon salt
- 2 tablespoons olive oil

Directions:

1. Pat dry zucchini slices and then spread them in an even layer on a baking sheet lined with parchment sheet.
2. Whisk together salt and oil, brush this mixture over zucchini slices on both sides and then bake for 2 hours or more until brown and crispy.
3. When done, let the chips cool for 10 minutes and then serve straight away.

Nutrition: Calories: 54 Cal Fat: 5 g Carbs: 1 g Protein: 0 g

333. Rosemary Beet Chips

Preparation Time: 10 minutes
Cooking Time: 20 minutes
Servings: 3

Ingredients:

- 3 large beets, scrubbed, thinly sliced
- 1/8 teaspoon ground black pepper
- ¼ teaspoon of sea salt
- 3 sprigs of rosemary, leaves chopped
- 4 tablespoons olive oil

Directions:

1. Spread beet slices in a single layer between two large baking sheets, brush the slices with oil, then season with spices and rosemary, toss until well coated, and bake for 20 minutes at 375 degrees F until crispy, turning halfway.
2. When done, let the chips cool for 10 minutes and then serve.

Nutrition: Calories: 79 Cal Fat: 4.7 g Carbs: 8.6 g Protein: 1.5 g Fiber: 2.5 g

334. Quinoa Broccoli Tots

Preparation Time: 10 minutes
Cooking Time: 20 minutes
Servings: 16

Ingredients:

- 2 tablespoons quinoa flour
- 2 cups steamed and chopped broccoli florets
- 1/2 cup nutritional yeast
- 1 teaspoon garlic powder

- 1 teaspoon miso paste
- 2 flax eggs
- 2 tablespoons hummus

Directions:

1. Place all the ingredients in a bowl, stir until well combined, and then shape the mixture into sixteen small balls.
2. Arrange the balls on a baking sheet lined with parchment paper, spray with oil and bake at 400 degrees F for 20 minutes until brown, turning halfway.
3. When done, let the tots cool for 10 minutes and then serve straight away.

Nutrition: Calories: 19 Cal Fat: 0 g Carbs: 2 g Protein: 1 g Fiber: 0.5 g

335. Spicy Roasted Chickpeas

Preparation Time: 10 minutes
Cooking Time: 20 minutes
Servings: 6

Ingredients:

- 30 ounces cooked chickpeas
- ½ teaspoon salt
- 2 teaspoons mustard powder
- ½ teaspoon cayenne pepper
- 2 tablespoons olive oil

Directions:

1. Place all the ingredients in a bowl and stir until well coated and then spread the chickpeas in an even layer on a baking sheet greased with oil.
2. Bake the chickpeas for 20 minutes at 400 degrees F until golden brown and crispy and then serve straight away.

Nutrition: Calories: 187.1 Cal Fat: 7.4 g Carbs: 24.2 g Protein: 7.3 g Fiber: 6.3 g

336. Nacho Kale Chips

Preparation Time: 10 minutes
Cooking Time: 14 hours
Servings: 10

Ingredients:

- 2 bunches of curly kale
- 2 cups cashews, soaked, drained
- 1/2 cup chopped red bell pepper
- 1 teaspoon garlic powder
- 1 teaspoon salt

- 2 tablespoons red chili powder
- 1/2 teaspoon smoked paprika
- 1/2 cup nutritional yeast
- 1 teaspoon cayenne
- 3 tablespoons lemon juice
- 3/4 cup water

Directions:

1. Place all the ingredients except for kale in a food processor and pulse for 2 minutes until smooth.
2. Place kale in a large bowl, pour in the blended mixture, mix until coated, and dehydrate for 14 hours at 120 degrees F until crispy.
3. If a dehydrator is not available, spread kale between two baking sheets and bake for 90 minutes at 225 degrees F until crispy, flipping halfway.
4. When done, let chips cool for 15 minutes and then serve.

Nutrition: Calories: 191 Cal Fat: 12 g Carbs: 16 g Protein: 9 g Fiber: 2 g

337. Roasted Brussels Sprouts With Cranberries

Preparation Time: 15-30 minutes
Cooking Time: 50 minutes
Servings: 4

Ingredients:

- 1 pound Brussels sprouts, halved
- 3 tbsp olive oil
- Salt and black pepper to taste
- 1 medium white onion, chopped
- ½ cup dried cranberries
- 1 lemon, juiced
- 1 tbsp chopped fresh basil

Directions:

1. Preheat the oven to 425 F.
2. Spread the Brussels sprouts on a roasting sheet, drizzle with olive oil, and season with salt and black pepper.
3. Mix the seasoning onto the vegetables and roast in the oven until light brown and tender, 20 to 25 minutes.
4. Transfer the Brussels sprouts to a large salad bowl and mix in the onion, cranberries, lemon juice, and basil. Serve immediately.

Nutrition: Calories 144 kcal Fats 10. 4g Carbs 12. 7g Protein 2. 1g

338. Roasted Garlic Asparagus with Dijon Mustard

Preparation Time: 15-30 minutes
Cooking Time: 35 minutes
Servings: 4

Ingredients:

- 2 tbsp plant butter
- 1 lb. asparagus, hard part trimmed
- 2 garlic cloves, minced
- 1 tsp Dijon mustard
- 1 tbsp freshly squeezed lemon juice

Directions:

1. Melt the butter in a large skillet and sauté the asparagus until softened with some crunch, 7 minutes. Mix in the garlic and cook until fragrant, 30 seconds.
2. Meanwhile, in a small bowl, quickly whisk the mustard, lemon juice and pour the mixture over the asparagus. Cook for 2 minutes and plate the asparagus. Serve warm.

Nutrition: Calories 77 Fats 6g Carbs 5. 2g Protein 2. 7g

339. Tofu Zucchini Kabobs

Preparation Time: 15-30 minutes
Cooking Time: 10 minutes
Servings: 4

Ingredients:

- 1 (14 oz) block extra-firm tofu, pressed and cut into 1-inch cubes
- 1 medium zucchini, cut into 2-inch rounds
- 1 tbsp olive oil
- 2 tbsp freshly squeezed lemon juice
- 1 tsp smoked paprika
- 1 tsp cumin powder
- 1 tsp garlic powder

Directions:

1. Preheat a grill to medium heat.
2. Meanwhile, thread the tofu and zucchini alternately on the wooden skewers.
3. In a small bowl, whisk the olive oil, lemon juice, paprika, cumin powder, and garlic powder. Brush

the skewers all around with the mixture and place them on the grill grate.

4. Cook on both sides until golden brown, 5 minutes. Serve afterward.

Nutrition: Calories 147 Fats 10. 3g Carbs 5g Protein 11. 9g

340. Chili Toasted Nuts

Preparation Time: 15-30 minutes
Cooking Time: 35 minutes
Servings: 4

Ingredients:

- 1 cup mixed nuts
- 1 tbsp plant butter, melted
- ¼ tsp hot sauce
- ¼ tsp garlic powder
- ¼ tsp onion powder

Directions:

1. Preheat the oven to 350 F and line a baking sheet with baking paper.
2. In a medium bowl, mix the nuts, butter, hot sauce, garlic powder, and onion powder. Spread the mixture on the baking sheet and toast in the oven for 10 minutes.
3. Remove the sheet, allow complete cooling, and serve.

Nutrition: Calories 267 Fats 28. 3g Carbs 4. 9g Protein 2. 7g

341. Chocolate Protein: Bites

Preparation Time: 10 minutes
Cooking Time: 20 minutes
Servings: 12

Ingredients:

- ½ cup chocolate protein powder
- 1 avocado, medium
- 1 tablespoon chocolate chips
- 1 tablespoon almond butter
- 1 tablespoon cocoa powder
- 1 teaspoon vanilla extract
- A pinch salt

Directions:

1 - Begin by blending avocado, almond butter, vanilla extract, and salt in a high-speed blender until you get a smooth mixture.

2 - Next, spoon in the protein powder, cocoa powder, and chocolate chips to the blender. Blend again until you get a smooth dough-like consistency mixture.

3 - Now, check for seasoning and add more sweetness if needed. Finally, with the help of a scooper, scoop out dough to make small balls.

Nutrition: Calories: 46 Fat: 2 g Carbohydrates: 2 g Protein: 2 g

342. Spicy Nuts and Seeds Snack Mix

Preparation Time: 5 minutes
Cooking Time: 10 minutes
Servings: 4
Ingredients:
- ¼ teaspoon garlic powder
- ¼ teaspoon nutritional yeast
- ½ teaspoon smoked paprika
- ¼ teaspoon sea salt
- ¼ teaspoon dried parsley
- ½ cup slivered almonds
- ½ cup cashew pieces
- ½ cup sunflower seeds
- ½ cup pepitas

Directions:
1 - Mix the garlic powder, nutritional yeast, paprika, salt, and parsley in a small bowl. Set aside. In a large skillet, add the almonds, cashews, sunflower seeds and pepitas. Heat over low fire until warm and glistening, 3 minutes.

2 - Turn the heat off and stir in the parsley mixture. Allow complete cooling and enjoy!

Nutrition: Calories: 385 Fat: 33 g Protein: 12 g Carbohydrates: 16 g

343. Lentil Cakes

Preparation Time: 10 minutes
Cooking Time: 10 minutes
Servings: 8
Ingredients:
- 2 teaspoons basil, dried
- 1 cup chopped yellow onion
- 1 cup leeks, chopped
- 1 cup canned red lentils, drained and rinsed
- 1 teaspoon coriander, ground
- ¼ cup chopped parsley
- 1 tablespoon curry powder
- ¼ cup chopped cilantro
- 2 tablespoons coconut flour
- 1 tablespoon olive oil

Directions:
1 - Put the lentils in your bowl and mash them well using a potato masher. Add the basil, onion, and the other ingredients except for the oil and stir. Shape medium cakes out of this mix.

2 - Warm up a pan with the oil over medium-high heat. Add the cakes and cook them for about 5 minutes on each side.

3 - Serve warm.

Nutrition: Calories: 142 Fat: 4 g Carbohydrates: 8 g Protein: 4.4 g

344. Balsamic Green Beans Bowls

Preparation Time: 10 minutes
Cooking Time: 25 minutes
Servings: 4
Ingredients:
- 1-pound green beans, trimmed and halved
- A pinch salt and black pepper
- 1 teaspoon turmeric powder
- 1 teaspoon sweet paprika
- 4 tablespoons balsamic vinegar
- 1 teaspoon Italian seasoning

Directions:
1 - Spread the green beans on a lined baking sheet. Add the rest of the ingredients. Toss and bake at 430°Fahrenheit for 25 minutes.

2 - Serve as a snack.

Nutrition: Calories: 210 Fat: 5.5 g Carbohydrates: 11 g Protein: 6.3 g

345. Kale Bowls

Preparation Time: 10 minutes
Cooking Time: 10 minutes
Servings: 4
Ingredients:
- 2 tablespoons almonds, chopped
- 2 tablespoons walnuts, chopped
- 2 bunches kale, trimmed and roughly chopped
- 1 cup cherry tomatoes, halved
- Salt and black pepper to taste
- 2 tablespoons avocado oil
- 1 lemon juice
- 1 cup jarred roasted peppers
- 1 teaspoon Italian seasoning

- ¼ teaspoon chili powder

Directions:

1 - Warm up a pan with the oil over medium heat. Add kale and cook for 5 minutes.

2 - Add the rest of the ingredients. Toss; cook for 5 minutes more. Divide into bowls and serve.

Nutrition: Calories: 143 Fat: 5.9 g Carbohydrates: 9 g Protein: 7 g

346.　Green Bean Fries

Preparation Time: 10 minutes
Cooking Time: 8 hours
Servings: 8

Ingredients:

- 1 cup avocado oil
- 5 pounds green beans, trimmed
- Salt and black pepper to taste
- 1 teaspoon garlic powder
- 1 teaspoon onion powder
- 1 teaspoon turmeric powder
- 1 teaspoon oregano, dried
- 1 teaspoon mint, dried

Directions:

1 - Mix the green beans with the oil, salt, pepper, and the other ingredients in a bowl and toss well.

2 - Put the green beans in your dehydrator and dry them for 8 hours at 135°Fahrenheit.

3 - Serve cold as a snack.

Nutrition: Calories: 100 Fat: 12 g Carbohydrates: 8 g Protein: 5 g

347.　Chili Walnuts

Preparation Time: 10 minutes
Cooking Time: 10 minutes
Servings: 4

Ingredients:

- ½ teaspoon chili flakes
- ½ teaspoon curry powder
- ½ teaspoon hot paprika
- A pinch cayenne peppers
- 14 ounces walnuts
- 2 teaspoons avocado oil

Directions:

1 - Put the walnuts on your lined baking sheet, add the chili and the other ingredients. Toss, introduce in the oven and bake at 400°Fahrenheit for 10 minutes.

2 - Divide the mix into bowls and serve as a snack.

Nutrition: Calories: 204 Fat: 3.2 g Carbohydrates: 7.4 g Protein: 7 g

348.　Seed and Apricot Bowls

Preparation Time: 10 minutes
Cooking Time: 10 minutes
Servings: 4

Ingredients:

- 6 ounces apricots, dried
- 1 cup sunflower seeds
- 2 tablespoons coconut, shredded
- 1 tablespoon sesame seeds
- 1 tablespoon avocado oil
- 3 tablespoons hemp seeds
- 1 tablespoon chia seeds

Directions:

1 - Spread the apricots, seeds, and the other ingredients on a lined baking sheet. Toss and cook at 430°Fahrenheit for 10 minutes.

2 - Cool down, divide into bowls and serve as a snack.

Nutrition: Calories: 200 Fat: 4.3 g Carbohydrates: 8 g Protein: 5 g

349.　Spiced Lentil Burgers

Preparation Time: 10 minutes
Cooking Time: 43 minutes
Servings: 4

Ingredients:

- ¼ cup minced onion
- 1 garlic clove, minced
- 2 tablespoons water
- 1 cup chopped boiled potatoes
- 1 cup cooked lentils
- 2 tablespoons minced fresh parsley
- 1 teaspoon onion powder
- 1 teaspoon minced fresh basil
- 1 teaspoon dried dill
- 1 teaspoon paprika

Directions:

1 - Preheat the oven to 350°Fahrenheit (180°Celsius).

2 - In a pot, sauté the onion and garlic in the water for about 3 minutes, or until soft.

3 - Combine the lentils and potatoes in a large bowl and mash them together well. Add the cooked onion and garlic and the remaining ingredients to the lentil-potato mixture and stir until well combined.

4 - Form the mixture into four patties and place it on a non-stick baking sheet. Bake in the oven for 20 minutes. Turnover and bake for an additional 20 minutes.

5 - Serve hot.

Nutrition: Calories: 101 Fat: 0.4 g Carbohydrates: 19.9 g Protein: 5.5 g Fiber 5.3 g

350. Filled Dough Pieces in Carrot Shape

Preparation Time: 30 minutes
Cooking Time: 0 minutes
Servings: 8

Ingredients:

- 400 ml vegetable stock
- 200 g red lentils
- 1 tablespoon almond butter
- 1 pack. Pizza dough
- salt and pepper
- 1 bunch of parsley

Directions:

1. Do not make funnels out of aluminum paper to hold the pizza dough in the shape of a carrot.
2. Roll out the dough, cut into strips and wrap around the funnels.
3. Then bake at 200 degrees Celsius for about 10 minutes until they are golden brown.
4. In the meantime, bring the broth to a boil and cook the lentils in it.
5. Season with almond butter, salt, and pepper and let cool slightly.
6. Fill the funnels with lentils and finally put a bunch of parsley on top.
7. These bites go perfectly with an Easter brunch.

Nutrition: Calories: 229 Fat: 9.4g Carbs: 11.5g Protein: 12.1g Fiber: 3.2g

351. Banana Cream Stuffed Strawberries

Preparation Time: 15-30 minutes
Cooking Time: 10 minutes
Servings: 4

Ingredients:

- 12 fresh strawberries, heads removed
- ¼ cup cashew cream
- ¼ tsp banana extract
- 1 tbsp unsweetened coconut flakes

Directions:

1. Use a teaspoon to scoop out some of the strawberries pulp to create a hole within.
2. In a small bowl, mix the cashew cream, banana extract, and maple syrup.
3. Spoon the mixture into the strawberries and garnish with the coconut flakes. Serve.

Nutrition: Calories 47 Fats 3. 38g Carbs 4. 11g Protein 0. 69g

352. Tahini String Beans

Preparation Time: 15-30 minutes
Cooking Time: 10 minutes
Servings: 4

Ingredients:

- 1 tbsp sesame oil
- 1 cup string beans, trimmed
- Salt to taste
- 2 tbsp pure tahini
- 2 tbsp coarsely chopped mint leaves
- ¼ tsp red chili flakes for topping

Directions:

1. Pour the string beans into a medium safe microwave dish, sprinkle with 1 tbsp of water, and steam in the microwave until softened, 1 minute.
2. Heat the sesame oil in a large skillet and toss in the string beans until well coated in the butter.
3. Season with salt and mix in the tahini and mint leaves. Cook for 1 to 2 minutes and turn the heat off.
4. Plate the string beans and serve.

Nutrition: Calories 79 kcal Fats 4. 3g Carbs 9. 5g Protein 1. 27g

353. Black Beans Burger

Preparation Time: 15 minutes
Cooking Time: 5 minutes
Servings: 5

Ingredients:

- 1 cup black beans, cooked
- 2 tablespoons bread crumbs
- 1 teaspoon salt
- 1/4 cup sweet corn, cooked
- 1 teaspoon turmeric
- 1 tablespoon fresh parsley, chopped

- 1/2 yellow sweet pepper, chopped
- 1/2 cup of water

Directions:
1. Mash the black beans until you get puree and combine them with salt, sweet corn, turmeric, parsley, and sweet pepper.
2. Mix it up carefully with the help of a spoon.
3. Add breadcrumbs and stir again.
4. Pour water into the instant pot bowl and insert the steamer rack.
5. Make the burgers from the black bean mixture and freeze them for 30 minutes.
6. Then wrap every burger in the foil and place it on the steamer rack.
7. Close the lid and cook on Manual mode (High pressure) for 5 minutes.
8. Then allow natural pressure release for 5 minutes.
9. Remove the foil from the burgers and transfer it to the plate. Garnish burgers with lettuce leaves if desired.

Nutrition: Calories: 155, Fat: 0.9, Fiber: 6.5, Carbs: 28.8, Protein: 9.2

354. Mushroom Burger

Preparation Time: 10 minutes
Cooking Time: 14 minutes
Servings: 4

Ingredients:
- 2 cups mushrooms, chopped
- 1 onion, diced
- 1/2 cup silken tofu
- 1/2 teaspoon salt
- 1/2 teaspoon chili flakes
- 1 tablespoon dried parsley
- 1 teaspoon dried dill
- 3 tablespoon flax meal
- 1/2 teaspoon olive oil

Directions:
1. Put mushrooms in the blender and grind.
2. Then transfer the vegetables to the instant pot together with onion, and olive oil.
3. Stir gently and close the lid. Cook **Ingredients:** on Sauté mode for 10 minutes.
4. Meanwhile, mash silken tofu until you get a puree. Mix it up with salt, chili flakes, dried parsley, and dried dill. Add flax meal and pulse for 10 seconds.

5. When the mushroom mixture is cooked transfer it to a bowl and combine it with the silken tofu.
6. Stir well.
7. Make the burgers.
8. Line the instant pot pan with baking paper and place burgers on it.
9. Close the lid and meal for 4 minutes on High. Then use quick pressure release.
10. Chill the burgers to room temperature before serving.

Nutrition: Calories: 47, Fat: 2.6, Fiber: 2.5, Carbs: 5.4, Protein: 2.6

355. Seitan Burgers

Preparation Time: 10 minutes
Cooking Time: 2 minutes
Servings: 1

Ingredients:
- 1 burger bun
- 1 teaspoon mustard
- 1 teaspoon soy sauce
- 1 seitan steak
- 1 teaspoon onion powder
- 1 teaspoon olive oil
- 1 tablespoon apple cider vinegar

Directions:
1. Make the sauce for seitan steak: mix up together soy sauce, onion powder, olive oil, and apple cider vinegar.
2. Brush seitan steak with sauce from each side and place in the instant pot.
3. Close the lid and cook on Manual mode (High pressure) for 2 minutes (quick pressure release).
4. Meanwhile, cut the burger bun into halves and spread with mustard.
5. Place seitan steak on the one half of the burger bun and cover with the second one.

Nutrition: Calories: 303, Fat: 8.8, Fiber: 2.8, Carbs: 24.9, Protein: 26.8

356. Maple Roasted Squash

Preparation Time: 15-30 minutes
Cooking Time: 40 minutes
Servings: 4

Ingredients:
- 1 large butternut squash, deseeded and cubed
- 2 tbsp olive oil

- 4 garlic cloves, minced
- ¼ cup pure maple syrup
- Salt and black pepper to taste
- 1 tsp red chili flakes
- 1 tsp coriander seeds

Directions:
1. Preheat the oven to 375 F.
2. In a medium bowl, toss the squash with the olive oil, garlic, maple syrup, salt, black pepper, red chili flakes, and coriander seeds.
3. Spread the mixture on a baking sheet and roast in the oven for 25 to 30 minutes or until the potatoes soften and golden brown.
4. Remove from the oven, plate, and serve warm.

Nutrition: Calories 126 kcal Fats 7. 1g Carbs 15. 6g Protein 1. 1g

357.   Carrot And Red Onion Sauté

Preparation Time: 15-30 minutes
Cooking Time: 20 minutes
Servings: 4
Ingredients:
- 2 beets, peeled and cut into wedges
- 3 small carrots, cut crosswise
- 2 tbsp plant butter
- 1 medium red onion, cut into wedges
- ½ tsp dried oregano
- 1/8 tsp salt

Directions:
1. Steam the beets and carrots in a medium safe microwave bowl until softened, 6 minutes.
2. Meanwhile, melt the butter in a large skillet and sauté the onion until softened, 3 minutes. Stir in the carrots, beets, oregano, and salt. Mix well and cook for 5 minutes. Dish the food into serving bowls and serve warm.

Nutrition: Calories 95 kcal Fats 6g Carbs 10. 2g Protein 1. 4g

358.   Avocado Tomato Bruschetta

Preparation Time: 10 minutes
Cooking Time: 0 minute
Servings: 4
Ingredients:
- 3 slices of whole-grain bread
- 6 chopped cherry tomatoes
- ½ of sliced avocado
- ½ teaspoon minced garlic
- ½ teaspoon ground black pepper
- 2 tablespoons chopped basil
- ½ teaspoon of sea salt
- 1 teaspoon balsamic vinegar

Directions:
1. Place tomatoes in a bowl, and then stir in vinegar until mixed. Top bread slices with avocado slices, then top evenly with tomato mixture, garlic, and basil, and season with salt and black pepper.
2. Serve straight away

Nutrition: Calories: 131 Cal Fat: 7.3 g Carbs: 15 g Protein: 2.8 g Fiber: 3.2 g

359.   Thai Snack Mix

Preparation Time: 15 minutes
Cooking Time: 90 minutes
Servings: 4
Ingredients:
- 5 cups mixed nuts
- 1 cup chopped dried pineapple
- 1 cup pumpkin seed
- 1 teaspoon garlic powder
- 1 teaspoon onion powder
- 2 teaspoons paprika
- 1 teaspoon of sea salt
- 1/4 cup coconut sugar
- 1/2 teaspoon red chili powder
- 1/2 teaspoon ground black pepper
- 1 tablespoon red pepper flakes
- 1/2 tablespoon red curry powder
- 2 tablespoons soy sauce
- 2 tablespoons coconut oil

Directions:
1. Switch on the slow cooker, add all the ingredients in it except for dried pineapple and red pepper flakes, stir until combined, and cook for 90 minutes at a high heat setting, stirring every 30 minutes.
2. When done, spread the nut mixture on a baking sheet lined with parchment paper and let it cool.
3. Then spread dried pineapple on top, sprinkle with red pepper flakes and serve.

Nutrition: Calories: 230 Cal Fat: 17.5 g Carbs: 11.5 g Protein: 6.5 g Fiber: 2 g

360. Broccoli Poppers

Preparation Time: 15 minutes
Cooking Time: 10 minutes
Servings: 4

Ingredients:

- 2 tablespoons plain almond milk yogurt
- ½ teaspoon red chili powder
- ¼ teaspoon ground cumin
- ¼ teaspoon ground turmeric
- Salt, as required
- 1 pound broccoli, cut into small florets
- 2 tablespoons chickpea flour

Directions:

1 - In a bowl, mix together the yogurt and spices.

2 - Add the broccoli and coat with marinade generously.

3 - Refrigerate for about 20 minutes.

4 - Remove from the refrigerator and sprinkle the broccoli florets with chickpea flour.

5 - Set the temperature of Air Fryer to 400 degrees F to preheat for 5 minutes.

6 - After preheating, arrange the broccoli florets into the greased Air Fryer Basket.

7 - Slide the basket into Air Fryer and set the time for 10 minutes.

8 - While cooking, toss the broccoli florets once halfway through.

9 - When cooking time is completed, transfer the broccoli poppers onto a platter.

10 - Serve hot.

Nutrition: Calories: 71/ Fat: 1.5g/ Carbohydrates: 11.7g/ Fiber: 4.2g / Sugar: 2.6g/ Protein: 4.7g

361. Cauliflower Poppers

Preparation Time: 10 minutes
Cooking Time: 8 minutes
Servings: 3

Ingredients:

- ½ of large head cauliflower, cut into bite-sized floret
- 2 tablespoons olive oil
- Salt and ground black pepper, as required

Directions:

1 - Drizzle the cauliflower florets with oil and sprinkle with salt and black pepper.

2 - Set the temperature of Air Fryer to 390 degrees F to preheat for 5 minutes.

3 - After preheating, place the cauliflower florets in a greased Air Fryer Basket in a single layer.

4 - Slide the basket into Air Fryer and set the time for 8 minutes.

5 - While cooking, shake the basket once halfway through.

6 - When cooking time is completed, transfer the cauliflower poppers onto a platter.

Nutrition: Calories: 91 Fat: 9.4g Carbohydrates: 2.3g Fiber: 1.1g Sugar: 1.1g Protein: 0.9g

362. Buffalo Cauliflower Bites

Preparation Time: 15 minutes
Cooking Time: 30 minutes
Servings: 4

Ingredients:

- ½ cup hot sauce
- 2 tablespoons coconut oil, melted
- 1 tablespoon olive oil
- 1 head cauliflower, cut into florets
- ½ cup almond flour
- 3 tablespoons dried parsley
- 1 teaspoon seasoning salt
- ½ tablespoon garlic powder

Directions:

1 - In a bowl, add hot sauce, coconut oil and oil and mix well.

2 - Add the cauliflower florets and toss to coat well.

3 - In another bowl, mix together the flour, parsley, seasoning salt and garlic powder.

4 - Add the cauliflower florets and toss to coat well.

5 - Set the temperature of Air Fryer to 350 degrees F to preheat for 5 minutes.

6 - After preheating, arrange the cauliflower florets into the greased Air Fryer Basket in 2 batches.

7 - Slide the basket into Air Fryer and set the time for 15 minutes.

8 - While cooking, shake the Air Fryer Basket twice.

9 - When cooking time is completed, transfer the cauliflower poppers onto a platter.

10 - Serve hot.

Nutrition: Calories: 193 Fat: 17.5g Carbohydrates: 8g Fiber: 3.4g Sugar: 2.7g Protein: 4.7g

363. Veggie Nuggets

Preparation Time: 20 minutes
Cooking Time: 45 minutes
Servings: 4

Ingredients:

- 2 cups potatoes, chopped finely

- 1 teaspoon extra-virgin olive oil
- 1 garlic clove, minced
- 4 cups fresh kale, tough ribs removed and chopped roughly
- 2 tablespoons unsweetened almond milk
- Salt and ground black pepper, as required

Directions:

1 - In a large saucepan of boiling water, add the potatoes and cook for about 30 minutes.

2 - Meanwhile, in a large skillet, heat the oil over medium-high heat and sauté the garlic for about 1 minute.

3 - Add the kale and sauté for about 2-3 minutes.

4 - Transfer the kale mixture into a large bowl.

5 - Drain the cooked potatoes and transfer into a bowl.

6 - Add the milk, salt, and pepper and mash with a potato masher, mash well.

7 - Transfer the mashed potatoes into the bowl of kale and mix well.

8 - Shape the potato mixture into 1-inch nuggets.

9 - Set the temperature of Air Fryer to 390 degrees F to preheat for 5 minutes.

10 - After preheating, arrange the nuggets into the greased Air Fryer Basket in a single layer.

11 - Slide the basket into Air Fryer and set the time for 15 minutes.

12 - While cooking, shake the Air Fryer Basket once after 6 minutes.

13 - When cooking time is completed, transfer the nuggets onto a platter.

14 - Serve hot.

Nutrition: Calories: 197 Fat: 17.2g Carbohydrates: 8g Fiber: 3.4g Sugar: 2.2g Protein: 4.7g

364. Fried Ravioli

Preparation Time: 15 minutes
Cooking Time: 8 minutes
Servings: 4

Ingredients:

- ¼ cup aquafaba (liquid from can of chickpeas)
- ½ cup vegan panko breadcrumbs
- 2 teaspoons nutritional yeast flakes
- 1 teaspoon dried oregano
- 1 teaspoon dried basil
- 1 teaspoon garlic powder
- Pinch of salt and ground black pepper
- 8 ounces frozen vegan ravioli, thawed

- Non-stick cooking spray

Directions:

1 - In a shallow dish, place the aquafaba.

2 - In another shallow dish, mix together the breadcrumbs, nutritional yeast, dried herbs, garlic powder, salt, and black pepper.

3 - Dip each ravioli into aquafaba and shake off the excess liquid.

4 - Then coat each ravioli with breadcrumb mixture.

5 - Spray each ravioli with cooking spray evenly.

6 - Set the temperature of Air Fryer to 390 degrees F to preheat for 5 minutes.

7 - After preheating, arrange the ravioli into the greased Air Fryer Basket in a single layer.

8 - Slide the basket into Air Fryer and set the time for 8 minutes.

9 - While cooking, flip the ravioli once after 6 minutes.

10 - When cooking time is completed, transfer the ravioli onto a platter.

11 - Serve hot.

Nutrition: Calories: 172 Fat: 4.2g Carbohydrates: 19.2g Fiber: 1.5g Sugar: 1g Protein: 6.4g

365. Tofu Bites

Preparation Time: 15 minutes
Cooking Time: 12 minutes
Servings: 4

Ingredients:

- 14 ounces extra-firm tofu, pressed, drained and cubed
- ½ cup cornmeal
- ½ cup quinoa flour
- 3 tablespoons nutritional yeast
- 2 tablespoons bouillon granules
- 1 tablespoon Dijon mustard
- 1 teaspoon onion powder
- 1 teaspoon garlic powder
- Salt and ground black pepper, as required
- ¾ cup unsweetened almond milk
- 1½ cups vegan panko breadcrumbs

Directions:

1 - In a shallow bowl, add cornmeal, flour, nutritional yeast, bouillon granules, mustard, onion powder, garlic powder, salt and black pepper and mix well.

2 - Add the almond milk into a large bowl and mix until well combined.

3 - In another shallow bowl, place the breadcrumbs.

4 - Dip tofu pieces into the flour mixture, then coat with breadcrumbs.

5 - Set the temperature of Air Fryer to 350 degrees F to preheat for 5 minutes.

6 - After preheating, arrange the tofu cubes into the greased Air Fryer Basket.

7 - Slide the basket into Air Fryer and set the time for 12 minutes.

8 - While cooking, flip the tofu cubes once halfway through.

9 - When cooking time is completed, transfer the tofu bites onto a platter.

10 - Serve hot.

Nutrition: Calories: 403 Fat: 11.1g Carbohydrates: 36.9g Fiber: 5g Sugar: 1.1g Protein: 19.6g

Chapter 22.　　Sides

366.　Peas with Lemon

Preparation Time: 2 minutes
Cooking Time: 3 minutes
Servings: 1

Ingredients:

- 2 cups frozen peas
- 2 garlic cloves
- 1 tablespoon nutritional yeast
- 1 tablespoon olive oil
- ¼ teaspoon sea salt
- Fresh ground pepper as needed
- ½ lemon zest

Directions:

1 - Rinse peas under warm running water and drain.
2 - Peel and mince garlic cloves.
3 - Add nutritional yeast and olive oil to a large skillet and place over medium heat.
4 - Sauté in minced garlic and peas, cooking for 2 minutes until completely warm but still vivid in color.
5 - Sprinkle black pepper, sea salt, and lemon zest
6 - Remove the garlic cloves from the peas before serving.
7 - It is a healthy side dish to have with a variety of grains.

Nutrition: Calories: 107 Fat: 6.6g Saturated Fat: 2.4g Carbohydrates: 9.1g Fiber: 3g Sugars: 3.4g

367.　Smashed Brussels Sprouts

Preparation Time: 10 minutes
Cooking Time: 30 minutes
Servings: 1

Ingredients:

- 1 ½ oz. stemless Brussels sprouts
- 3 tablespoons extra-virgin olive oil
- 1 tablespoon sea salt
- 1/3 cup cashew cheese
- ¼ teaspoon garlic powder
- ¼ teaspoon onion powder
- Ground black pepper as needed

Directions:

1 - Set the oven to 450 degrees Fahrenheit.
2 - Bring a pot of water to boil after adding 1 tablespoon of sea salt to it.
3 - Cut off the rough ends of the Brussels sprouts and boil them for 8 minutes, until tender yet vivid in color.
4 - Drain the water and let them steam in a colander for some time.
5 - Dry them with a clean kitchen towel and transfer to a large bowl.
6 - Add olive oil, sea salt, onion, garlic and black pepper powder to the bowl.
7 - Toss to combine well.
8 - Transfer the sprouts to a parchment-lined baking tray.
9 - Smash them slightly with a small skillet until they are a little mashed, but not overly mushy.
10 - Top with some cashew cheese and bake for 25 minutes, or until nicely brown and crispy.
11 - Remove from the oven once baked and season with salt if necessary.
12 - Serve them right away to enjoy the crispiness.

Nutrition: Calories: 154 Fat: 8g Cholesterol: 2mg Sodium: 248 mg Carbohydrates: 16g Fiber 7g Protein 7g Sugars 4g

368.　Quick Baked Potatoes

Preparation Time: 5 minutes
Cooking Time: 30 minutes
Servings: 1

Ingredients:

- 4 medium russet potatoes
- Extra-virgin olive oil as needed
- Sea Salt & pepper to taste

Directions:

1 - Set the oven to 450 degrees Fahrenheit.
2 - Slice the potatoes in half after washing them.
3 - Prepare a baking sheet with parchment paper.
4 - Apply enough olive oil to coat the potatoes and place them on the baking sheet.
5 - Sprinkle sea salt over them.
6 - Fork prick the potatoes several times on top, cut side down.
7 - Bake for 25 to 35 minutes, depending on the size of the potatoes, until the potatoes are tender and lightly browned from around the edges.
8 - To check if they are done, prick them with a fork.
9 - If necessary, add another sprinkle of salt.
10 - Serve as a side dish with any meal.

Nutrition: Calories:168 Fat: 0.2g Saturated Fat 0.1g Carbohydrates 38.5g Fiber 2.8g Sugars 1.3g

369. Crispy Breaded Cauliflower

Preparation Time: 10 minutes
Cooking Time: 30 minutes
Servings: 4

Ingredients:

- 1 medium head chopped cauliflower florets
- ½ cup gluten-free breadcrumbs
- ½ cup cornmeal
- 1 tablespoon peanut butter
- 1 tablespoon maple syrup
- 1 teaspoon cumin
- 1 teaspoon garlic powder
- ¼ teaspoon turmeric
- ½ teaspoon sea salt
- 1 tablespoon refined coconut oil
- 1 teaspoon smoked paprika
- 2 tablespoons tamari
- ½ tablespoon hot sauce

Directions:

1 - Preheat the oven to 400F.
2 - Place cauliflower florets in a large bowl.
3 - Mix the dry ingredients in a small bowl.
4 - Place a saucepan over medium flame and whisk in all the wet ingredients for 2 minutes, or until well-combined and slightly darkened.
5 - Stir in the sauce to the cauliflower bowl and make sure the florets are evenly coated.
6 - Take half of the dry mixture and add to the bowl of cauliflower and mix well.
7 - Add the remaining dry mixture to ensure each floret is covered properly.
8 - Use your hands to transfer the breaded cauliflower florets onto a parchment lined baking sheet.
9 - Put in the oven for 30 minutes and do not forget to flip after 15 minutes.
10 - Remove from oven when done and serve immediately with your favorite dip.
Nutrition: Calories: 151 Fat: 6.4g Saturated Fat: 3.5g Carbohydrates: 20.9g Fiber: 4g Sugars: 7.1g

370. "Delicata" Squash Tahini Fries

Preparation Time: 5 minutes
Cooking Time: 25 minutes
Servings: 4

Ingredients:

- 4 "delicata" squash
- Extra-virgin olive oil as needed
- ½ teaspoon kosher salt
- 2 garlic cloves
- ¼ cup lemon tahini sauce
- Black pepper as needed
- 2 tablespoons vegan butter

Directions:

1 - Heat the oven to 450°F.
2 - Wash, cut in half lengthwise, and scoop out the seeds of the squash.
3 - Slice each half into 1/2-inch pieces.
4 - Drizzle olive oil over the slices and place in a bowl.
5 - Stir in kosher salt and freshly ground black pepper as needed.
6 - Place the squash in a single layer on a baking sheet covered with parchment paper.
7 - Bake for about 25 minutes until tender and nicely browned.
8 - Start preparing the buffalo sauce.
9 - Start by melting the butter in a saucepan and mince the garlic.
10 - Stir tahini sauce into butter and garlic.
11 - Serve breaded squash fresh out of the oven with buffalo sauce.
Nutrition: Calories: 74 Fat: 3.6g Saturated Fat: 0.3g Cholesterol: 0 mg Sodium: 584.6mg Carbohydrates: 11.2g Fiber: 1.6g Sugars: 0g Protein: 0.9g

371. Coconut Mushroom Dumplings

Preparation Time: 10minutes
Cooking Time: 12minutes
Servings: 4

Ingredients:

- 1 lb. ground mushroom
- 2 scallions, chopped
- 1 small cucumber, deseeded and grated
- 4 garlic cloves, minced
- 1 tsp freshly pureed ginger
- 1 tsp red chili flakes
- 2 tbsp tamari sauce
- 2 tbsp sesame oil
- 3 tbsp coconut oil, for frying

Directions:

1. In a medium bowl, combine the mushroom, scallions, cucumber, garlic, ginger, red chili flakes, tamari sauce, and sesame oil. Using your

hands, form 1-inch oval shapes out of the mixture and place them on a plate.
2. Heat the coconut oil in a medium skillet over medium heat; fry the dumplings for 12 minutes until brown on both sides and cooked
3. Transfer to a paper towel-lined plate to drain grease and serve with creamy spinach puree.

Nutrition: Calories:439, Total Fat:31.9g, Saturated Fat:12.2g, Total Carbs:9g, Dietary Fiber:4g, Sugar:1g, Protein:36g, Sodium:574mg

372. Balsamic Beans Salad

Preparation Time: 10 minutes
Cooking Time: 00 minutes
Servings: 4

Ingredients:
- 1 cup of frozen green beans
- 1/4 cup chopped almonds
- 1/2 cup chopped green onions
- 3/4 cup mayonnaise
- 2 tablespoons balsamic vinegar
- Black pepper to taste

Directions:
1. Place beans in a colander, and run warm water over them until they are thawed. Place in a large bowl.
2. Toast almonds in a skillet over medium heat. Then combine with beans.
3. Stir in onions, and mayonnaise. Mix in balsamic vinegar, and season with pepper. Cover, and refrigerator.

Nutrition: Calories145, Total Fat 10.9g, Saturated Fat 2.6g, Cholesterol 14mg, Sodium 263mg, Total Carbohydrate 9.4g, Dietary Fiber 1.5g, Total Sugars 3.1g, Protein 3.3g, Calcium 67mg, Iron 1mg, Potassium 94mg, Phosphorus 44mg

373. Kale and Cauliflower Salad

Preparation Time: 10 minutes
Cooking Time: 00 minutes
Servings: 4

Ingredients:
- ½ cup lemon juice
- 1 tablespoon olive oil
- 1 teaspoon maple syrup
- 1/8 teaspoon salt
- ¼ teaspoon ground black pepper

- 1 bunch kale, cut into bite-size pieces
- ½ cup roasted cauliflower
- ½ cup dried cranberries

Directions:
1. Whisk lemon juice, olive oil, maple syrup, salt, and black pepper in a large bowl. Add kale, cauliflower, and cranberries; toss to combine.

Nutrition: Calories 76, Total Fat 5g, Saturated Fat 1.2g, Cholesterol 2mg, Sodium 131mg, Total Carbohydrate 5.9g, Dietary Fiber 1.3g, Total Sugars 2.8g, Protein 1.8g, Calcium 59mg, Iron 1mg, Potassium 146mg, Phosphorus 88mg

374. Kale and Cucumber Salad

Preparation Time: 05 minutes
Cooking Time: 10 minutes
Servings: 4

Ingredients:
- 2 tablespoons olive oil
- 3 tablespoons lemon juice
- 2 tablespoons water
- 1 tablespoon minced garlic
- 1 tablespoon soy sauce
- 2 teaspoons maple syrup
- 8 cups thinly sliced kale, packed
- 1 cucumber, peeled and sliced

Directions:
1. Combine olive oil, lemon juice, water, garlic, soy sauce, and maple syrup in a small bowl. Stir until smooth.
2. Place kale and cucumbers in a large bowl. Pour dressing over kale; toss until combined.
3. Marinate for a minimum of 20 minutes, tossing occasionally.
4. Serve.

Nutrition: Calories 80, Total Fat 2.9g, Saturated Fat 0.4g, Cholesterol 0mg, Sodium 115mg, Total Carbohydrate 13g, Dietary Fiber 1.1g, Total Sugars 5.6g, Protein 2g, Calcium 78mg, Iron 1mg, Potassium 231mg, Phosphorus156mg

375. Broccoli and Black Bean Chili

Preparation Time: 15 minutes
Cooking Time: 15 minutes
Servings: 2

Ingredients:

- ½ tablespoon coconut oil
- 1 cup broccoli
- 1 cup chopped red onions
- ½ tablespoon paprika
- 1/2 teaspoon salt
- ¼ cup tomatoes
- 1 cup black beans drained, rinsed
- ¼ chopped green chills
- ½ cup of water

Directions:
1. In the Instant Pot, select Sauté; adjust to normal. Heat coconut oil in Instant Pot. Add broccoli, onions, paprika, and salt; cook 8 to 10 minutes, stirring occasionally, until thoroughly cooked. Select Cancel.
2. Stir in tomatoes, black beans, chills, and water. Secure lid set pressure valve to Sealing. Select Manual, cook on High pressure 5 minutes. Select Cancel. Keep the pressure valve in the Sealing position to release pressure naturally.

Nutrition: Calories 408, Total Fat 5. 3g, Saturated Fat 3. 4g, Cholesterol 0mg, Sodium 607mg, Total Carbohydrate 70. 7g, Dietary Fiber 18. 1g, Total Sugars 6g, Protein 23. 3g

376.   Potato and Chickpea Curry

Preparation Time: 05 minutes
Cooking Time: 10 minutes
Servings: 2

Ingredients:
- ½ tablespoon coconut oil
- 1 small onion chopped
- 2 teaspoons paprika
- ½ teaspoon garlic powder
- ¼ teaspoon salt
- ¼ teaspoon chipotle chili powder
- ¼ teaspoon ground cumin
- 1 cup vegetable broth
- 1 cup chickpea rinsed and drained
- ¼ cup potatoes peeled and cut into 1/2-inch pieces
- ½ cup diced tomatoes

Directions:
1. Press Sauté, heat coconut oil in Instant Pot. Add chopped onions; cook 3 minutes or until softened. Add paprika, garlic powder, salt,

chipotle chili powder, and ground cumin; cook and stir for 1 minute. Stir in broth, scraping up browned bits from the bottom of Instant Pot. Add chickpea, potatoes, and diced tomatoes; mix well.
2. Secure lid and move pressure release valve to the Sealing position. Press Manual or Pressure Cook; cook at High Pressure for 4 minutes.
3. When cooking is complete, press Cancel and use Quick-release.
4. Press Sauté; cook and stir for 3 to 5 minutes or until thickened to desired consistency. Serve with desired toppings.

Nutrition: Calories 575, Total Fat 11. 3g, Saturated Fat 3. 8g, Cholesterol 0mg, Sodium 679mg, Total Carbohydrate 96. 2g, Dietary Fiber 25. 1g, Total Sugars 13. 8g, Protein 26. 7g

377.   Vegetarian Chili

Preparation Time: 15 minutes
Cooking Time: 20 minutes
Servings: 2

Ingredients:
- 1 tablespoon avocado oil
- ½ teaspoon garlic powder
- 1 cup chopped onion
- ½ cup chopped carrots
- ¼ cup chopped green bell pepper
- ¼ cup chopped red bell pepper
- 1 tablespoon chili powder
- ½ cup chopped fresh mushrooms
- ½ cup whole peeled tomatoes with liquid, chopped
- ¼ cup black beans
- ¼ cup kidney beans
- ¼ cup pinto beans
- ¼ cup whole kernel corn
- ½ tablespoon cumin seed
- 1/2 tablespoons dried basil
- 1/2 tablespoon garlic minced

Directions:
1. Select the Sauté setting on the Instant Pot, add avocado oil, cook and stir the garlic minced, onions, and carrots in the Instant Pot until tender. Mix in the green bell pepper, red bell pepper, and chili powder. Season with chili

powder. Continue cooking for 2 minutes, or until the peppers are tender.

2. Mix the mushrooms into the Instant pot. Stir in the tomatoes with liquid, black beans, kidney beans, pinto beans, and corn. Season with cumin seed, basil, and garlic powder.

3. Select Pressure Cook or Manual, and adjust the pressure to High and the time to 12 minutes. After cooking, let the pressure release naturally for 10 minutes, then quickly release any remaining pressure.

Nutrition: Calories 348, Total Fat 3. 3g, Saturated Fat 0. 6g, Cholesterol 0mg, Sodium 77mg, Total Carbohydrate 65g, Dietary Fiber 16. 5g, Total Sugars 9. 5g, Protein 19. 1g

378. Coconut Curry Chili

Preparation Time: 15 minutes
Cooking Time: 30 minutes
Servings: 2
Ingredients:

- 1 cup tomatoes
- 2 cups of water
- 1 tablespoon minced garlic
- ½ cup garbanzo beans
- ½ cup red kidney beans
- 1/2 cup chopped zucchini
- ¼ cup mango
- 1 1/2 tablespoons curry powder
- 1cup onions, chopped
- Salt and ground black pepper to taste
- ½ cup of coconut milk

Directions:

1. In the Instant Pot, add all ingredients like tomatoes, water, garlic, garbanzo beans, kidney beans, zucchini, mango, curry powder, onions, salt, and black pepper.

2. Select Pressure Cook or Manual, and adjust the pressure to High and the time to 12 minutes. After cooking, let the pressure release naturally for 10 minutes, then quickly release any remaining pressure.

3. Stir coconut milk.

4. Serve.

Nutrition: Calories 548, Total Fat 18. 6g, Saturated Fat 13. 2g, Cholesterol 0mg, Sodium 46mg, Total

Carbohydrate 78g, Dietary Fiber 21. 1g, Total Sugars 16. 6g, Protein 24g

379. Spicy Butternut Squash Chili

Preparation Time: 15 minutes
Cooking Time: 30 minutes
Servings: 2
Ingredients:

- ½ teaspoon crushed red pepper flakes, or to taste
- 1 teaspoon garlic powder
- ½ large onion, diced
- 1 green bell pepper, chopped
- 1 red bell pepper, chopped
- ½ cup kidney beans
- ½ cup black beans
- ½ cup pinto beans,
- 1 cup tomato paste
- 2 tomatoes, diced
- ½ cup butter squash diced
- ½ cup green peas
- ½ teaspoons chili powder
- 1 teaspoon cumin
- Salt and pepper to taste

Directions:

1. In the Instant Pot, combine red pepper flakes, garlic powder, onion, kidney beans, black beans, pinto beans, tomato paste, diced tomatoes, and butter squash.

2. Add the green and red bell pepper and water and cook for 5 minutes. Season with chili powder, cumin, and salt.

3. Stir the green peas, salt, and pepper into the Instant pot. Select Pressure Cook or Manual, and adjust the pressure to High and the time to 12 minutes. After cooking, let the pressure release naturally for 10 minutes, then quickly release any remaining pressure.

4. Serve and enjoy.

Nutrition: Calories 620, Total Fat 2. 9g, Saturated Fat 0. 6g, Cholesterol 0mg, Sodium 37mg, Total Carbohydrate 117. 2g, Dietary Fiber 29. 3g, Total Sugars 16. 1g, Protein 37g

380. Creamy White Beans and Chickpeas Chili

Preparation Time: 05 minutes

Cooking Time: 35 minutes
Servings: 2
Ingredients:

- 1 teaspoon coconut oil
- 1 onion finely diced
- ½ teaspoon garlic powder
- 2 cups vegetable broth
- ½ cup chickpeas
- ½ cup navy beans
- ½ tablespoon chili powder
- ½ cumin powder
- ½ teaspoon kosher salt
- ¼ teaspoon black pepper
- 1/2 cup butter
- 3 tablespoon coconut flour
- 1 cup coconut milk warmed
- ¼ cup coconut cream
- ½ tablespoon lime juice

Directions:

1. Add coconut oil to the Instant Pot. Using the display panel select the Sauté function.
2. When oil gets hot, add onion to the pot and sauté until soft, 3-4 minutes. Add garlic powder and cook for 1-2 minutes more.
3. Add broth to the pot and deglaze by using a wooden spoon to scrape the brown bits from the bottom of the pot.
4. Add chickpeas, beans, chili and cumin powder, salt, and pepper, and stir to combine.
5. Turn the pot off by selecting Cancel, then secure the lid, making sure the vent is closed.
6. Using the display panel select the Manual or Pressure Cook function. Use the + /- keys and program the Instant Pot for 15 minutes.
7. When the time is up, let the pressure naturally release for 10 minutes, then quickly release the remaining pressure.
8. In a medium bowl, melt butter, then whisk in flour until well combined. Stir into the pot and simmer 3-5 minutes until thickened, returning to Sauté mode as needed.
9. Stir in coconut milk, coconut cream, and lime juice. Adjust seasonings.

Nutrition: Calories 1086, Total Fat 71. 3g, Saturated Fat 47. 6g, Cholesterol 122mg, Sodium 1764mg, Total Carbohydrate 86. 3g, Dietary Fiber 32. 3g, Total Sugars 14. 5g, Protein 32. 1g

381. Potato Chili

Preparation Time: 10 minutes
Cooking Time: 25 minutes
Servings: 2
Ingredients:

- 1/2 teaspoon olive oil
- 1/2 cup onion chopped
- 1/2 teaspoon garlic powder
- 1/2 teaspoon chili powder
- 1/2 teaspoon ground cumin
- 1 cup diced tomatoes
- 1/2 cup black beans rinsed and drained
- 1 medium red bell pepper seeded and diced
- 1 medium potato peeled and diced
- 1 teaspoon kosher salt
- 1/4 cup frozen corn kernels

Directions:

1. Select Sauté and add the olive oil to the Instant Pot. Add the onions and garlic powder. Sauté for 2 minutes, or until the garlic powder is fragrant and the onion is soft and translucent.
2. Add the chili powder and ground cumin, followed by the tomatoes, black beans, red bell pepper, potato, corn, and salt. Stir well.
3. Cover, lock the lid and flip the steam release handle to the Sealing position. Select Pressure Cook High and set the cooking time for 15 minutes. When the cooking time is complete, allow the pressure to release naturally for about 20 minutes.
4. Remove the lid and ladle the chili into serving bowls. Serve hot.

Nutrition: Calories 207, Total Fat 2. 1g, Saturated Fat 0. 3g, Cholesterol 0mg, Sodium 1207mg, Total Carbohydrate 41. 4g, Dietary Fiber 8. 8g, Total Sugars 7. 7g, Protein 8. 2g

382. Beans Baby Potato Curry

Preparation Time: 10 minutes
Cooking Time:30 minutes
Servings: 2
Ingredients:

- 1 small onion, chopped
- ½ teaspoon garlic, chopped finely
- 1 cup baby potatoes
- 1/2 tablespoon curry powder

- 2 cups of water
- 1/2 cup pinto beans
- 1/2 cup coconut milk
- 1/2 tablespoon maple syrup
- Salt & pepper to taste
- 1/2 teaspoon chili pepper flakes
- 1 tablespoon arrowroot powder

Directions:

1. Set your Instant Pot to Sauté. Once hot, add a few drops of water and cook the onions until translucent, then add the garlic and cook for one minute longer. Press the Keep Warm/Cancel button.
2. Add everything to the Instant Pot except the arrowroot powder.
3. Set the Instant Pot to 20 minutes on Manual High pressure and allow the pressure to release naturally after this time.
4. Press Keep Warm/Cancel, remove the lid, and press Sauté. Put the arrowroot into a small bowl or cup and mix into it a few tablespoons of water to make a thickness but pour slurry. Pour it into the Instant Pot stirring as you go.
5. Add salt and pepper to taste then cook for about 5 minutes until they are tender and the gravy has thickened.
6. Serve immediately.

Nutrition: Calories342, Total Fat 2. 3g, Saturated Fat 1g, Cholesterol 5mg, Sodium 58mg, Total Carbohydrate 67. 2g, Dietary Fiber 12. 1g, Total Sugars 10g, Protein 14. 2g

383.   Butter Tofu with Soy Bean and Chickpeas

Preparation Time: 10 minutes
Cooking Time: 30 minutes
Servings: 2

Ingredients:

- 2 large ripe tomatoes
- 1/2 teaspoon garlic powder
- 1/2 teaspoon ginger powder
- 1/2 tablespoon hot green chili
- 1 cup of water
- 1/4 teaspoon garam masala
- 1/8 teaspoon paprika
- 1/4 teaspoon salt

- 1/4 cup of soybeans
- 1/2 cup chickpeas
- 1/2 teaspoon maple syrup
- 1/2 cup coconut cream
- Cilantro for garnish

Directions:

1. Blend the tomatoes, garlic powder, ginger powder, hot green chili with water until smooth.
2. Add pureed tomato mixture to the Instant Pot. Add soybeans, chickpeas, spices, and salt. Close the lid and cook on Manual for 8 to 10 minutes. Quick-release after 10 minutes.
3. Start the Instant Pot on Sauté. Add the coconut cream, Garam masala, maple syrup, and mix in. Bring to a boil, taste, and adjust salt. Add more paprika and salt if needed.
4. Serve with cilantro garnishing

Nutrition: Calories 242, Total Fat 1. 3g, Saturated Fat 1. 5g, Cholesterol 5mg, Sodium 38mg, Total Carbohydrate 47. 2g, Dietary Fiber 10. 1g, Total Sugars 10g, Protein 14. 2g.

384.   Black Eyed Peas Curry with Jaggery

Preparation Time: 10 minutes
Cooking Time: 30 minutes
Servings: 2

Ingredients:

- 1/4 cup dried black-eyed peas, soaked in water for about 1-2 hours
- 2 cups of water
- 1 dried curry leaves
- 1/8 teaspoon mustard seeds
- 1/2 teaspoon garlic powder
- 1/2 small onion, finely chopped
- 2 tablespoons tomato paste
- 1/2 teaspoon ground cumin
- 1 teaspoon ground coriander
- 1/4 teaspoon ground turmeric
- 1 tablespoon jaggery
- 1 tablespoon fresh lemon juice
- Chili powder, to taste (optional
- 1 tablespoon avocado oil
- Salt to taste
- Fresh cilantro, finely chopped

Directions:

1. Select the Sauté button into the Instant Pot and add avocado oil.
2. Once the oil is hot, add the mustard seeds and curry leaves. Fry for a few seconds until fragrant.
3. Add the onions and garlic powder. Sauté until fragrant and the onions start to become translucent. Be sure not to burn either. If you see this happening add more oil or turn down the sauté heat.
4. Quickly add the tomato paste, ground cumin, and ground coriander. Combine and cook for a minute mixing frequently.
5. Drain the soaked black-eyed peas and add them into the Instant Pot.
6. Mix in the water, turmeric powder, chili powder, jaggery, fresh lemon juice, and salt.
7. Close the Instant Pot lid, select the Pressure Cook button to cook on High. Set the timer for about 13-15 minutes.
8. When the time is up, allow the pressure to release naturally.
9. Once the pressure has been released, remove the lid, and press the Sauté (normally Low) button again on the Instant Pot. The black-eyed peas should be fully cooked.
10. Simmer for a few more minutes until the curry becomes thick.
11. Add salt to taste. Also, feel free to adjust the amount of lemon juice and jaggery as needed.
12. Turn the Instant Pot off. Add freshly chopped cilantro and serve hot.

Nutrition: Calories79, Total Fat 0. 9g, Saturated Fat 0. 2g, Cholesterol 0mg, Sodium 75mg, Total Carbohydrate 18g, Dietary Fiber 4. 7g, Total Sugars 8. 2g, Protein 4g

385. Jackfruit with Beans Curry

Preparation Time: 10 minutes
Cooking Time: 20 minutes
Servings: 2
Ingredients:

- 1/2 tablespoon coconut oil
- 1/2 tablespoon curry powder
- 1/4 teaspoon paprika
- 1/2 teaspoon cumin seeds
- 1/4 teaspoon turmeric powder
- 1 sprig fresh rosemary
- 1/2 cup onion, finely chopped
- 1 teaspoon garlic powder
- 1 teaspoon ginger powder
- 1 celery, chopped
- 1 cup jackfruit, drained and rinsed
- 1/2 cup pinto beans
- 1/2 medium zucchini, diced
- 1/2 cup coconut milk
- 1 cups vegetable broth
- 1/4 cup parsley leaves, chopped
- Salt, to taste

Directions:

1. Plug your Instant Pot and press the Sauté mode button. Add coconut oil, once heated add dry spices, curry powder, paprika, cumin seeds, turmeric powder, rosemary, and cook for a minute stirring constantly.
2. Add onions, garlic powder, ginger powder, and celery, and cook for 2 minutes or until onions are soft. Add jackfruit, pinto beans, zucchini and stir to coat.
3. Add salt, coconut milk, and vegetable broth.
4. Close the Instant Pot lid and press Manual mode for 10 minutes. When finished, allow Instant Pot to natural release for 10 minutes. Carefully release the knob to release the remaining pressure. Remove lid, stir in parsley leaves, and check seasonings.

Nutrition: Calories320, Total Fat 5. 5g, Saturated Fat 3. 5g, Cholesterol 1mg, Sodium 582mg, Total Carbohydrate 50. 7g, Dietary Fiber 17. 6g, Total Sugars 7g, Protein 17. 5g

386. Black Bean Meatball Salad

Preparation Time: 10 minutes
Cooking Time: 25 minutes
Servings: 4
Ingredients:
For the Meatballs:

- 1/2 cup quinoa, cooked
- 1 cup cooked black beans
- 3 cloves of garlic, peeled
- 1 small red onion, peeled
- 1 teaspoon ground dried coriander
- 1 teaspoon ground dried cumin

- 1 teaspoon smoked paprika

For the Salad:

- 1 large sweet potato, peeled, diced
- 1 lemon, juiced
- 1 teaspoon minced garlic
- 1 cup coriander leaves
- 1/3 cup almonds
- 1/3 teaspoon ground black pepper
- ½ teaspoon salt
- 1 1/2 tablespoons olive oil

Directions:

1. Prepare the meatballs and for this, place beans and puree in a blender, pulse until pureed, and place this mixture in a medium bowl.
2. Add onion and garlic, process until chopped, add to the bean mixture, add all the spices, stir until combined, and shape the mixture into uniform balls.
3. Bake the balls on a greased baking sheet for 25 minutes at 350 degrees F until browned.
4. Meanwhile, spread sweet potatoes on a baking sheet lined with baking paper, drizzle with ½ tablespoon oil, toss until coated, and bake for 20 minutes with the meatballs.
5. Prepare the dressing, and for this, place the remaining ingredients for the salad in a food processor and pulse until smooth.
6. Place roasted sweet potatoes in a bowl, drizzle with the dressing, toss until coated, and then top with meatballs.
7. Serve straight away.

Nutrition: Calories: 140 Cal Fat: 8 g Carbs: 8 g Protein: 10 g Fiber: 4 g

387.   Kale Slaw

Preparation Time: 10-75 minutes
Cooking Time: 15 minutes
Servings: 4

Ingredients:

- 1 small bunch kale, chopped
- ½ small head cabbage, shredded
- ¼ onion, thinly sliced
- ¼ cup tender herbs (cilantro, basil, parsley, chives)
- ¼ cup olive oil
- 4 tablespoons lemon juice

- 2 garlic cloves, minced
- salt, pepper, and chili flakes

Directions:

1. Combine kale, cabbage, herbs, and onions in a large bowl.
2. Add olive oil, lemon juice, minced garlic, salt, pepper and mix well.
3. Add chili flakes, toss well before serving.

Nutrition: Calories: 140 Cal Fat: 0.9 g Carbs: 27.1 g Protein: 6.3 g Fiber: 6.2 g

388.   Sweet Potatoes

Preparation Time: 29 minutes
Cooking Time: 15-120 minutes
Servings: 4

Ingredients:

- 4 Sweet Potatoes, scrubbed and rinsed
- 1 1/2 Cups Water
- Optional Toppings:
- Scrambled Tofu, Avocado, Tomatoes
- Vegan Butter, Coconut Sugar, Cinnamon
- Arugula, Olive Oil, Lemon, Sea Salt

Directions:

1. Add water to the instant pot.
2. Place the steaming tray inside and put potatoes on top.
3. Cover with lid and seal.
4. Pressure cooks for 18 minutes in manual mode.
5. When done cooking, allow pressure to release on its own (about 15 minutes).
6. Remove the lid.
7. Serve immediately with desired toppings. Enjoy!

Nutrition: Calories: 140 Cal Fat: 0.9 g Carbs: 27.1 g Protein: 6.3 g Fiber: 6.2 g

389.   Baked Sweet Potatoes with Corn Salad

Preparation Time: 15-30 minutes
Cooking Time: 35 minutes
Servings: 4

Ingredients:

For the baked sweet potatoes:

- 3 tbsp olive oil
- 4 medium sweet potatoes, peeled and cut into ½-inch cubes
- 2 limes, juiced

- Salt and black pepper to taste
- ¼ tsp cayenne pepper
- 2 scallions, thinly sliced

For the corn salad:
- 1 (15 oz) can sweet corn kernels, drained
- ½ tbsp, plant butter, melted
- 1 large green chili, deseeded and minced
- 1 tsp cumin powder

Directions:

For the baked sweet potatoes:

1. Preheat the oven to 400 F and lightly grease a baking sheet with cooking spray.
2. In a medium bowl, add the sweet potatoes, lime juice, salt, black pepper, and cayenne pepper. Toss well and spread the mixture on the baking sheet. Bake in the oven until the potatoes soften, 20 to 25 minutes.
3. Remove from the oven, transfer to a serving plate, and garnish with the scallions.

For the corn salad:

1. In a medium bowl, mix the corn kernels, butter, green chili, and cumin powder. Serve the sweet potatoes with the corn salad.

Nutrition: Calories 372 Fats 20. 7g Carbs 41. 7g Protein 8. 9g

390. Cashew Siam Salad

Preparation Time: 10 minutes
Cooking Time: 3 minutes
Servings: 4

Ingredients:

Salad:
- 4 cups baby spinach, rinsed, drained
- ½ cup pickled red cabbage

Dressing:
- 1-inch piece ginger, finely chopped
- 1 tsp. chili garlic paste
- 1 tbsp. soy sauce
- ½ tbsp. rice vinegar
- 1 tbsp. sesame oil
- 3 tbsp. avocado oil

Toppings:
- ½ cup raw cashews, unsalted
- ¼ cup fresh cilantro, chopped

Directions:

1. Put the spinach and red cabbage in a large bowl. Toss to combine and set the salad aside.
2. Toast the cashews in a frying pan over medium-high heat, stirring occasionally until the cashews are golden brown. This should take about 3 minutes. Turn off the heat and set the frying pan aside.
3. Mix all the dressing ingredients in a medium-sized bowl and use a spoon to mix them into a smooth dressing.
4. Pour the dressing over the spinach salad and top with the toasted cashews.
5. Toss the salad to combine all ingredients and transfer the large bowl to the fridge. Allow the salad to chill for up to one hour – doing so will guarantee a better flavor. Alternatively, the salad can be served right away, topped with the optional cilantro. Enjoy!

Nutrition: Calories 236 Carbohydrates 6. 1 g Fats 21. 6 g Protein 4. 2 g

391. Chickpea Curry

Preparation Time: 10 minutes
Cooking Time: 30 minutes
Servings: 2

Ingredients:

- ½ cup dried chickpeas rinsed
- 2 cups of water
- 1 tablespoon vegetable oil
- ½ teaspoon cumin seeds
- 1 small onion finely diced
- ½ teaspoon ginger powder
- ½ teaspoon garlic powder
- ½ tablespoon coriander powder
- 1 teaspoon salt
- ¼ teaspoon turmeric powder
- 1 tomato cored and finely diced,
- ½ cup parsley fresh, chopped
- 1/4 teaspoon garam masala

Directions:

1. In a bowl, combine the chickpeas and 2 cups of warm water and let soak for at least 4 hours or up to overnight. Drain the chickpeas and set them aside.
2. Select the High Sauté setting on the Instant Pot and heat the vegetable oil. Add the cumin seeds directly to the hot oil at the bottom edges of the

Instant Pot and cook until they start to sizzle, about 1 minute. Add the chopped onions and cook, stirring occasionally, until translucent, about 5 minutes. Add the ginger powder and garlic powder and sauté until aromatic, about 1 minute. Add the coriander powder, salt, turmeric powder, and chickpeas; pour in the 2 cups water, and stir well.

3. Secure the lid and set the Pressure Release to Sealing. Press the Cancel button to reset the cooking program, then select the Pressure Cook or Manual setting and set the cooking time for 35 minutes at High Pressure.

4. Let the pressure release naturally; this will take 10 to 20 minutes. Open the pot and stir in the tomatoes and garam masala. Select the High Sauté setting and cook until the tomatoes soften about 5 minutes. Press the Cancel button to turn off the Instant Pot. Ladle into bowls, sprinkle with the parsley, and serve.

Nutrition: Calories 202, Total Fat 9. 2g, Saturated Fat 1. 4g, Cholesterol 0mg, Sodium 1186mg, Total Carbohydrate 27. 9g, Dietary Fiber 7. 8g, Total Sugars 7. 3g, Protein 8. 2g

392. Easy Lentil and Vegetable Curry

Preparation Time: 10 minutes
Cooking Time: 45 minutes
Servings: 2
Ingredients:

- 3 ½ cups water
- ½ tablespoon butter
- ¼ teaspoon cumin seeds
- ½ teaspoon coriander seeds
- ¼ teaspoon turmeric powder
- ¼ teaspoon paprika
- ½ teaspoon garam masala
- ½ teaspoon garlic powder
- ¼ teaspoon ginger powder
- ¼ cup onion, finely chopped
- 2 cups chopped veggies of your choice (red pepper, carrot, cabbage, broccoli, etc.)
- ¼ cup dried red lentils
- 1 1/2 cups vegetable stock
- ½ coconut milk

- ¼ cup green peas
- 1 teaspoon lime juice
- ¼ teaspoon of sea salt
- ¼ teaspoon ground pepper

Directions:

1. Select the High Sauté setting on the Instant Pot and heat the butter. Add the cumin seeds directly to the melted butter at the bottom edges of the Instant Pot and cook until they start to sizzle, about 1 minute. Add the onion and cook, stirring occasionally, until translucent, about 5 minutes. Add the ginger powder and garlic powder and sauté until aromatic, about 1 minute. Add the coriander seeds, salt, paprika, turmeric powder, and chopped vegetables and red lentils; pour in the 1 1/2 cups water, and stir well.

2. Secure the lid and set the Pressure Release to Sealing. Press the Cancel button to reset the cooking program, then select the Pressure Cook or Manual setting and set the cooking time for 35 minutes at High Pressure.

3. Let the pressure release naturally; this will take 10 to 20 minutes. Open the Instant Pot and stir in the green peas and garam masala milk. Select the High Sauté setting and cook for 2 minutes. Press the Cancel button to turn off the Instant Pot. Ladle into bowls, sprinkle with the cilantro and lime juice, serve.

Nutrition: Calories 200, Total Fat 4. 2g, Saturated Fat 2. 4g, Cholesterol 8mg, Sodium 331mg, Total Carbohydrate 31. 3g, Dietary Fiber 11. 9g, Total Sugars 5. 8g, Protein 9. 8g

393. Herbed Lentil Chili

Preparation Time: 10 minutes
Cooking Time: 20 minutes
Servings: 2
Ingredients:

- 1 tablespoon coconut oil
- 1 small onion chopped
- ½ teaspoon garlic powder
- 1 zucchini chopped
- 1 leek chopped
- ½ tablespoon paprika
- ¼ teaspoon cumin powder
- ¼ teaspoon coriander powder
- ½ teaspoon dried basil

- ¼ teaspoon dry mustard
- 1 cup crushed tomatoes
- ½ cup dry lentils
- 1 1/2 cups low sodium vegetable broth
- Salt to taste
- ¼ teaspoon pepper

Directions:

1. Select the "Sauté" setting on Instant Pot. Add coconut oil and let heat up. Add onions, garlic powder, zucchinis, and leeks. Sauté until onions are softened and lightly browned, about 4 minutes. Add paprika, cumin powder, coriander powder, basil, mustard and stir well for a minute or two. Add tomatoes, lentils, broth, salt to taste, and pepper.
2. Select "Cancel", then close the lid. Turn steam release handle to "Sealing" position. Select "Bean/Chili" and set the time for 14 minutes. Press "Cancel" and let Instant Pot naturally release pressure until float valve drops down and lid unlocks; alternatively, press "Cancel" and let Instant Pot naturally release for 10 minutes; then turn steam release valve to "Venting" until float valve drops down and lid unlocks.

Nutrition: Calories 296, Calories from Fat 27, Fat 3g, Sodium 596mg, Potassium 935mg, Carbohydrates 49g, Fiber 22g, Sugar 6g, Protein 18g

394.   Garbanzo Beans with Kale

Preparation Time: 05 minutes
Cooking Time: 30 minutes
Servings: 2

Ingredients:

- ½ cup dried garbanzo beans rinsed
- 2 cups of water
- ½ cup tomato paste
- ¼ teaspoon garlic powder
- ¼ teaspoon ginger powder
- ½ tablespoon curry powder
- ¼ teaspoon cinnamon powder
- ¼ teaspoon salt
- ¼ teaspoon ground black pepper
- 2 cups fresh kale

Directions:

1. Add garbanzo beans and water to the Instant Pot. Lock lid.

2. Press the beans button and cook for the default time of 30 minutes. When the timer beeps, let the pressure release naturally for 10 minutes. Quick-release any additional pressure until the float valve drops and then unlock the lid. Drain any extra liquid.
3. Stir in remaining ingredients. Switch to Low Pressure and simmer for 4 minutes to heat through and wilt kale.
4. Transfer mixture to a serving dish and serve warm.

Nutrition: Calories 129, Total Fat 1. 8g, Saturated Fat 0. 1g, Cholesterol 0mg, Sodium 395mg, Total Carbohydrate 26. 6g, Dietary Fiber 6. 1g, Total Sugars 8. 1g, Protein 7. 1g

395.   Three-Lentil Curry

Preparation Time: 10 minutes
Cooking Time: 25 minutes
Servings: 2

Ingredients:

- ½ tablespoon coconut oil
- 1 teaspoon garlic powder
- 1 teaspoon ginger powder
- ½ tablespoon garam masala
- 1 teaspoon cumin powder
- ¼ teaspoon turmeric powder
- ¼ teaspoon table salt
- ¼ teaspoon paprika
- 1 cinnamon stick 4-inch stick
- 2 green cardamom pods
- 1 bay leaf
- ½ cup red tomatoes chopped
- ¼ cup red lentils
- ¼ cup brown lentils
- ¼ cup green lentils
- ¼ cup
- 4 cups of water
- 1/2 cup coconut cream

Directions:

1. Press Sauté, set the time for 5 minutes.
2. Add coconut oil to the Instant Pot. Add the garlic powder, ginger powder, garam masala, cumin powder, turmeric powder, salt, paprika, cinnamon stick, cardamom pods, and bay leaves. Stir until fragrant, about 1 minute. Add the

tomatoes and cook, stirring often, until it just begins to break down, 1 to 2 minutes.

3. Turn off the Sauté function. Stir in the red lentils, brown lentils, and green lentils until coated in the spices. Stir in the water and lock the lid onto the Instant Pot.

4. Press Pressure Cook on Max Pressure for 16 minutes with the Keep Warm setting off.

5. Use the Quick-release method to bring the Instant Pot pressure back to normal. Unlatch the lid and open the Instant Pot. Remove and discard the cinnamon stick, cardamom pods, and bay leaves. Stir in the cream until uniform, then set the lid askew over the Instant Pot for 5 minutes to blend the flavors. Stir again before serving.

Nutrition: Calories 340, Total Fat 21. 1g, Saturated Fat 16. 3g, Cholesterol 0mg, Sodium 390mg, Total Carbohydrate 30. 8g, Dietary Fiber 10. 8g, Total Sugars 5. 7g, Protein 10. 4g

396. Baked Beans with Mustard

Preparation Time: 05 minutes
Cooking Time: 15 minutes
Servings: 2
Ingredients:

- 1/2 cup kidney beans rinsed and drained
- 1/2 cup pinto beans rinsed and drained
- 1/2 cup chickpea beans rinsed and drained
- 1 cup of water
- 1/2 cup tomato paste
- 1 teaspoon maple syrup
- 1/2 tablespoon ground mustard
- 1 teaspoon paprika

Directions:

1. Add the kidney beans, pinto beans, chickpeas beans, water, tomato paste, maple syrup, ground mustard, and paprika. Lock the lid into place and turn the valve to "Sealing." Select Manual or Pressure Cook and adjust the pressure to High.

2. Set the time for 8 minutes. When cooking ends, let the pressure release naturally for 15 minutes, then turn the valve to "Venting" to quickly release the remaining pressure. Unlock and remove the lid and stir well before serving.

Nutrition: Calories 268, Total Fat 2. 7g, Saturated Fat 0. 3g, Cholesterol 0mg, Sodium 555mg, Total Carbohydrate 50. 6g, Dietary Fiber 13g, Total Sugars 11. 8g, Protein 14g

397. Garden Salad Wraps

Preparation time: 15 minutes
Cooking time: 10 minutes
Servings: 4
Ingredients:

- 6 tbsps. extra-virgin olive oil
- 1 lb. extra-firm tofu, drained, patted dry, and cut into ½-inch strips
- 1 tbsp. soy sauce
- ¼ cup apple cider vinegar
- 1 tsp. yellow or spicy brown mustard
- ½ tsp. salt
- ¼ tsp. freshly ground black pepper
- 3 cups shredded romaine lettuce
- 3 ripe Roma tomatoes, finely chopped
- 1 large carrot, shredded
- 1 medium English cucumber, peeled and chopped
- 1/3 cup minced red onion
- ¼ cup sliced pitted green olives
- 4 (10-inch) whole-grain flour tortillas or lavash flatbread

Directions:

1. Warm-up 2 tablespoons of the oil in a large skillet over medium heat. Add the tofu and cook until golden brown. Sprinkle with soy sauce and set aside to cool.

2. In a small bowl, combine the vinegar, mustard, salt, and pepper with the remaining 4 tablespoons oil, stirring to blend well. Set aside.

3. Combine the lettuce, tomatoes, carrot, cucumber, onion, and olives in a large bowl. Put on the dressing then toss to coat.

4. To assemble wraps, place 1 tortilla on a work surface and spread with about one-quarter of the salad. Place a few strips of tofu on the tortilla and roll up tightly. Slice in half.

Nutrition: Calories: 85; Carbs: 17g; Fat: 0g; Protein: 46g

398. Black Sesame Wonton Chips

Preparation time: 5 minutes
Cooking time: 5 minutes
Servings: 24 chips
Ingredients:

- 12 vegan wonton wrappers
- Toasted sesame oil
- 1/3 cup black sesame seeds
- Salt to taste

Directions:

1 - Preheat the oven to 450°F. Oil a baking sheet then set aside. Cut the wonton wrappers in half crosswise, oil them with sesame oil, then arrange them in a single layer on your prepared baking sheet.

2 - Sprinkle wonton wrappers with sesame seeds and salt. Bake until crisp and golden brown. Cool completely before serving.

Nutrition: Calories: 180; Carbs: 31g; Fat: 1g; Protein: 10g.

399. Marinated Mushroom Wraps

Preparation time: 15 minutes
Cooking time: 0 minutes
Servings: 2

Ingredients:

- 3 tbsps. soy sauce
- 3 tbsps. fresh lemon juice
- 1½ tbsps. toasted sesame oil
- 2 portobello mushroom caps, cut into ¼-inch strips
- 1 ripe Hass avocado, pitted and peeled
- 2 (10-inch) whole-grain flour tortillas
- 2 cups fresh baby spinach leaves
- 1 medium red bell pepper, cut into ¼ inch strips
- 1 ripe tomato, chopped
- Salt and freshly ground black pepper

Directions:

1 - In a medium bowl, combine the soy sauce, 2 tablespoons of the lemon juice, and the oil. Add the portobello strips, toss to combine, and marinate for 1 hour or overnight.

2 - Drain the mushrooms and set them aside. Mash your avocado with the remaining 1 tablespoon of lemon juice.

3 - To assemble wraps, place 1 tortilla on a work surface and spread with some of the mashed avocado. Top with a layer of baby spinach leaves.

4 - In the lower third of each tortilla, arrange strips of the soaked mushrooms and some of the bell pepper strips.

5 - Sprinkle with the tomato and salt and black pepper to taste. Roll up tightly and cut in half diagonally. Repeat with the remaining ingredients and serve.

Nutrition: Calories: 112; Carbs: 5g; Fat: 7g; Protein: 1g.

400. Tamari Toasted Almonds

Preparation time: 2 minutes
Cooking time: 8 minutes
Servings: ½ cup

Ingredients:

- ½ cup raw almonds, or sunflower seeds
- 2 tbsps. tamari, or soy sauce
- 1 tsp. toasted sesame oil

Directions:

1 - Heat a dry skillet to medium-high heat, then add the almonds, stirring frequently to keep them from burning.

2 - Once the almonds are toasted—7-8 minutes for almonds, or 34 minutes for sunflower seeds—pour the tamari and sesame oil into the hot skillet and stir to coat.

3 - You can turn off the heat, and as the almonds cool the tamari mixture will stick and dry onto the nuts.

Nutrition: Calories: 89; Fat: 8g; Carbs: 3g; Protein: 4g.

401. Avocado and Tempeh Bacon Wraps

Preparation time: 10 minutes
Cooking time: 8 minutes
Servings: 4

Ingredients:

- 2 tbsps. extra-virgin olive oil
- 8 oz. tempeh bacon, homemade or store-bought
- 4 (10-inch) soft flour tortillas or lavash flatbread
- ¼ cup vegan mayonnaise, homemade or store-bought
- 4 large lettuce leaves
- 2 ripe Hass avocados, pitted, peeled, and cut into ¼-inch slices
- 1 large ripe tomato, cut into ¼-inch slices

Directions:

1 - Heat-up the oil in a large skillet over medium heat. Add the tempeh bacon and cook until browned on both sides, about 8 minutes. Remove from the heat and set aside.

2 - Place 1 tortilla on a work surface. Spread with some of the mayonnaise and one-fourth of the lettuce and tomatoes.

3 - Thinly slice the avocado and place the slices on top of the tomato. Add the reserved tempeh bacon and roll up tightly. Repeat with remaining ingredients and serve.

Nutrition: Calories: 315; Carbs: 22g; Fat: 20g; Protein: 14g.

402. Kale Chips

Preparation time: 5 minutes
Cooking time: 25 minutes
Servings: 2
Ingredients:
- 1 large bunch kale
- 1 tbsp. extra-virgin olive oil
- ½ tsp. chipotle powder
- ½ tsp. smoked paprika
- ¼ tsp. salt

Directions:
1 - Preheat the oven to 275°F. Prepare a large baking sheet lined using parchment paper. In a large bowl, stem the kale and tear it into bite-size pieces. Add the olive oil, chipotle powder, smoked paprika, and salt.

2 - Toss the kale with tongs or your hands, coating each piece well. Spread the kale over the parchment paper in a single layer.

3 - Bake within 25 minutes, turning halfway through, until crisp. Cool for 10 to 15 minutes before dividing and storing in 2 airtight containers.

Nutrition: Calories: 100; Carbs: 9g; Fat: 7g; Protein: 4g.

403. Tempeh-Pimiento Cheese Ball

Preparation time: 5 minutes
Cooking time: 30 minutes
Servings: 8
Ingredients:
- 8 oz. tempeh, cut into ½ -inch pieces
- 1 (2 oz.) jar chopped pimientos, drained
- ¼ cup nutritional yeast
- ¼ cup vegan mayonnaise, homemade or store-bought
- 2 tbsps. soy sauce
- ¾ cup chopped pecans

Directions:
1 - Cook the tempeh within 30 minutes in a medium saucepan of simmering water. Set aside to cool. In a food processor, combine the cooled tempeh, pimientos, nutritional yeast, mayo, and soy sauce. Process until smooth.

2 - Transfer the tempeh mixture to a bowl and refrigerate until firm and chilled for at least 2 hours or overnight.

3 - Toast the pecans in a dry skillet over medium heat until lightly toasted. Set aside to cool.

4 - Shape the tempeh batter into a ball, then roll it in the pecans, pressing the nuts lightly into the tempeh mixture so they stick. Refrigerate within 1 hour before serving.

Nutrition: Calories: 170; Carbs: 6g; Fat: 14g; Protein: 5g.

404. Peppers and Hummus

Preparation time: 15 minutes
Cooking time: 0 minutes
Servings: 4
Ingredients:
- One 15 oz. can chickpeas, drained and rinsed
- Juice of 1 lemon, or 1 tbsp. prepared lemon juice
- ¼ cup tahini
- 3 tbsps. extra-virgin olive oil
- ½ tsp. ground cumin
- 1 tbsp. water
- ¼ tsp. paprika
- 1 red bell pepper, sliced
- 1 green bell pepper, sliced
- 1 orange bell pepper, sliced

Directions:
1 - Combine chickpeas, lemon juice, tahini, 2 tablespoons of the olive oil, the cumin, and water in a food processor.

2 - Process on high speed until blended for about 30 seconds. Scoop the hummus into a bowl and drizzle with the remaining tablespoon of olive oil. Sprinkle with paprika and serve with sliced bell peppers.

Nutrition: Calories: 170; Carbs: 13g; Fat: 12g; Protein: 4g.

405. Roasted Chickpeas

Preparation time: 5 minutes
Cooking time: 25 minutes
Servings: 1 cup
Ingredients:
- 1 (14 oz.) can chickpeas, rinsed & drained; 1½ cups cooked

- 2 tbsps. tamari, or soy sauce
- 1 tbsp. nutritional yeast
- 1 tsp. smoked paprika, or regular paprika
- 1 tsp. onion powder
- ½ tsp. garlic powder

Directions:

1 - Preheat the oven to 400°F. Toss the chickpeas with all the other fixings, and spread them out on a baking sheet.

2 - Bake for 20-25 minutes, tossing halfway through. Bake these at a lower temperature until fully dried and crispy if you want to keep them longer.

3 - You can easily double the batch, and if you dry them out, they will keep about a week in an airtight container.

Nutrition: Calories: 121; Fat: 2g; Carbs: 20g; Protein: 8g.

406. Seed Crackers

Preparation time: 5 minutes
Cooking time: 50 minutes
Servings: 20

Ingredients:

- ¾ cup pumpkin seeds (pepitas)
- ½ cup sunflower seeds
- ½ cup sesame seeds
- ¼ cup chia seeds
- 1 tsp. minced garlic (about 1 clove)
- 1 tsp. tamari or soy sauce
- 1 tsp. vegan Worcestershire sauce
- ½ tsp. ground cayenne pepper
- ½ tsp. dried oregano
- ½ cup water

Directions:

1 - Preheat the oven to 325°F. Prepare a rimmed baking sheet lined using parchment paper.

2 - In a large bowl, combine the pumpkin seeds, sunflower seeds, sesame seeds, chia seeds, garlic, tamari, Worcestershire sauce, cayenne, oregano, and water.

3 - Transfer to the prepared baking sheet and spread it out to all sides. Bake for 25 minutes. Remove the pan, then flip the seed "dough" over so the wet side is up.

4 - Bake for another 20-25 minutes until the sides are browned. Cool completely before breaking up into 20 pieces. Divide evenly among 4 glass jars and close tightly with lids.

Nutrition: Calories: 339; Fat: 29g; Protein: 14g; Carbs: 17g.

407. Tomato and Basil Bruschetta

Preparation time: 10 minutes
Cooking time: 6 minutes
Servings: 12

Ingredients:

- 3 tomatoes, chopped
- ¼ cup chopped fresh basil
- 1 tbsp. extra-virgin olive oil
- Pinch of sea salt
- 1 baguette, cut into 12 slices
- 1 garlic clove, sliced in half

Directions:

1 - Combine the tomatoes, basil, olive oil, and salt in a small bowl, and stir to mix. Set aside. Preheat the oven to 425°F.

2 - Put your baguette slices in a single layer on your baking sheet and toast in the oven until brown for about 6 minutes.

3 - Flip the bread slices over once during cooking. Remove from the oven and rub the bread on both sides with the sliced clove of garlic. Top with the tomato-basil mixture and serve immediately.

Nutrition: Calories: 102; Carbs: 17g; Fat: 3g; Protein: 0g.

408. Refried Bean and Salsa Quesadillas

Preparation time: 5 minutes
Cooking time: 6 minutes
Servings: 4

Ingredients:

- 1 tbsp. canola oil, + more for frying
- 1½ cups cooked or 1 (15.5 oz.) can pinto beans, drained and mashed
- 1 tsp. chili powder
- 4 (10-inch) whole-wheat flour tortillas
- 1 cup tomato salsa, homemade or store-bought
- ½ cup minced red onion (optional)

Directions:

1 - In a medium saucepan, heat the oil over medium heat. Add the mashed beans and chili powder and cook, stirring, until hot, about 5 minutes. Set aside.

2 - To assemble, place 1 tortilla on a work surface and spoon about ¼cup of the beans across the bottom half. Top the beans with the salsa and onion, if using. Fold the top half of the tortilla over the filling and press slightly.

3 - In a large skillet heat a thin layer of oil over medium heat. Place folded quesadillas, 1 or 2 at a time, into the hot skillet and heat until hot, turning once, about 1 minute per side. Cut quesadillas into 3 or 4 wedges and arrange on plates. Serve immediately.
Nutrition: Calories: 487; Carbs: 65g; Fat: 18g; Protein: 20g.

409. Jicama and Guacamole

Preparation time: 15 minutes
Cooking time: 0 minutes
Servings: 4
Ingredients:
- Juice of 1 lime, or 1 tbsp. prepared lime juice
- 2 hass avocados, peeled, pits removed, and cut into cubes
- ½ tsp. sea salt
- ½ red onion, minced
- 1 garlic clove, minced
- ¼ cup chopped cilantro (optional)
- 1 jicama bulb, peeled and cut into matchsticks

Directions:
1 - In a medium bowl, squeeze the lime juice over the top of the avocado and sprinkle with salt. Lightly mash the avocado with a fork. Stir in the onion, garlic, and cilantro, if using.
2 - Serve with slices of jicama to dip in guacamole. To store, place plastic wrap over the bowl of guacamole and refrigerate. The guacamole will keep for about 2 days.
Nutrition: Calories: 145; Carbs: 0g; Fat: 10g; Protein: 9g.

410. Quick & Easy Cilantro Lime Rice

Preparation Time: 10 minutes
Cooking Time: 15 minutes
Servings: 4
Ingredients:
- 1 cup long-grain brown rice
- ½ teaspoon kosher salt
- 1 tablespoon coconut oil
- 2 tablespoons lime juice
- ½ teaspoon garlic powder
- ¼ cup finely chopped cilantro
- 1 teaspoon lime zest

Directions:

1 - Add 2 cups of water to a saucepan and add your rice.
2 - Bring the water to a boil, cover and allow it to simmer until the water has completely vanished.
3 - Mix lime juice, zest and cilantro in a small bowl.
4 - Remove the cover from the rice and add salt and garlic powder.
5 - Put the cover back and let it steam for 10 minutes.
6 - Uncover and mix in the coconut oil and the cilantro mix from the small bowl.
7 - Serve it immediately with any meal.
Nutrition: Calories: 271 Fat: 0.4g Saturated Fat: 0.1g Trans Fat: 0g Cholesterol: 0mg Sodium: 787mg Potassium: 82mg Carbohydrates: 60g Fiber: 0.3g Sugars: 0.3g Protein: 5g

411. Simple Homemade Marinara Sauce

Preparation Time: 10 minutes
Cooking Time: 20 minutes
Servings: 4
Ingredients:
- 1 yellow chopped onion
- 1 tablespoon extra-virgin olive oil
- 3 minced garlic cloves
- 1 teaspoon dried basil
- 1 teaspoon dried oregano
- ½ teaspoon ground black pepper
- Sea salt as needed
- 28oz. whole San Marzano tomatoes

Directions:
1 - Heat olive oil in a saucepan over a medium flame.
2 - Sauté onion and garlic until translucent.
3 - Stir in the juicy tomatoes, oregano, basil, salt and mix well.
4 - Mash up the tomatoes with a potato masher in the saucepan.
5 - Continue cooking the sauce until it simmers.
6 - Then, turn the flame to a simmer for 20 minutes and cover. Stir frequently!
7 - Serve the marinara chunky or puree it with a hand blender for a smoother consistency.
Nutrition: Calories: 55 Fat: 4g Carbohydrates: 4g Fiber: 2g Sugar: 1g Protein: 1g

412. A Classic Hummus Recipe

Preparation Time: 17 minutes

Cooking Time: 1 hour
Servings: 4
Ingredients:
- 1 cup dry chickpeas
- 2 teaspoons baking soda
- 1 teaspoon fine sea salt
- 1 teaspoon ground cumin
- 1 cup tahini
- ½ cup lemon juice
- 2 garlic cloves
- 4-6 tablespoons ice-cold water
- 1 tablespoon extra-virgin olive oil

Directions:
1 - Soak chickpeas in a large bowl with 1 teaspoon of baking soda and plenty of water as they will expand in size.
2 - Keep them soaked for 12 hours or overnight at room temperature.
3 - Drain the water and rinse under cold water.
4 - Cook the chickpeas in a medium pan with another 1 teaspoon baking powder added with enough water.
5 - Let it boil over high heat and remove any film that covers the surface.
6 - Lower the flame to low-medium, sprinkle some salt, and allow it to simmer half covered, until fully cooked and it starts to crumble.
7 - Chickpeas can easily take 1-2 hours to cook. You only need to keep them filled with water. Meanwhile, start preparing the tahini sauce.
8 - Combine garlic, lemon juice, cumin and salt in a fast blender and blend until smooth.
9 - After a rest of 10 minutes, add tahini and give it a blend until you reach a creamy consistency.
10 - Gradually add water, 2 tablespoons at a time to thin out the sauce.
11 - It will turn lighter and creamier.
12 - Drain the chickpeas and add to the sauce and blend until smooth.
13 - Do not forget to scrape the sides.
14 - As the blender runs, drizzle in olive oil to create a lightweight texture.
15 - Place the hummus into a wide bowl and use the back of the spoon to flatten it.
16 - Serve it with crackers.
Nutrition: Calories: 292 Fat: 19g Carbohydrates: 23g Fiber: 7g Sugar: 2g Protein: 10g

413. Vegan Cheesy Queso Dip

Preparation Time: 5 minutes
Cooking Time: 20 minutes
Servings: 3
Ingredients:
- 1 cup raw cashews
- 1 cup cubed butternut squash
- 1 cup unsweetened plant-based milk
- 1 tablespoon nutritional yeast
- 1 seeded & quartered orange bell pepper
- 2 cups &1 teaspoon waters
- ½ teaspoon salt
- ¼ teaspoon smoked paprika
- 1 teaspoon tapioca flour
- ½ teaspoon onion powder
- ½ teaspoon garlic powder

Directions:
1 - Combine squash, cashews, bell pepper and 2 cups of water in a medium pan.
2 - Bring to a boil and reduce the heat to medium.
3 - Cook until the squash and cashews turn soft.
4 - Once done, drain and add to a blender.
5 - Put in nutritional yeast, plant-based milk, onion powder, smoked paprika, and garlic powder.
6 - Blend until creamy and smooth.
7 - Return the squash mixture back to the saucepan and slowly allow it to boil over medium heat.
8 - Mix often and cook for 3 minutes.
9 - In a separate bowl, combine tapioca flour and 1 teaspoon of water to create a slurry.
10 - Transfer the slurry to the squash sauce and cook, while stirring steadily, until the sauce turns thick and creamy.
Nutrition: Calories: 85 Fat: 6g Carbohydrates: 7g Protein: 3g Fiber: 1g Sodium: 109mg

414. Lemonish Steamed Green Beans

Preparation Time: 5 minutes
Cooking Time: 5 minutes
Servings: 4
Ingredients:
- 1oz. fresh trimmed green beans
- 1 tablespoon fresh lemon juice & zest
- 1 tablespoon extra-virgin olive oil
- ½ teaspoon kosher salt

- Fresh ground black pepper
- 1 1/3 cups water

Directions:
1 - Add 1 ½ cups of water into a pot.
2 - Once it starts boiling, put in green beans.
3 - Cover and give steam for 4-5 minutes or until fork tender.
4 - Drain the water and add the beans to a mixture of olive oil, lemon juice, zest, salt and a generous sprinkling of black pepper.
5 - Serve along with your favorite dishes.
Nutrition: Calories: 67 Fat 3.8g Saturated Fat 0.6g Carbohydrates 8.5g Fiber 3.2g Sugars 3.8g

415. Marinated Mushrooms

Preparation time: 10 minutes
Cooking time: 7 minutes
Servings: 6
Ingredients:
- 12 oz. small button mushrooms
- 1 tsp. minced garlic
- ¼ tsp. dried thyme
- ½ tsp. sea salt
- ½ tsp. dried basil
- ½ tsp. red pepper flakes
- ¼ tsp. dried oregano
- ½ tsp. maple syrup
- ¼ cup apple cider vinegar
- ¼ cup and 1 tsp. olive oil
- 2 tbsps. chopped parsley

Directions:
1 - Take a skillet pan, place it over medium-high heat, add 1 teaspoon oil and when hot, add mushrooms and cook for 5 minutes until golden brown.
2 - Meanwhile, prepare the marinade and for this, place the remaining ingredients in a bowl and whisk until combined.
3 - When mushrooms have cooked, transfer them into the bowl of marinade and toss until well coated. Serve straight away
Nutrition: Calories: 103; Fat: 9g; Carbs: 2g; Protein: 1g.

416. Hummus Quesadillas

Preparation time: 5 minutes
Cooking time: 15 minutes
Servings: 1
Ingredients:
- 1 tortilla, whole wheat
- ¼ cup diced roasted red peppers
- 1 cup baby spinach
- 1/3 tsp. minced garlic
- ¼ tsp. salt
- ¼ tsp. ground black pepper
- ¼ tsp. olive oil
- ¼ cup hummus

Directions:
1 - Put your large pan on medium heat, add oil and when hot, add red peppers and garlic, season with salt and black pepper, and cook for 3 minutes until sauté.
2 - Then stir in spinach, cook for 1 minute, remove the pan from heat and transfer the mixture to a bowl.
3 - Prepare quesadilla and for this, spread hummus on one-half of the tortilla, then spread spinach mixture on it, cover the filling with the other half of the tortilla and cook in a pan for 3 minutes per side until browned. When done, cut the quesadilla into wedges and serve.
Nutrition: Calories: 187; Fat: 9g; Carbs: 16.3g; Protein: 10.4g.

417. Vegan Fat Bombs

Preparation time: 15 minutes
Cooking time: 0 minutes
Servings: 8
Ingredients:
- 8-oz cream cheese, softened to room temperature
- 1 tsp. kosher salt
- 1 cup keto-friendly dark chocolate chips
- ½ cup keto-friendly peanut butter
- ¼ cup coconut oil, + 2 tbsps.

Directions:
1 - With parchment paper, line a baking sheet. Mix well salt, coconut oil, peanut butter, and cream cheese in a bowl until combined thoroughly.
2 - Place in the freezer for 15 minutes to firm up. Then with a spoon, roll into golf ball-sized balls. In a microwave-safe cup, melt chocolate in 30-second intervals until melted fully.
3 - With a fork, drizzle melted chocolate all over each ball. Store in a tightly lidded container in the fridge and enjoy as a snack.
Nutrition: Calories: 313; Protein: 7.2g; Carbs: 12.4g; Fat: 27.2g.

418. Fudgy Choco-Peanut Butter

Preparation time: 15 minutes
Cooking time: 0 minutes
Servings: 32

Ingredients:

- 4 oz. cream cheese (softened)
- 2 tbsps. unsweetened cocoa powder
- ½ cup butter
- ½ cup natural peanut butter
- ½ tsp. vanilla extract
- ¼ cup powdered erythritol

Directions:

1 - In a microwave-safe bowl, mix peanut butter and butter. Microwave for 10-second intervals until melted. While mixing every after sticking in the microwave.

2 - Mix in vanilla extract, cocoa powder, erythritol, and cream cheese. Thoroughly mix. Line an 8x8-inch baking pan with foil and evenly spread the mixture.

3 - Place in the fridge to set and slice into 32 equal squares. Store in a tightly lidded container in the fridge and enjoy as a snack.

Nutrition: Calories: 65; Protein: 1.5g; Carbs: 1.0g; Fat: 6.0g.

419. Vegan Fudgy Granola Bar

Preparation time: 15 minutes
Cooking time: 25 minutes
Servings: 16

Ingredients:

- 1 pinch salt
- 1 ½ cups sliced almonds
- ½ cup flaked coconut (unsweetened)
- ½ cup pecans
- ½ cup sunflower seeds
- ½ cup dried, unsweetened cranberries (chopped)
- ½ cup butter
- ½ cup powdered erythritol
- ½ tsp. vanilla extract

Directions:

1 - With parchment paper line a square baking dish and preheat the oven to 300°F. In a food processor, pulse sunflower seeds, pecans, coconut, and almonds until crumb-like.

2 - In a bowl, add a pinch of salt and cranberries. Stir in crumb mixture and mix well. In a microwave-safe mug, melt butter in 20-second intervals. Whisk in

vanilla extract and erythritol. Pour over granola crumbs and mix well.

3 - Press mixture as compact as you can on the prepared dish. Pop in the oven and bake for 25 minutes. Let it cool and cut into 16 equal squares.

Nutrition: Calories: 180; Protein: 4.0g; Carbs: 5.0g; Fat: 17.0g.

420. Cinnamon Muffins

Preparation time: 15 minutes
Cooking time: 15 minutes
Servings: 12

Ingredients:

- 1 tbsp. cinnamon
- 1 tsp. baking powder
- ½ cup almond flour
- ½ cup coconut oil
- ½ cup almond butter
- ½ cup pumpkin puree
- 2 scoops vanilla protein powder

Glaze Ingredients:

- 1 tbsp. granulated sweetener of choice
- 2 tsp. lemon juice
- ¼ cup coconut butter
- ¼ cup coconut milk of choice

Directions:

1 - Line 12 muffin tins with muffin liners and preheat oven to 350°F. Whisk well cinnamon, baking powder, flour, and protein powder in a medium bowl.

2 - Whisk in coconut oil, almond butter, and pumpkin puree. Mix well. Evenly divide into prepared muffin tins.

3 - Bake in the oven for 13 minutes or until cooked through. Move it to a wire rack and let it cool. Meanwhile, mix all glaze ingredients in a small bowl and drizzle over the cooled muffin.

Nutrition: Calories: 112; Protein: 5.0g; Carbs: 3.0g; Fat: 9.0g.

421. Vegan Avocado & Spinach Dip

Preparation time: 15 minutes
Cooking time: 0 minutes
Servings: 12

Ingredients:

- 1 garlic clove crushed
- 1 tbsp. lime juice
- ½ cup fresh spinach leaves in boiling water within 2 minutes, squeezed, drained

- ½ tsp. sea salt
- ¼ cup fresh coriander chopped
- 2 large ripe avocados about 2 cups of mashed avocado
- 3 tbsps. Extra Virgin Avocado Oil
- ¾ cup dairy-free coconut yogurt

Directions:

1 - With a paper towel, pat dry blanched spinach leaves. In a blender or food processor, puree pepper, salt, avocado oil, lime juice, coconut yogurt, coriander, crushed garlic, and ripe avocado.

2 - Transfer to a bowl and whisk in spinach leaves. Serve and enjoy.

Nutrition: Calories: 91; Protein: 1.1g; Carbs: 3.1g; Fat: 8.8g.

422. Carrot Cake Balls

Preparation time: 15 minutes
Cooking time: 0 minutes
Servings: 15

Ingredients:

- ½ cup coconut flour
- ½ cup + 1 tbsp. water
- 2 tbsps. unsweetened applesauce
- ½ tsp. vanilla extract
- 1 tsp. cinnamon
- 4 tbsps. Lakanto Classic Monkfruit Sweetener
- 1 medium carrot, finely chopped or shredded
- 4 tbsps. reduced-fat shredded coconut

Directions:

1 - In a mixing bowl, whisk well vanilla extract, applesauce, water, and coconut flour. Stir in shredded carrots, Lakanto, and cinnamon. Mix well.

2 - Place dough in the fridge for 15 minutes. Place shredded coconut in a bowl. Evenly divide the dough into 15 equal parts and roll into balls.

3 - Roll balls in a bowl of shredded coconut. Store in lidded containers and enjoy as a snack.

Nutrition: Calories: 24; Protein: 1.0g; Carbs: 3.0g; Fat: 1.0g.

423. Nori Snack Rolls

Preparation time: 5 minutes
Cooking time: 10 minutes
Servings: 4

Ingredients:

- 2 tbsps. almond, cashew, peanut, or other nut butter
- 2 tbsps. tamari, or soy sauce
- 4 standard nori sheets
- 1 mushroom, sliced
- 1 tbsp. pickled ginger
- ½ cup grated carrots

Directions:

1 - Preheat the oven to 350°F. Mix the nut butter and tamari until smooth and very thick. Layout your nori sheet, rough side up, the long way.

2 - Spread a thin line of the tamari mixture on the far end of the nori sheet, from side to side. Lay the mushroom slices, ginger, and carrots in a line at the other end (the end closest to you).

3 - Fold the vegetables inside the nori, rolling toward the tahini mixture, which will seal the roll. Repeat to make 4 rolls.

4 - Put on a baking sheet and bake within 8-10 minutes, or until the rolls are slightly browned and crispy at the ends. Let the rolls cool for a few minutes, then slice each roll into 3 smaller pieces.

Nutrition: Calories: 79; Fat: 5g; Carbs: 6g; Protein: 4g.

424. Risotto Bites

Preparation time: 15 minutes
Cooking time: 20 minutes
Servings: 12

Ingredients:

- ½ cup panko bread crumbs
- 1 tsp. paprika
- 1 tsp. chipotle powder or ground cayenne pepper
- 1½ cups cold Green Pea Risotto
- Nonstick cooking spray

Directions:

1 - Preheat the oven to 425°F. Line a baking sheet with parchment paper. On a large plate, combine the panko, paprika, and chipotle powder. Set aside.

2 - Roll 2 tablespoons of the risotto into a ball. Gently roll in the bread crumbs, and place on the prepared baking sheet. Repeat to make a total of 12 balls.

3 - Spritz the tops of the risotto bites with nonstick cooking spray and bake for 15-20 minutes until they begin to brown.

4 - Cool completely before storing in a large airtight container in a single layer (add a piece of parchment paper for a second layer), or in a plastic freezer bag.
Nutrition: Calories: 100; Fat: 2g; Protein: 6g; Carbs: 17g.

425. Garden Patch Sandwiches on Multigrain Bread

Preparation time: 15 minutes
Cooking time: 0 minutes
Servings: 4
Ingredients:
- 1 lb. extra-firm tofu, drained and patted dry
- 1 medium red bell pepper, finely chopped
- 1 celery rib, finely chopped
- 3 green onions, minced
- ¼ cup shelled sunflower seeds
- ½ cup vegan mayonnaise, homemade or store-bought
- ½ tsp. salt
- ½ tsp. celery salt
- ¼ tsp. freshly ground black pepper
- 8 slices whole-grain bread
- 4 (¼-inch) slices ripe tomato
- 4 lettuce leaves

Directions:
1 - Crumble your tofu then place it in a large bowl. Add the bell pepper, celery, green onions, and sunflower seeds. Stir in the mayonnaise, salt, celery salt, and pepper and mix until well combined.
2 - Toast the bread, if desired. Spread the mixture evenly onto 4 slices of the bread. Put on top the tomato slice, lettuce leaf, and the remaining bread. Slice the sandwiches diagonally in half then serve.
Nutrition: Calories: 130; Carbs: 17g; Fat: 7g; Protein: 2g.

426. Steamed Broccoli

Preparation Time: 5 minutes
Cooking Time: 5 minutes
Servings: 4
Ingredients:
- 2 large heads broccoli
- ¼ cup thinly sliced green onions
- 2 tablespoons extra-virgin olive oil
- ½ teaspoon kosher salt
- Freshly ground black pepper as needed

- 1 ½ cup water
Directions:
1 - Cut broccoli into florets.
2 - Add 1 ½ cup water into a saucepan.
3 - Once it starts boiling, put in the florets.
4 - Cover and give steam for 4-5 minutes or until fork tender.
5 - Drain the water and add the broccoli to a mixture of olive oil, salt, onion and a generous sprinkling of ground black pepper.
6 - Serve along with your favorite dishes.
7 - Carefully remove the broccoli to a bowl. Toss with the olive oil, kosher salt, and drained red onions.
8 - Top with freshly ground black pepper.
Nutrition: Calories: 147 Total Fat: 9.6g Saturated Fat: 2.5g Carbohydrate: 12.6g Fiber: 4.6g Sugar: 3.7g Proteins 6.2g

427. Best Sauteed Kale

Preparation Time: 5 minutes
Cooking Time: 3 minutes
Servings: 4
Ingredients:
- 2 bunches Tuscan kale
- 2 garlic cloves
- 2 tablespoons extra-virgin olive oil
- ¼ teaspoon kosher salt
- Fresh ground pepper
- Lemon wedges

Directions:
1 - Wash and dry the kale leaves.
2 - De-stem and roughly chop.
3 - Peel and mince the garlic cloves.
4 - Pour olive oil to a large skillet over medium-high heat.
5 - Once hot, add minced garlic and kale, cook for 3 minutes.
6 - Stir often until droopy and turn bright green in color.
7 - Take off from heat and sprinkle kosher salt and fresh ground pepper.
8 - Discard the garlic cloves and serve with your favorite dishes and lemon wedges

Nutrition: Calories: 118 Fat: 8.1g Saturated Fat: 1.1g Carbohydrates: 10.4g Fiber: 4.1g Sugars: 2.6g

Chapter 23.　　Smoothies

428.　Chocolate and Peanut Butter Smoothie

Preparation Time: 5 minutes
Cooking Time: 0 minutes
Servings: 4

Ingredients:
- 1 tablespoon unsweetened cocoa powder
- 1 tablespoon peanut butter
- 1 banana
- 1 teaspoon maca powder
- ½ cup unsweetened soy milk
- ¼ cup rolled oats
- 1 tablespoon flaxseeds
- 1 tablespoon maple syrup
- 1 cup water

Directions:
1 - Add all the ingredients to a blender, then process until the mixture is smooth and creamy. Add water or soy milk if necessary.
2 - Serve immediately.

Nutrition: Calories: 474; Fat: 16 g; Carbs: 27 g; Fiber: 18 g; Proteins: 13 g.

429.　Golden Milk

Preparation Time: 5 minutes
Cooking Time: 0 minutes
Servings: 4

Ingredients:
- ¼ teaspoon ground cinnamon
- ½ teaspoon ground turmeric
- ½ teaspoon grated fresh ginger
- 1 teaspoon maple syrup
- 1 cup unsweetened coconut milk
- Ground black pepper to taste
- 2 tablespoons water

Directions:
1 - Combine all the ingredients in a saucepan. Stir to mix well.
2 - Heat over medium heat for 5 minutes. Keep stirring during the heating.
3 - Allow to cool for 5 minutes, then pour the mixture into a blender.
4 - Pulse until creamy and smooth. Serve immediately.

Nutrition: Calories: 577; Fat: 57.3 g; Carbs: 19.7 g; Fiber: 6.1 g; Proteins: 5.7 g.

430.　Mango Agua Fresca

Preparation Time: 5 minutes
Cooking Time: 0 minutes
Servings: 2

Ingredients:
- 2 fresh mangoes, diced
- 1 ½ cups water
- 1 teaspoon fresh lime juice
- Maple syrup to taste
- 2 cups ice
- 2 slices fresh lime for garnish
- 2 fresh mint sprigs for garnish

Directions:
1 - Put the mangoes, lime juice, maple syrup and water into a blender.
1 - Process until creamy and smooth.
2 - Divide the beverage into two glasses, then garnish each glass with ice, lime slice and mint sprig before serving.

Nutrition: Calories: 230; Fat: 1.3 g; Carbs: 57.7 g; Fiber: 5.4 g; Proteins: 2.8 g.

431.　Fruity Smoothie

Preparation Time: 10 minutes
Cooking Time: 0 minute
Servings: 1

Ingredients:
- ¾ cup soy yogurt
- ½ cup pineapple juice
- 1 cup pineapple chunks
- 1 cup raspberries, sliced
- 1 cup blueberries, sliced

Directions:
1 - Process the ingredients in a blender.
2 - Chill before serving.

Nutrition: Calories: 279; Total Fat 2 g; Saturated Fat: 0 g; Cholesterol: 4 mg; Sodium: 149 mg; Total Carbohydrates: 56 g; Dietary Fibers: 7 g; Proteins: 12 g; Total Sugars: 46 g; Potassium: 719 mg.

432.　Pineapple, Banana & Spinach Smoothie

Preparation Time: 10 minutes

Cooking Time: 0 minute

Servings: 1

Ingredients:

- ½ cup almond milk
- ¼ cup soy yogurt
- 1 cup spinach
- 1 cup banana
- 1 cup pineapple chunks
- 1 tablespoon chia seeds

Directions:

1 - Add all the ingredients to a blender.

2 - Blend until smooth.

3 - Chill in the refrigerator before serving.

Nutrition: Calories: 297; Total Fat: 6 g; Saturated Fat: 1 g; Cholesterol: 4 mg; Sodium: 145 mg; Total Carbohydrates: 54 g; Dietary Fiber: 10 g; Proteins: 13 g; Total Sugars: 29 g; Potassium: 1038 mg.

433. Kale & Avocado Smoothie

Preparation Time: 10 minutes

Cooking Time: 0 minute

Servings: 1

Ingredients:

- 1 ripe banana
- 1 cup kale
- 1 cup almond milk
- ¼ avocado
- 1 tablespoon chia seeds
- 2 teaspoons maple syrup
- 1 cup ice cubes

Directions:

1 - Blend all the ingredients until smooth.

Nutrition: Calories: 343; Total Fat: 14 g; Saturated Fat: 2 g; Cholesterol: 0 mg; Sodium: 199 mg; Total Carbohydrates: 55 g; Dietary Fiber 12 g; Proteins: 6 g; Total Sugars: 29 g; Potassium: 1051 mg.

434. Coconut & Strawberry Smoothie

Preparation Time: 10 minutes

Cooking Time: 0 minutes

Servings: 1

Ingredients:

- 1 cup strawberries, frozen & thawed slightly
- 1 ripe banana, sliced & frozen
- ½ cup coconut milk, light
- ½ cup vegan yogurt
- 1 tablespoon chia seeds

- 1 teaspoon lime juice, fresh
- 4 ice cubes

Directions:

1 - Blend everything until smooth, and serve immediately.

Nutrition: Calories: 278; Proteins: 14 g; Fat: 2 g; Carbs: 57 g.

435. Pumpkin Chia Smoothie

Preparation Time: 5 minutes

Cooking Time: 0 minutes

Servings: 1

Ingredients:

- 3 tablespoons pumpkin puree
- 1 tablespoon MCT oil
- ¾ cup coconut milk, full fat
- ½ avocado, fresh
- 1 teaspoon vanilla, pure
- ½ teaspoon pumpkin pie spice

Directions:

1 - Combine all ingredients together until blended.

Nutrition: Calories: 726; Proteins: 5.5 g; Fat: 69.8 g; Carbs: 15 g.

436. Cantaloupe Smoothie Bowl

Preparation Time: 5 minutes

Cooking Time: 0 minutes

Servings: 2

Ingredients:

- ¾ cup carrot juice
- 4 cups cantaloupe, frozen & cubed
- Mellon balls or berries to serve
- Pinch sea salt

Directions:

1 - Blend everything together until smooth.

Nutrition: Calories: 135; Proteins: 3 g; Fat: 1 g; Carbs: 32 g.

437. Kiwi Clementine Smoothie

Preparation time: 10 minutes

Cooking time: 2 hours

Servings: 2

Ingredients:

- 2 kiwis, peeled and diced
- 2 clementine, peeled and diced
- 1 banana, peeled and sliced
- 1 cup of coconut water
- 2 cups baby spinach

- 1/4 cup Greek yogurt

Directions:

1 - Ready all the fruits and vegetables then put them in a blender jug.

2 - Toss in the rest of the smoothie ingredients.

3 - Hit the pulse button to blend the smoothie until smooth.

4 - Chill the smoothie for 2 hours in the refrigerator.

5 - Serve chilled and fresh.

Nutrition: Calories 182 Fat 1.6 g Carbohydrates 40.1 g Protein 6.4 g

438. Cucumber Medjool Smoothie

Preparation time: 10 minutes

Cooking time: 2 hours

Servings: 2

Ingredients

- 1 cup of water
- 1/2 cucumber, peeled and cubed
- 1 frozen banana, peeled and sliced
- 1 cup mixed berries, frozen
- 1 teaspoon spirulina powder
- 1 Medjool date, pitted
- 1 handful baby spinach

Directions:

1 - Ready all the fruits and vegetables then put them in a blender jug.

2 - Toss in the rest of the smoothie ingredients.

3 - Hit the pulse button to blend the smoothie until smooth.

4 - Chill the smoothie for 2 hours in the refrigerator.

5 - Serve chilled and fresh.

Nutrition: Calories 165 Fat 0.6 g Carbohydrates 40 g Protein 3.8 g

439. Strawberry Ceylon Smoothie

Preparation time: 10 minutes

Cooking time: 2 hours

Servings: 2

Ingredients

- 1 ripe banana, peeled and sliced
- 1 cup almond milk
- 1/2 cup strawberries, fresh
- 1 cup baby spinach, fresh
- 1 teaspoon spirulina powder
- 1 tablespoon hemp seeds
- 1 teaspoon vanilla extract
- 1 teaspoon Ceylon cinnamon powder

- 1 teaspoon baobab powder

Directions:

1 - Ready all the fruits and vegetables then put them in a blender jug.

2 - Toss in the rest of the smoothie ingredients.

3 - Hit the pulse button to blend the smoothie until smooth.

4 - Chill the smoothie for 2 hours in the refrigerator.

5 - Serve chilled and fresh.

Nutrition: Calories 135 Fat 3.4 g Carbohydrates 23.4 g Protein 3.8 g

440. Jalapeno Smoothie

Preparation time: 10 minutes

Cooking time: 2 hours

Servings: 2

Ingredients

- 2 bananas, peeled and sliced
- 2 cups baby spinach
- 1 cup mango chunks, frozen
- 1/2 teaspoon jalapeno pepper, chopped
- 1 cup of water

Directions:

1 - Ready all the fruits and vegetables then put them in a blender jug.

2 - Toss in the rest of the smoothie ingredients.

3 - Hit the pulse button to blend the smoothie until smooth.

4 - Chill the smoothie for 2 hours in the refrigerator.

5 - Serve chilled and fresh.

Nutrition: Calories 157 Fat 0.5 g Carbohydrates 40.1g Protein 20g

441. Pomegranate Green Smoothie

Preparation time: 10 minutes

Cooking time: 2 hours

Servings: 3

Ingredients

- 1/2 banana, peeled and sliced
- 1/2 mango, peeled and cubed
- 1 cup raspberries, frozen
- 1 cup strawberries, frozen
- 2 cups of coconut water
- 1 tablespoon chia seeds
- 1 tablespoon pomegranate powder
- 1 pinch cinnamon
- 1 teaspoon spirulina powder
- 1/2 teaspoon chlorella powder

Directions:

1 - Ready all the fruits and put them in a blender jug.
2 - Toss in the rest of the smoothie ingredients.
3 - Hit the pulse button to blend the smoothie until smooth.
4 - Chill the smoothie for 2 hours in the refrigerator.
5 - Serve chilled and fresh.
Nutrition: Calories 190 Fat 4.1 g Carbohydrates 36.4 g Protein 5.6 g

442.   Popeye's Spirulina Smoothie

Preparation time: 10 minutes
Cooking time: 2 hours
Servings: 2
Ingredients
- 1 handful spinach
- 2 kiwi fruit, peeled
- 1 cup mango chunks
- 1/2 cup fresh orange juice
- 1 teaspoon spirulina powder
- 3 tablespoons unsweetened vanilla powder

Directions:

1 - Ready all the fruits and vegetables then put them in a blender jug.
2 - Toss in the rest of the smoothie ingredients.
3 - Hit the pulse button to blend the smoothie until smooth.
4 - Chill the smoothie for 2 hours in the refrigerator.
5 - Serve chilled and fresh.
Nutrition: Calories 203 Fat 1.2 g Carbohydrates 34.4 g Protein 15.1 g

443.   Psyllium Husk Smoothie

Preparation time: 10 minutes
Cooking time: 2 hours
Servings: 2
Ingredients
- 1 cup of coconut water
- 1 banana, peeled and sliced
- 1 handful kale, chopped
- 1 cup pineapple chunks
- 1 teaspoon psyllium husk
- 1/2 teaspoon spirulina powder

Directions:

1 - Ready all the fruits and vegetables then put them in a blender jug.
2 - Toss in the rest of the smoothie ingredients.

3 - Hit the pulse button to blend the smoothie until smooth.
4 - Chill the smoothie for 2 hours in the refrigerator.
5 - Serve chilled and fresh.
Nutrition: Calories 149 Fat 0.6 g Carbohydrates 38 g Protein 3.3 g

444.   Walnut Spinach Smoothie

Preparation time: 10 minutes
Cooking time: 2 hours
Servings: 2
Ingredients
- 1 cup almond milk
- 1 tablespoon ground flaxseed
- 1 scoop vanilla protein powder
- 1/4 cup walnuts, raw
- 1/4 teaspoon cinnamon
- 1/4 teaspoon vanilla extract
- 2 handfuls baby spinach
- 4 ice cubes

Directions:

1 - Ready all the fruits and vegetables then put them in a blender jug.
2 - Toss in the rest of the smoothie ingredients.
3 - Hit the pulse button to blend the smoothie until smooth.
4 - Chill the smoothie for 2 hours in the refrigerator.
5 - Serve chilled and fresh.
Nutrition: Calories 292 Fat 14.1 g Carbohydrates 20.9 g Protein 21.9 g

445.   Spirulina Orange Smoothie

Preparation time: 10 minutes
Cooking time: 2 hours
Servings: 2
Ingredients
- 1 orange, peeled and diced
- 1 cup mango, frozen and diced
- 1 frozen banana
- 1/2 teaspoon spirulina powder
- 1/2 cup almond milk

Directions:

1 - Ready all the fruits and put them in a blender jug.
2 - Toss in the rest of the smoothie ingredients.
3 - Hit the pulse button to blend the smoothie until smooth.
4 - Chill the smoothie for 2 hours in the refrigerator.
5 - Serve chilled and fresh.

Nutrition: Calories 165 Fat 1.4 g Carbohydrates 39.1 g Protein

446.   Cocoa Spinach Smoothie

Preparation time: 10 minutes
Cooking time: 2 hours
Servings: 2
Ingredients
- 1/2 cup mixed berries frozen
- 1 cup coconut cream
- 3 1/2 oz. spinach, chopped
- 1/4 cup cocoa powder
- 1 tablespoon granulated erythritol

Directions:
1 - Ready all the fruits and vegetables then put them in a blender jug.
2 - Toss in the rest of the smoothie ingredients.
3 - Hit the pulse button to blend the smoothie until smooth.
4 - Chill the smoothie for 2 hours in the refrigerator.
5 - Serve chilled and fresh.
Nutrition: Calories 189 Fat 13.6 g Carbohydrates 24.8 g Protein 5 g

447.   Berry & Cauliflower Smoothie

Preparation Time: 10 minutes
Cooking Time: 0 minutes
Servings: 2
Ingredients:
- 1 cup rice cauliflower, frozen
- 1 cup banana, sliced & frozen
- ½ cup mixed berries, frozen
- 2 cups almond milk, unsweetened
- 2 teaspoons maple syrup, pure & optional

Directions:
1 - Blend until mixed well.
Nutrition: Calories: 149; Proteins: 3 g; Fat: 3 g; Carbs: 29 g.

448.   Green Mango Smoothie

Preparation Time: 5 minutes
Cooking Time: 0 minutes
Servings: 1
Ingredients:
- 2 cups spinach
- 1-2 cups coconut water
- 2 mangos, ripe, peeled and diced

Directions:

1.   Blend everything together until smooth.
Nutrition: Calories: 417; Proteins: 7.2 g; Fat: 2.8 g; Carbs: 102.8 g.

449.   Chia Seed Smoothie

Preparation Time: 5 minutes
Cooking Time: 0 minutes
Servings: 3
Ingredients:
- ¼ teaspoon cinnamon
- 1 tablespoon ginger, fresh & grated
- Pinch cardamom
- 1 tablespoon chia seeds
- 2 Medjool dates, pitted
- 1 cup alfalfa sprouts
- 1 cup water
- 1 banana
- ½ cup coconut milk, unsweetened

Directions:
1 - Blend everything together until smooth.
Nutrition: Calories: 477; Proteins: 8 g; Fat: 29 g; Carbs: 57 g.

450.   Mango Smoothie

Preparation Time: 5 minutes
Cooking Time: 0 minutes
Servings: 3
Ingredients:
- 1 carrot, peeled and chopped
- 1 cup strawberries
- 1 cup water
- 1 cup peaches, chopped
- 1 banana, frozen and sliced
- 1 cup mango, chopped

Directions:
1 - Blend everything together until smooth.
Nutrition: Calories: 376; Proteins: 5 g; Fat: 2 g; Carbs: 95 g.

451.   Max Power Smoothie

Preparation Time: 5 minutes
Cooking Time: 0 minutes
Servings: 4
Ingredients:
- 1 banana
- ¼ cup rolled oats or 1 scoop plant protein powder
- 1 tablespoon flaxseed or chia seeds

- 1 cup raspberries or other berries
- 1 cup chopped mango (frozen or fresh)
- ½ cup non-dairy milk (optional)
- 1 cup water

Directions:
1 - Purée everything in a blender until smooth, adding more water (or non-dairy milk) if needed.
Nutrition: Calories: 550; Fat: 9 g; Carbs: 116 g; Fiber: 29 g; Proteins: 13 g.

452. Chai Chia Smoothie
Preparation Time: 5 minutes
Cooking Time: 0 minutes
Servings: 3
Ingredients:
- 1 banana
- ½ cup coconut milk
- 1 cup water
- 1 cup alfalfa sprouts (optional)
- 1 to 2 soft Medjool dates, pitted
- 1 tablespoon chia seeds, or ground flax or hemp hearts ¼ teaspoon ground cinnamon
- A pinch of ground cardamom
- 1 tablespoon grated fresh ginger or ¼ teaspoon ground ginger

Directions:
1 - Purée everything in a blender until smooth, adding more water (or coconut milk) if needed.
Nutrition: Calories: 477; Fat: 29 g; Carbs: 57 g; Fiber: 14 g; Proteins: 8 g.

453. Trope-Kale Breeze
Preparation Time: 5 minutes
Cooking Time: 0 minutes
Servings: 4
Ingredients:
- 1 cup chopped pineapple (frozen or fresh)
- 1 cup chopped mango (frozen or fresh)
- ½ to 1 cup kale, chopped
- ½ avocado
- ½ cup coconut milk
- 1 cup water (or coconut water)
- 1 teaspoon matcha green tea powder (optional)

Directions:
1 - Purée everything in a blender until smooth, add more water (or coconut milk) if needed.

Nutrition: Calories: 566; Fat: 36 g; Carbs: 66 g; Fiber: 12 g; Proteins: 8 g.

454. Hydration Station
Preparation Time: 5 minutes
Cooking Time: 0 minutes
Servings: 4
Ingredients:
- 1 banana
- 1 orange, peeled and divided, or 1 cup pure orange juice
- 1 cup strawberries (frozen or fresh)
- 1 cup chopped cucumber
- ½ cup coconut water
- 1 cup water
- ½ cup ice

Directions:
1 - Purée everything in a blender until smooth, adding more water if needed.
2 - Add bonus boosters, as desired, and purée until blended.
Nutrition: Calories: 320; Fat: 3 g; Carbs: 76 g; Fiber: 13 g; Proteins: 6 g.

455. Mango Madness
Preparation Time: 5 minutes
Cooking Time: 0 minutes
Servings: 4
Ingredients:
- 1 banana
- 1 cup chopped mango (frozen or fresh)
- 1 cup chopped peach (frozen or fresh)
- 1 cup strawberries
- 1 carrot, peeled and chopped (optional)
- 1 cup water

Directions:
1 - Purée everything in a blender until smooth, adding more water if needed.
Nutrition: Calories: 376; Fat: 2 g; Carbs: 95 g; Fiber: 14 g; Proteins: 5 g.

456. Chocolate PB Smoothie
Preparation Time: 5 minutes
Cooking Time: 0 minutes
Servings: 4
Ingredients:
- 1 banana

- ¼ cup rolled oats, or 1 scoop plant protein powder
- 1 tablespoon flaxseed or chia seeds
- 1 tablespoon unsweetened cocoa powder
- 1 tablespoon peanut butter, or almond or sunflower seed butter
- 1 tablespoon maple syrup (optional)
- 1 cup alfalfa sprouts or spinach, chopped (optional) ½ cup non-dairy milk (optional)
- 1 cup water

Directions:

1 - Purée everything in a blender until smooth, add more water (or non-dairy milk) if needed. Add bonus boosters, as desired, and purée until blended.

Nutrition: Calories: 474; Fat: 16 g; Carbs: 79 g; Fiber: 18 g; Proteins: 13 g.

457. Pink Panther Smoothie

Preparation Time: 5 minutes
Cooking Time: 0 minutes
Servings: 3

Ingredients:

- 1 cup strawberries
- 1 cup chopped melon (any kind)
- 1 cup cranberries or raspberries
- 1 tablespoon chia seeds
- ½ cup coconut milk or other non-dairy milk
- 1 cup water

Directions:

1 - Purée everything in a blender until smooth, add more water (or coconut milk) if needed.

Nutrition: Calories: 459; Fat: 30 g; Carbs: 52 g; Fiber: 19 g; Proteins: 8 g.

458. Banana Nut Smoothie

Preparation Time: 5 minutes
Cooking Time: 0 minutes
Servings: 3

Ingredients:

- 1 banana
- 1 tablespoon almond butter, or sunflower seed butter
- ¼ teaspoon ground cinnamon
- A pinch of ground nutmeg
- 1 to 2 tablespoons dates, or maple syrup
- 1 tablespoon ground flaxseed, or chia or hemp hearts
- ½ cup non-dairy milk (optional)

- 1 cup water

Directions:

1 - Purée everything in a blender until smooth, add more water (or non-dairy milk) if needed.

Nutrition: Calories: 343; Fat: 14 g; Carbs: 55 g; Fiber: 8 g; Proteins: 6 g.

459. Light Ginger Tea

Preparation Time: 5 minutes
Cooking Time: 10 minutes
Servings: 2

Ingredients:

- 1 small ginger knob, sliced into four 1-inch chunks
- 4 cups water
- Juice of 1 large lemon
- Maple syrup to taste

Directions:

1 - Add the ginger knob and water in a saucepan, then simmer over medium heat for 10 to 15 minutes.

2 - Turn off the heat, then mix in the lemon juice. Strain the liquid to remove the ginger, then fold in the maple syrup and serve.

Nutrition: Calories: 32; Fat: 0.1 g; Carbs: 8.6 g; Fiber: 0.1 g; Proteins: 0.1 g.

460. Kale Smoothie

Preparation Time: 5 minutes
Cooking Time: 0 minutes
Servings: 2

Ingredients:

- 2 cups chopped kale leaves
- 1 banana, peeled
- 1 cup frozen strawberries
- 1 cup unsweetened almond milk
- 4 Medjool dates, pitted and chopped

Directions:

1 - Put all the ingredients in a food processor, then blitz until glossy and smooth.

2 - Serve immediately or chill in the refrigerator for 1 hour before serving.

Nutrition: Calories: 663; Fat: 10 g; Carbs: 142.5 g; Fiber: 19 g; Proteins: 17.4 g.

461. Hot Tropical Smoothie

Preparation Time: 5 minutes
Cooking Time: 0 minutes
Servings: 4

Ingredients:

- 1 cup frozen mango chunks
- 1 cup frozen pineapple chunks
- 1 small tangerine, peeled and pitted
- 4 cups spinach leaves
- 1 cup coconut water
- ¼ teaspoon cayenne pepper, optional

Directions:

1 - Add all the ingredients to a food processor, then blitz until the mixture is smooth and combined well.

2 - Serve immediately or chill in the refrigerator for 1 hour before serving.

Nutrition: Calories: 283, Fat: 1.9 g; Carbs: 67.9 g; Fiber: 10.4 g; Proteins: 6.4 g.

462. Berry Smoothie

Preparation Time: 5 minutes
Cooking Time: 0 minutes
Servings: 4

Ingredients:

- 1 cup berry mix (strawberries, blueberries and cranberries)
- 4 Medjool dates, pitted and chopped
- 1 ½ cups unsweetened almond milk, plus more as needed

Directions:

1 - Add all the ingredients to a blender, then process until the mixture is smooth and well mixed.

2 - Serve immediately or chill in the refrigerator for 1 hour before serving.

Nutrition: Calories: 473; Fat: 4 g; Carbs: 103.7 g; Fiber: 9.7 g; Proteins: 14.8 g.

463. Cranberry and Banana Smoothie

Preparation Time: 5 minutes
Cooking Time: 0 minutes
Servings: 4

Ingredients:

- 1 cup frozen cranberries
- 1 large banana, peeled
- 4 Medjool dates, pitted and chopped
- 1 ½ cups unsweetened almond milk

Directions:

1 - Add all the ingredients to a food processor, then process until the mixture is glossy and well mixed.

2 - Serve immediately or chill in the refrigerator for 1 hour before serving.

Nutrition: Calories: 616; Fat: 8 g; Carbs: 132.8 g; Fiber: 14.6 g; Proteins: 15.7 g.

464. Pumpkin Smoothie

Preparation Time: 5 minutes
Cooking Time: 0 minutes
Servings: 2

Ingredients:

- ½ cup pumpkin purée
- 4 Medjool dates, pitted and chopped
- 1 cup unsweetened almond milk
- ¼ teaspoon vanilla extract
- ¼ teaspoon ground cinnamon
- ½ cup ice
- A pinch of ground nutmeg

Directions:

1 - Add all the ingredients to a blender, then process until the mixture is glossy and well mixed.

2 - Serve immediately.

Nutrition: Calories: 417; Fat: 3 g; Carbs: 94.9 g; Fiber: 10.4 g; Proteins: 11.4 g.

465. Green Milk Shake

Preparation time: 5 minutes
Cooking time: 2 minutes
Servings: 1

Ingredients:

- Coconut oil (1 Tbsp.)
- Mix salad (2 c.)
- Water (1 c.)
- Coconut flakes (1 Tbsp.)
- Stevia (1 packet)
- Almond milk (1 c.)

Directions:

1 - Prepare all ingredients to a blender and mix until well combined.

Nutrition: Calories 309 Carbohydrates 19g Fat 23g Protein 10g

466. Greens and Raspberry Shake

Preparation time: 5 minutes
Cooking time: 3 minutes
Servings: 1

Ingredients:

- Spinach (1 c.)
- Raspberries (.25 c.)
- Macadamia oil (1 Tbsp.)
- Almond milk (1 c.)

- Water (1 c.)
- Stevia (1 packet

Directions:

1 - Prepare ingredients to a blender and mix until well combined.

Nutrition: Calories 292 Carbohydrates 17g Fat 22g Protein 9g

467.   Melon Delight

Preparation time: 5 minutes
Cooking time: 2 minutes
Servings: 1

Ingredients:

- Water 11/2 cup)
- Chia seeds (1 Tbsp.)
- Coconut flakes (1 Tbsp.)
- Coconut oil (1 Tbsp.)
- Plant-based yogurt (1/4 c.)
- Melon slices (1/2 cup)
- Stevia (1 packet)

Directions:

1 - Prepare all ingredients to a blender and mix until well combined.

Nutrition: Calories 141 Carbohydrates 20g Fat 6g Protein 1g

468.   Nutty Berry Shake

Preparation time: 10 minutes
Cooking time: 2 minutes
Servings: 1

Ingredients:

- Water (1 1/2 cup)
- Chia seeds (1 Tbsp.)
- Pepitas (1 Tbsp.)
- Hemp seeds (1 Tbsp.)
- Chopped strawberries (1/4 c.)
- Blackberry (1/4 c.)
- Boysenberries (1/4 c.)
- Stevia (1 packet)
- Plant-based yogurt (1/2 cup)

Directions:

1 - Set all ingredients to a blender and mix until well combined.

Nutrition: Calories 160 Carbohydrates 18g Fat 10g Protein 6g

469.   Rosemary Lemon Smoothie

Preparation time: 5 minutes

Cooking time: 2 minutes
Servings: 1

Ingredients:

- Water (1 1/2 c)
- Ground flaxseed (1 Tbsp.)
- Pepitas (1 Tbsp.)
- Lemon juice (1 Tbsp.)
- Rosemary (1 stalk)
- Olive oil (1 Tbsp.)
- Stevia (1 packet)
- Garden greens (1 c.)
- Plant-based yogurt (1/2 cup)

Directions:

1 - Prepare all ingredients to a blender and mix until well combined.

Nutrition: Calories 131 Carbohydrates 21g Fat 6g Protein 3g

470.   Basil Delight

Preparation time: 10 minutes
Cooking time: 2 minutes
Servings: 1

Ingredients:

- Water (1 1/2 cup)
- Hemp seeds (1 Tbsp.)
- Basil leaves (10)
- Chopped walnuts (2 Tbsp.)
- Chopped pine nuts (2 Tbsp.)
- Olive oil (1 Tbsp.)
- Stevia (1 packet)
- Mix salad greens (1 c.)
- Plant-based yogurt (1/2 cup)

Directions:

1 - Prepare all ingredients to a blender and mix until well combined.

Nutrition: Calories: 160 Carbohydrates 18g Fat 4g Protein 18g

471.   Blueberry Kale Shake

Preparation time: 5 minutes
Cooking time: 2 minutes
Servings: 1

Ingredients:

- Water (1 1/2 cup)
- Ground flaxseed (1 Tbsp.)
- Pepitas (1 Tbsp.)
- MCT oil (1 Tbsp.)
- Blueberries (1/4c.)

- Stevia (1 packet)
- Kale greens (1 c.)
- Plant-based yogurt (1/2)

Directions:

1 - Prepare and mix all the ingredients into a blender until well combined.

Nutrition: Calories 219 Carbohydrates 31g Fat 9g Protein 6g

472.   Green Yogurt Smoothie

Preparation time: 10 minutes

Cooking time: 2 hours

Servings: 3

Ingredients

- 3 kiwis, peeled and cubed
- 1 banana, sliced
- 2 cups spinach, chopped
- 1 cup almond milk
- 2 teaspoons coconut shreds
- 1 cup plain Greek yogurt

Directions:

1 - Ready all the fruits and vegetables, then put them in a blender jug.

2 - Put in the rest of the smoothie ingredients.

3 - Hit the pulse button to blend the smoothie until smooth.

4 - Chill the smoothie for 2 hours in the refrigerator.

5 - Serve chilled and fresh.

Nutrition: Calories 134 Fat 2.3 g Carbohydrates 27.1 g Protein 3.9 g

473.   Creamy Kiwi Smoothie

Preparation time: 10 minutes

Cooking time: 2 hours

Servings: 3

Ingredients

- 6 kiwis, peeled and chopped
- 1 cup Greek-style yogurt
- 1 cup of coconut milk
- 1 drop green food coloring

Directions:

1 - Ready all the kiwis and put them in a blender jug.

2 - Put in the rest of the smoothie ingredients.

3 - Hit the pulse button to blend the smoothie until smooth.

4 - Chill the smoothie for 2 hours in the refrigerator.

5 - Serve chilled and fresh.

Nutrition: Calories 212 Fat 9.9 g Carbohydrates 26.6 g Protein 6.8 g

474.   Cilantro Ginger Smoothie

Preparation time: 10 minutes

Cooking time: 2 hours

Servings: 4

Ingredients

- 1 apple, cored and chopped
- 1 kiwi, peeled and quartered
- 2 cups tender kale leaves, chopped
- 1/2 cup cilantro leaves, chopped
- 1 1/4-inch ginger slice, peeled and chopped
- 1 cup of distilled water

Directions:

1 - Ready all the fruits and vegetables, then put them in a blender jug.

2 - Add in the rest of the smoothie ingredients.

3 - Hit the pulse button to blend the smoothie until smooth.

4 - Chill the smoothie for 2 hours in the refrigerator.

5 - Serve chilled and fresh.

Nutrition: Calories 119 Fat 0.5 g Carbohydrates 28.9 g Protein 2.9 g

475.   Broccoli Mango Smoothie

Preparation time: 10 minutes

Cooking time: 2 hours

Servings: 3

Ingredients

- 1/2 cup broccoli florets, raw
- 1 banana, peeled and frozen
- 1 cup mango chunks
- 3/4 cup strawberries, frozen
- 1/2 cup spinach, chopped
- 1 cup pineapple juice
- 3/4 cup water

Directions:

1 - Ready all the fruits and vegetables, then put them in a blender jug.

2 - Add in the rest of the smoothie ingredients.

3 - Hit the pulse button to blend the smoothie until smooth.

4 - Chill the smoothie for 2 hours in the refrigerator.

5 - Serve chilled and fresh.

Nutrition: Calories 147 Fat 0.5 g Carbohydrates 35.3 g Protein 2.4 g

476.   Dandelion Smoothie

Preparation time: 10 minutes
Cooking time: 2 hours
Servings: 3
Ingredients:

- 2 cups dandelion greens, fresh
- 2 cups orange juice
- 2 cups strawberries
- 2 kiwis, peeled and cubed
- 1 banana, peeled and sliced
- 1 lemon, juiced

Directions:

1 - Ready all the fruits and vegetables, then put them in a blender jug.
2 - Add the rest of the smoothie ingredients.
3 - Hit the pulse button to blend the smoothie until smooth.
4 - Chill the smoothie for 2 hours in the refrigerator.
5 - Serve chilled and fresh.
Nutrition: Calories 193 Fat 1.3 g Carbohydrates 46.2 g Protein 4 g

477.   Zespri Ginger Smoothie

Preparation time: 10 minutes
Cooking time: 2 hours
Servings: 3
Ingredients:

- 1 cup Greek yogurt
- 1 cup baby spinach, chopped
- 1 cup oat milk
- 1 cup grapes
- 1/2 teaspoon ginger, grated
- 2 Zespri kiwi fruit
- 2 dates, pitted

Directions:

1 - Ready all the fruits and vegetables, then put them in a blender jug.
2 - Toss in the rest of the smoothie ingredients.
3 - Hit the pulse button to blend the smoothie until smooth.
4 - Chill the smoothie for 2 hours in the refrigerator.
5 - Serve chilled and fresh.
Nutrition: Calories 110 Fat 0 g Carbohydrates 26 g Protein: 2g

478.   Thai Iced Tea

Preparation Time: 5 minutes
Cooking Time: 10 minutes

Servings: 4
Ingredients:

- 4 cups of water
- 1 can of light coconut milk (14 oz.)
- ¼ cup of maple syrup
- ¼ cup of muscovado sugar
- 1 teaspoon of vanilla extract
- 2 tablespoons of loose-leaf black tea

Directions:

1. In a large saucepan, over medium heat brings the water to a boil.
2. Turn off the heat and add in the tea, cover and let steep for five minutes.
3. Strain the tea into a bowl or jug. Add the maple syrup, muscovado sugar, and vanilla extract. Give it a good whisk to blend all the ingredients.
4. Set in the refrigerator to chill. Upon serving, pour ¾ of the tea into each glass, top with coconut milk, and stir.

Tips:

Add a shot of dark rum to turn this iced tea into a cocktail.
You could substitute the coconut milk for almond or rice milk too.
Nutrition: Calories 844 Carbohydrates: 2.3g Protein: 21.6g Fat: 83.1g

479.   Hot Chocolate

Preparation Time: 5 minutes
Cooking Time: 15 minutes
Servings: 2
Ingredients:

- Pinch of brown sugar
- 2 cups of milk, soy or almond, unsweetened
- 2 tablespoons of cocoa powder
- ½ cup of vegan chocolate

Directions:

1. In a medium saucepan, over medium heat gently brings the milk to a boil. Whisk in the cocoa powder.
2. Remove from the heat, add a pinch of sugar and chocolate. Give it a good stir until smooth, serve, and enjoy.

Tips:

You may substitute the almond or soy milk for coconut milk too.

Nutrition: Calories 452 Carbs: 29.8g Protein: 15.2g Fat: 30.2g

480.   Chai and Chocolate Milkshake

Preparation Time: 5 minutes
Cooking Time: 15 minutes
Servings: 2
Ingredients:

- 1 and ½ cups of almond milk, sweetened or unsweetened
- 3 bananas, peeled and frozen 12 hours before use
- 4 dates, pitted
- 1 and ½ teaspoons of chocolate powder, sweetened or unsweetened
- ½ teaspoon of vanilla extract
- ½ teaspoon of cinnamon
- ¼ teaspoon of ground ginger
- Pinch of ground cardamom
- Pinch of ground cloves
- Pinch of ground nutmeg
- ½ cup of ice cubes

Directions:

1. Add all the ingredients to a blender except for the ice-cubes. Pulse until smooth and creamy, add the ice-cubes, pulse a few more times and serve.

Tips:

The dates provide enough sweetness to the recipe; however, you are welcome to add maple syrup or maple syrup for a sweeter drink.

Nutrition: Calories 452 Carbs: 29.8g Protein: 15.2g Fat: 30.2g

481.   Lemon Infused Water

Preparation Time: 10 minutes
Cooking Time: 2 hours
Servings: 12
Ingredients:

- 2 cups of coconut sugar
- 2 cups of lemon juice
- 3 quarts of water

Directions:

1. Pour water into a 6-quarts slow cooker and stir the sugar and lemon juice properly.
2. Then plug in the slow cooker and let it cook on a high heat setting for 2 hours or until it is heated thoroughly.

3. Serve the drink hot or cold.

Nutrition: Calories 523 Carbohydrates: 4.6g Protein: 47.9g Fat: 34.8g

482.   Soothing Ginger Tea Drink

Preparation Time: 5 minutes
Cooking Time: 2 hours 20 minutes
Servings: 8
Ingredients:

- 1 tablespoon of minced ginger root
- 2 tablespoons of maple syrup
- 15 green tea bags
- 32 fluid ounce of white grape juice
- 2 quarts of boiling water

Directions:

1. Pour water into a 4-quarts slow cooker, immerse tea bags, cover the cooker, and let stand for 10 minutes.
2. After 10 minutes, remove and discard tea bags and stir in the remaining ingredients.
3. Return cover to the slow cooker, let cook at high heat setting for 2 hours or until heated through.
4. When done, strain the liquid and serve hot or cold.

Nutrition: Calories 232 Carbs: 7.9g Protein: 15.9g Fat: 15.1g

483.   Ginger Cherry Cider

Preparation Time: 1 hour 5 minutes
Cooking Time: 3 hours
Servings: 16
Ingredients:

- 2 knobs of ginger, each about 2 inches
- 6-ounce of cherry gelatin
- 4 quarts of apple cider

Directions:

1. Using a 6-quarts slow cooker, pour the apple cider and add the ginger.
2. Stir, then cover the slow cooker with its lid. let it cook for 3 hours at the high heat setting or until it is heated thoroughly.
3. Then add and stir the gelatin properly, then continue cooking for another hour.
4. When done, remove the ginger and serve the drink hot or cold.

Nutrition: Calories 78 Carbs: 13.2g Protein: 2.8g Fat: 1.5g

484. Colorful Infused Water

Preparation Time: 5 minutes
Cooking Time: 1 hour
Servings: 8

Ingredients:

- 1 cup of strawberries, fresh or frozen
- 1 cup of blueberries, fresh or frozen
- 1 tablespoon of baobab powder
- 1 cup of ice cubes
- 4 cups of sparkling water

Directions:

1. In a large water jug, add in the sparkling water, ice cubes, and baobab powder. Give it a good stir.
2. Add in the strawberries and blueberries and cover the infused water, store in the refrigerator for one hour before serving.

Tips: Store for 12 hours for optimum taste and nutritional benefits.

Instead of using strawberries and blueberries, add slices of lemon and six mint leaves, one cup of mangoes or cherries, or half a cup of leafy greens such as kale and/or spinach.

Nutrition: Calories 163 Carbs: 4.1g Protein: 1.7g Fat: 15.5g

485. Hibiscus Tea

Preparation Time: 1 Minute
Cooking Time: 5 minutes
Servings: 2

Ingredients:

- 1 tablespoon of raisins, diced
- 6 Almonds, raw and unsalted
- ½ teaspoon of hibiscus powder
- 2 cups of water

Directions:

1. Bring the water to a boil in a small saucepan, add in the hibiscus powder and raisins. Give it a good stir, cover, and let simmer for a further two minutes.
2. Strain into a teapot and serve with a side helping of almonds.
3. As an alternative to this tea, do not strain it and serve with the raisin pieces still swirling around in the teacup.
4. You could also serve this tea chilled for those hotter days.

5. Double or triple the recipe to provide you with iced-tea to enjoy during the week without having to make a fresh pot each time.

Nutrition: Calories 139 Carbohydrates: 2.7g Protein: 8.7g Fat: 10.3

486. Lemon and Rosemary Iced Tea

Preparation Time: 5 minutes
Cooking Time: 10 minutes
Servings: 4

Ingredients:

- 4 cups of water
- 4 earl grey tea bags
- ¼ cup of sugar
- 2 lemons
- 1 sprig of rosemary

Directions:

1. Peel the two lemons and set the fruit aside.
2. In a medium saucepan, over medium heat combines the water, sugar, and lemon peels. Bring this to a boil.
3. Remove from the heat and place the rosemary and tea into the mixture. Cover the saucepan and steep for five minutes.
4. Add the juice of the two peeled lemons to the mixture, strain, chill, and serve.

Tips: Skip the sugar and use maple syrup to taste.

Do not squeeze the tea bags as they can cause the tea to become bitter.

Nutrition: Calories 229 Carbs: 33.2g Protein: 31.1g Fat: 10.2g

487. Apple Kiwi Smoothies

Preparation time: 10 minutes
Cooking time: 2 hours
Servings: 3

Ingredients

- 1 banana, peeled
- 1 green apple, cored and chopped
- 3 kiwis, peeled and cubed
- 1 cup coconut cream
- 1 cup of water
- 2 cups spinach, chopped

Directions:

1 - Ready all the fruits and vegetables, then put them in a blender jug.

2 - Toss in the rest of the smoothie ingredients.

3 - Hit the pulse button to blend the smoothie until smooth.

4 - Chill the smoothie for 2 hours in the refrigerator.

5 - Serve chilled and fresh.

Nutrition: Calories 183 Fat 1.7 g Carbohydrates 36.9 g Protein 6.7 g

488.   Kiwi Peach Smoothie

Preparation time: 10 minutes

Cooking time: 2 hours

Servings: 2

Ingredients

- 3 handfuls leafy greens
- 2 kiwis, peeled
- 1 1/2 cups peach, cored, peeled, and cubed
- 1 1/2 banana, frozen
- 1 1/2 tablespoons chia seeds
- 1 cup almond milk
- 3 ice cubes

Directions:

1 - Ready all the fruits and vegetables then put them in a blender jug.

2 - Toss in the rest of the smoothie ingredients.

3 - Hit the pulse button to blend the smoothie until smooth.

4 - Chill the smoothie for 2 hours in the refrigerator.

5 - Serve chilled and fresh.

Nutrition: Calories 250 Fat 3.3 g Carbohydrates 51.9 g Protein 6.8 g

489.   Super Smoothie

Preparation Time: 5 minutes

Cooking Time: 0 minutes

Servings: 4

Ingredients:

- 1 banana, peeled
- 1 cup chopped mango
- 1 cup raspberries
- ¼ cup rolled oats
- 1 carrot, peeled
- 1 cup chopped fresh kale
- 2 tablespoons chopped fresh parsley
- 1 tablespoon flaxseeds
- 1 tablespoon grated fresh ginger
- ½ cup unsweetened soy milk
- 1 cup water

Directions:

1 - Put all the ingredients in a food processor, then blitz until glossy and smooth.

2 - Serve immediately or chill in the refrigerator for 1 hour before serving.

Nutrition: Calories: 550; Fat: 39 g; Carbs: 31 g; Fiber: 15 g; Proteins: 13 g.

490.   Kiwi and Strawberry Smoothie

Preparation Time: 5 minutes

Cooking Time: 0 minutes

Servings: 3

Ingredients:

- 1 kiwi, peeled
- 5 medium strawberries
- ½ frozen banana
- 1 cup unsweetened almond milk
- 2 tablespoons hemp seeds
- 2 tablespoons peanut butter
- 1 to 2 teaspoons maple syrup
- ½ cup spinach leaves
- Handful broccoli sprouts

Directions:

1 - Put all the ingredients in a food processor, then blitz until creamy and smooth.

2 - Serve immediately or chill in the refrigerator for 1 hour before serving.

Nutrition: Calories: 562; Fat: 28.6 g; Carbs: 63.6 g; Fiber: 15.1 g; Proteins: 23.3 g.

491.   Banana and Chai Chia Smoothie

Preparation Time: 5 minutes

Cooking Time: 0 minutes

Servings: 3

Ingredients:

- 1 banana
- 1 cup alfalfa sprouts
- 1 tablespoon chia seeds
- ½ cup unsweetened coconut milk
- 1 to 2 soft Medjool dates, pitted
- ¼ teaspoon ground cinnamon
- 1 tablespoon grated fresh ginger
- 1 cup water
- A pinch of ground cardamom

Directions:

1 - Add all the ingredients to a blender, then process until the mixture is smooth and creamy. Add water or coconut milk if necessary.

2 - Serve immediately.

Nutrition: Calories: 477; Fat: 41 g; Carbs: 31 g; Fiber: 14 g; Proteins: 8 g

Chapter 24.   Dessert

492. Walnut Brownies
Preparation Time: 15 minutes
Cooking Time: 22 minutes
Servings: 6
Ingredients:
- 1 tablespoon ground flaxseed
- 3 tablespoons water
- ½ cup vegan chocolate, roughly chopped
- 1/3 cup coconut oil
- 5 tablespoon white sugar
- 1 teaspoon vanilla extract
- Pinch of salt
- 5 tablespoons self-rising flour
- ¼ cup walnuts, chopped

Directions:
1 - In a small bowl, add flaxseed and water and mix well.
2 - Set aside for about 5 minutes.
3 - In a microwave-safe bowl, add the chocolate and coconut oil and microwave on high heat for about 2 minutes, stirring after every 30 seconds.
4 - Remove from microwave and set aside to cool.
5 - In another bowl, add the sugar, flaxseed mixture, vanilla extract, and salt and whisk until creamy and light.
6 - Add the chocolate mixture and whisk until well combined
7 - Add the flour and walnuts and mix until well combined.
8 - Line a baking pan with greased parchment paper.
9 - Place mixture into the prepared pan evenly and with the back of spatula, smooth the top surface.
10 - Set the temperature of Air Fryer to 355 degrees F to preheat for 5 minutes.
11 - After preheating, arrange the baking pan into the Air Fryer Basket.
12 - Slide the basket into Air Fryer and set the time for 20 minutes.
13 - When cooking time is completed, remove the baking pan and place onto a wire rack to cool completely.
14 - Cut into desired sized squares and serve.
Nutrition: Calories: 281 Fat: 19.8g Carbohydrates: 24.2g Fiber: 1.3g Sugar: 17.4g Protein: 3.2g

493. Plum Crisp
Preparation Time: 10 minutes
Cooking Time: 40 minutes
Servings: 2
Ingredients:
- 1½ cups plums, pitted and sliced
- ¼ cup white sugar, divided
- 1½ teaspoons cornstarch
- 3 tablespoons flour
- ¼ teaspoon ground cinnamon
- Pinch of salt
- 1½ tablespoons cold coconut oil, chopped
- 3 tablespoons rolled oats

Directions:
1. - In a bowl, place plum slices, 1 teaspoon of sugar and cornstarch and toss to coat well
2 - Divide the plum mixture into 2 lightly greased (8-ounce) ramekins.
3 - In a bowl, mix together the flour, remaining sugar, cinnamon and salt.
4 - With a pastry blender, cut in the coconut oil until a crumbly mixture forms.
5 - Add the oats and gently stir to combine.
6 - Place the oat mixture over plum slices into each ramekin.
7 - Set the temperature of Air Fryer to 350 degrees F to preheat for 5 minutes.
8 - After preheating, arrange the ramekins into the Air Fryer Basket.
9 - Slide the basket into Air Fryer and set the time for 40 minutes.
10 - When cooking time is completed, place the ramekins onto a wire rack to cool for about 10 minutes.
11 - Serve warm.
Nutrition: Calories: 305 Fat: 11g Carbohydrates: 52.1g Fiber: 2g Sugar: 30.4g Protein: 2.6g

494. Apple Crumble
Preparation Time: 20 minutes
Cooking Time: 25 minutes
Servings: 6
Ingredients:
- For the filling
- 4 to 5 apples, cored and chopped (about 6 cups)
- ½ cup unsweetened applesauce, or ¼ cup water
- 2 to 3 tablespoons unrefined sugar (coconut, date, maple syrup)

- 1 teaspoon ground cinnamon
- Pinch sea salt
- For the crumble
- 2 tablespoons almond butter, or cashew or sunflower seed butter
- 2 tablespoons maple syrup
- 1½ cups rolled oats
- ½ cup walnuts, finely chopped
- ½ teaspoon ground cinnamon
- 2 to 3 tablespoons unrefined granular sugar (coconut, date, sucanat)

Directions:

1 - Preparing the Ingredients.

2 - Preheat the oven to 350°F. Put the apples and applesauce in an 8-inch-square baking dish, and sprinkle with the sugar, cinnamon, and salt. Toss to combine.

3 - In a medium bowl, mix together the nut butter and maple syrup until smooth and creamy. Add the oats, walnuts, cinnamon, and sugar and stir to coat, using your hands if necessary. (If you have a small food processor, pulse the oats and walnuts together before adding them to the mix.)

4 - Sprinkle the topping over the apples, and put the dish in the oven.

5 - Bake for 20 to 25 minutes, or until the fruit is soft and the topping is lightly browned.

Nutrition: Calories 195 Fat 7 g Carbohydrates 6 g Sugar 2 g Protein 24 g Cholesterol 65 mg

495.   Cashew-Chocolate Truffles

Preparation Time: 15 minutes
Cooking Time: 0 minutes
Servings: 12

Ingredients:

- 1 cup raw cashews, soaked in water overnight
- ¾ cup pitted dates
- 2 tablespoons coconut oil
- 1 cup unsweetened shredded coconut, divided
- 1 to 2 tablespoons cocoa powder, to taste

Directions:

1 - Preparing the Ingredients.

2 - In a food processor, combine the cashews, dates, coconut oil, ½ cup of shredded coconut, and cocoa powder. Pulse until fully incorporated; it will resemble chunky cookie dough. Spread the remaining ½ cup of shredded coconut on a plate.

3 - Form the mixture into tablespoon-size balls and roll on the plate to cover with the shredded coconut. Transfer to a parchment paper–lined plate or baking sheet. Repeat to make 12 truffles.

4 - Place the truffles in the refrigerator for 1 hour to set. Transfer the truffles to a storage container or freezer-safe bag and seal.

Nutrition: Calories 160 Fat 1 g Carbohydrates 1 g Sugar 0.5 g Protein 22 g Cholesterol 60 mg

496.   Banana Chocolate Cupcakes

Preparation Time: 20 minutes
Cooking Time: 20 minutes
Servings: 1

Ingredients:

- 3 medium bananas
- 1 cup non-dairy milk
- 2 tablespoons almond butter
- 1 teaspoon apple cider vinegar
- 1 teaspoon pure vanilla extract
- 1¼ cups whole-grain flour
- ½ cup rolled oats
- ¼ cup coconut sugar (optional)
- 1 teaspoon baking powder
- ½ teaspoon baking soda
- ½ cup unsweetened cocoa powder
- ¼ cup chia seeds, or sesame seeds
- Pinch sea salt
- ¼ cup dark chocolate chips, dried cranberries, or raisins (optional)

Directions:

1- Preparing the Ingredients.

2 - Preheat the oven to 350°F. Lightly grease the cups of two 6-cup muffin tins or line with paper muffin cups.

3 - Put the bananas, milk, almond butter, vinegar, and vanilla in a blender and purée until smooth. Or stir together in a large bowl until smooth and creamy.

4 - Put the flour, oats, sugar (if using), baking powder, baking soda, cocoa powder, chia seeds, salt, and chocolate chips in another large bowl, and stir to combine. Mix together the wet and dry ingredients, stirring as little as possible. Spoon into muffin cups, and bake for 20 to 25 minutes. Take the cupcakes out of the oven and let them cool fully before taking out of the muffin tins, since they'll be very moist.

Nutrition: Calories 295 Fat 17 g Carbohydrates 4 g Sugar 0.1 g Protein 29 g Cholesterol 260 mg

497. Minty Fruit Salad

Preparation Time: 15 minutes
Cooking Time: 5 minutes
Servings: 4
Ingredients:
- ¼ cup lemon juice (about 2 small lemons)
- 4 teaspoons maple syrup or agave syrup
- 2 cups chopped pineapple
- 2 cups chopped strawberries
- 2 cups raspberries
- 1 cup blueberries
- 8 fresh mint leaves

Directions:
Preparing the Ingredients.
1 - Beginning with 1 mason jar, add the ingredients in this order:
2 - 1 tablespoon of lemon juice, 1 teaspoon of maple syrup, ½ cup of pineapple, ½ cup of strawberries, ½ cup of raspberries, ¼ cup of blueberries, and 2 mint leaves.
3 - Repeat to fill 3 more jars. Close the jars tightly with lids.
4 - Place the airtight jars in the refrigerator for up to 3 days.
Nutrition: Calories 339 Fat 17.5 g Carbohydrates 2 g Sugar 2 g Protein 44 g Cholesterol 100 mg

498. Banana Cake

Preparation Time: 15 minutes
Cooking Time: 30 minutes
Servings: 5
Ingredients:
- 1 cup self-rising flour
- ½ teaspoon ground cinnamon
- Pinch of salt
- 1/3 cup brown sugar
- 3½ tablespoons coconut oil, softened
- 1 banana, peeled and mashed
- ¼ cup unsweetened applesauce
- 2 tablespoons maple syrup

Directions:
1 - In a bowl, sift together the flour, cinnamon and salt.
2 - In another bowl, add the brown sugar and coconut oil and with an electric mixer, beat until creamy.
3 - Add the banana, applesauce and maple syrup and beat until smooth.
4 - Add the flour mixture and beat until smooth.

5 - Place the mixture into a greased small fluted tube pan and with a spatula, smooth the top surface.
6 - Set the temperature of Air Fryer to 320 degrees F to preheat for 5 minutes.
7 - After preheating, arrange the cake pan into the Air Fryer Basket.
8 - Slide the basket into Air Fryer and set the time for 30 minutes.
9 - When cooking time is completed, remove the cake pan and place onto a wire rack for about 10 minutes.
10 - Carefully invert the cake onto the wire rack to cool completely before serving.
11 - Cut into desired sized slices and serve.
Nutrition: Calories: 258 Fat: 9.9g Carbohydrates: 40.9g Fiber: 1.6g Sugar: 18.3g Protein: 2.9g

499. Spiced Pumpkin Cake

Preparation Time: 15 minutes
Cooking Time: 25 minutes
Servings: 4
Ingredients:
- ¼ cup coconut flour
- 2 tablespoons stevia blend
- 1 teaspoon baking powder
- ¾ teaspoon pumpkin pie spice
- ¼ teaspoon ground cinnamon
- 1/8 teaspoon salt
- ¼ cup canned pumpkin
- ½ cup unsweetened applesauce
- 2 tablespoons unsweetened almond milk
- 1 teaspoon vanilla extract

Directions:
1 - In a bowl, mix together the flour, stevia, baking powder, spices, and salt.
2 - In another large bowl, add the pumpkin, applesauce, almond milk, and vanilla extract. Beat until well combined.
3 - Then, add in the flour mixture and mix until just combined
4 - Line a cake pan with greased parchment paper.
5 - Place the mixture evenly into the prepared pan.
6 - Set the temperature of Air Fryer to 350 degrees F to preheat for 5 minutes.
7 - After preheating, arrange the pan into an Air Fryer Basket.
8 - Slide the basket into Air Fryer and set the time for 25 minutes or until a toothpick inserted in the center comes out clean.

9 - When cooking time is completed, remove the cake pan and place onto a wire rack for about 10 minutes.
10 - Carefully invert the cake onto the wire rack to cool completely before serving.
11 - Cut into desired sized slices and serve.
Nutrition: Calories: 55/ Fat: 1g Carbohydrates: 10.8g Fiber: 4g Sugar: 3.7g Protein: 1.3g

500. Chocolate Bark

Preparation Time: 5 Minutes
Cooking Time: 5 Minutes
Servings: 1
Ingredients:
- ¼ cup dried cranberries
- 3 tablespoons chopped pistachios
- 3 tablespoons chopped almonds
- 3 tablespoons pumpkin seeds
- 3 tablespoons sunflower seeds
- 1 (8-ounce / 227-g) bag vegan dark chocolate chips
- Pink Himalayan salt, to taste

Directions:
1. Line an 8-inch square baking pan with parchment paper. Spread out the cranberries, pistachios, almonds, pumpkin seeds, and sunflower seeds on the baking pan.
2. In a small nonstick saucepan on low heat, gently heat the chocolate chips, stirring continuously, until they are melted and smooth.
3. Pour the melted chocolate evenly over the nuts, seeds, and dried fruit in the baking pan. Let cool to room temperature. Sprinkle with salt. Break the bark into pieces and remove it from the baking pan.

Nutrition: Calories: 275 Fats: 18g Carbs: 30g Proteins: 4g Fibers: 4g

501. Vanilla Rice Pudding with Cherries

Preparation Time: 5 Minutes
Cooking Time: 30 Minutes
Servings: 1
Ingredients:
- 1/2 cup short-grain brown rice
- ¾ cups coconut milk, plus more as needed
- ½ cups water
- 1 tablespoon unrefined sugar or pure maple syrup, plus more as needed
- 1 teaspoon vanilla extract
- Salt, to taste
- ¼ cup dried cherries or ½ cup fresh or frozen pitted cherries

Directions:
1. Combine the rice, milk, water, sugar, vanilla, and salt in the Instant Pot.
2. Lock the lid. Select the Manual mode and set the cooking time for 30 minutes at High Pressure.
3. When the timer beeps, perform a natural pressure release for 20 minutes, then release any remaining pressure. Carefully remove the lid.
4. Stir in the cherries and rest the lid back on (no need to lock it), and let sit for about 10 minutes.
5. Serve with more milk or sugar, as needed.

Nutrition: Calories: 150 Fats: 8g Carbs: 17g Proteins: 5g Fibers: 5g

502. Chocolate Chip Banana Cookies

Preparation Time: 5 Minutes
Cooking Time: 10 Minutes
Servings: 1
Ingredients:
- 2 bananas
- 1 cup rolled oats
- 1 teaspoon ground flaxseed
- 1 teaspoon vanilla extract
- ¼ cup vegan mini chocolate chips
- ¼ cup chopped walnuts

Directions:
1. Preheat the oven to 350ºF (180ºC). Line a baking sheet with parchment paper or a silicone liner.
2. In a food processor, combine the bananas, oats, flaxseed, and vanilla and blend until very well combined. Use a wooden spoon to stir in the chocolate chips and walnuts.
3. Scoop the batter into 9 cookies, spacing them out on the prepared baking sheet. Bake for 8 to 12 minutes, or until the bottoms are light brown. Enjoy right after they cool or store in a reusable container at room temperature.

Nutrition: Calories: 122 Fats: 5g Carbs: 17g Proteins: 2g Fibers: 2g

503. Cherry-Chocolate Ice Cream

Preparation Time: 15 Minutes
Cooking Time: 0 Minutes
Servings: 1

Ingredients:

- 1 frozen banana
- 1 teaspoon pure vanilla extract
- 1 tablespoons maple syrup
- 1 tablespoons coconut cream
- 1 tablespoon unsweetened almond milk (or any nut milk)
- 1/4 cup frozen dark sweet cherries
- 1/8 cup dairy-free dark chocolate chips

Directions:

1. In a food processor, combine the bananas, vanilla, maple syrup, coconut cream, and almond milk. Blend until it reaches a batter-like consistency, occasionally stopping to scrape down the sides of the bowl.
2. Scoop out about 1 cup of the banana mixture and place in a freezer-safe container. Add the cherries to the food processor with the remaining banana mixture, and blend until the mixture is pink, but you can still see some chunks. Add the chocolate chips and blend again until just combined.
3. Transfer the mixture to the container with the plain banana ice cream and gently stir to create white and pink swirls. Cover and freeze until solid, about 1 hour.

Nutrition: Calories: 252 Fats: 10g Carbs: 38g Proteins: 2g Fibers: 2g

504. Raw Cacao Mint Cheesecake

Preparation Time: 10 Minutes
Cooking Time: 0 Minutes
Servings: 1

Ingredients:
Almond Base:

- ½ cups raw almonds
- 1 Medjool dates, pitted
- 1 tablespoon cacao powder
- 1 tablespoon vegan butter, melted (or coconut oil)

Chocolate Layer:

- ½ cups raw cashews
- 3 tablespoons maple syrup
- 2 tablespoons cacao powder
- ¼ cup coconut oil, melted
- ¼ teaspoon peppermint extract
- ¼ cup cacao nibs (or dark chocolate chips)

Mint Layer:

- 1½ cups raw cashews
- 1 cup mint leaves
- ¼ cup maple syrup
- 2 tablespoons coconut oil, melted

Optional Garnish:

- Cacao nibs
- Mint leaves

Directions:

1. Line the bottom of a springform pan with parchment paper. Place the cashews for the mint layer in a heatproof bowl and add boiling water to cover. Let soak 10 minutes and then drain. Set aside until ready to use.
2. In a food processor, combine all ingredients for the almond base and blend until creamy. Press the mixture down in the pan and smooth out the top with a spatula. Place in the freezer while you make the next layer.
3. Without rinsing the food processor, add all ingredients for the chocolate layer, except the cacao nibs. Blend until smooth, then use a spatula to stir in the cacao nibs. Take the pan out of the freezer and add this layer. Smooth it out evenly, and then return to the freezer while you make the top layer.
4. Rinse the food processor bowl and blade (this is to remove any chocolate residue and ensure that the top layer will be light green in color). Place all ingredients for the mint layer in the food processor and blend until smooth. Add to the pan and smooth it out evenly. Return to the freezer until ready to serve. Take out to thaw 10 minutes before serving and garnish with cacao nibs and mint leaves, if desired.

Nutrition: Calories: 271 Fats: 19g Carbs: 19g Proteins: 6g Fibers: 2g

505. Watermelon Strawberry Ice Pops

Preparation Time: 5 Minutes
Cooking Time: 0 Minutes
Servings: 1

Ingredients:

- 1 cup diced watermelon
- 1 strawberry, tops removed
- 1 tablespoon freshly squeezed lime juice

Directions:

1. In a blender, combine the watermelon, strawberries, and lime juice. Blend for 1 to 2 minutes, or until well combined.
2. Pour evenly into 6 ice-pop molds, insert ice-pop sticks, and freeze for at least 6 hours before serving.

Nutrition: Calories: 61 Fats: 0g Carbs: 15g Proteins: 1g Fibers: 1g

506. Peppermint Chocolate Nice Cream

Preparation Time: 5 Minutes
Cooking Time: 0 Minutes
Servings: 1

Ingredients:

- 3 frozen ripe bananas, broken into thirds
- 3 tablespoons plant-based milk
- 2 tablespoons cocoa powder
- 1/8 teaspoon peppermint extract

Directions:

1. In a food processor, combine the bananas, milk, cocoa powder, and peppermint.
2. Process on medium speed for 30 to 60 seconds, or until the bananas have been blended into smooth soft-serve consistency, and serve. (If you notice any banana pieces stuck toward the top and sides of the food processor, you may need to stop and scrape them down with a spatula, then pulse until smooth.)

Nutrition: Calories: 173 Fats: 2g Carbs: 43g Proteins: 3g Fibers: 6g

507. Apple Crisp with Oats

Preparation Time: 10 Minutes
Cooking Time: 35 Minutes
Servings: 1

Ingredients:

- 1 medium apples, cored and cut into ¼-inch pieces
- 1/8 cup apple juice
- 1/4 teaspoon vanilla extract
- 1/4 teaspoon ground cinnamon, divided
- 1/2 cups rolled oats
- 1/8 cup maple syrup

Directions:

1. Preheat the oven to 375°F (190°C).
2. In a large bowl, combine the apple slices, apple juice, vanilla, and ½ teaspoon of cinnamon. Mix well to thoroughly coat the apple slices.
3. Layer the apple slices on the bottom of a round or square baking dish. Take any leftover liquid and pour it over the apple slices.
4. In a large bowl, stir together the oats, maple syrup, and the remaining ½ teaspoon of cinnamon until the oats are completely coated.
5. Sprinkle the oat mixture over the apples, being sure to spread it out evenly so that none of the apple slices are visible.
6. Bake for 35 minutes, or until the oats begin to turn golden brown, and serve.

Nutrition: Calories: 213 Fats: 2g Carbs: 47g Proteins: 4g Fibers: 6g

508. Carrot Mug Cake

Preparation Time: 10 minutes
Cooking Time: 20 minutes
Servings: 1

Ingredients:

- ¼ cup whole-wheat pastry flour
- 1 tablespoon coconut sugar
- ¼ teaspoon baking powder
- 1/8 teaspoon ground cinnamon
- 1/8 teaspoon ground ginger
- Pinch of ground cloves
- Pinch of ground allspice
- Pinch of salt
- 2 tablespoons plus 2 teaspoons unsweetened almond milk
- 2 tablespoons carrot, peeled and grated
- 2 tablespoons walnuts, chopped
- 1 tablespoon raisins
- 2 teaspoons unsweetened applesauce

Directions:

1 - In a bowl, mix together the flour, sugar, baking powder, spices and salt.

2 - Add the remaining ingredients and mix until well combined.

3 - Place the mixture into a lightly greased ramekin.

4 - Set the temperature of Air Fryer to 350 degrees F to preheat for 5 minutes.

5 - After preheating, arrange the ramekin into an Air Fryer Basket.

6 - Slide the basket into Air Fryer and set the time for 20 minutes or until a toothpick inserted in the center comes out clean.

7 - When cooking time is completed, place the ramekin onto a wire rack to cool slightly before serving.

Nutrition: Calories: 303 Fat: 10.2g Carbohydrates: 48.7g Fiber: 3.2g Sugar: 19.4g Protein: 7.6g

509.   Pineapple Bites

Preparation Time: 10 minutes
Cooking Time: 10 minutes
Servings: 4

Ingredients:
- ½ of pineapple
- ¼ cup desiccated coconut

Directions:

1 - With a sharp knife, remove the outer peel of pineapple and then, cut into 1-2-inch-thick sticks lengthwise.

2 - Add the desiccated coconut in a shallow dish.

3 - Coat the pineapple sticks evenly with coconut.

4 - Set the temperature of Air Fryer to 390 degrees F to preheat for 5 minutes.

5 - After preheating, place the pineapple sticks into the greased Air Fryer Basket in a single layer.

6 - Slide the basket into Air Fryer and set the time for 10 minutes.

7 - When cooking time is completed, transfer the pineapple sticks onto a platter.

8 - Serve warm.

Nutrition: Calories: 74 Fat: 1.8g Carbohydrates: 15.6g Fiber: 2g Sugar: 11.5g Protein: 0.8g

510.   Fried Banana Slices

Preparation Time: 15 minutes
Cooking Time: 15 minutes
Servings: 8

Ingredients:
- 1/3 cup white rice flour, divided
- 2 tablespoons all-purpose flour
- 2 tablespoons cornflour
- 2 tablespoons desiccated coconut
- ½ teaspoon baking powder
- ½ teaspoon ground cardamom

- Pinch of salt
- Water, as required
- ¼ cup sesame seeds
- 4 medium ripe bananas, peeled

Directions:

1 - In a shallow bowl, mix together 2 tablespoons of rice flour, all-purpose flour, cornflour, coconut, baking powder, cardamom, and salt.

2 - Gradually add enough water and mix until a thick and smooth mixture forms.

3 - In a second bowl, place the remaining rice flour.

4 - In a third bowl, place the sesame seeds.

5 - Cut each banana into half and then cut each half in 2 pieces lengthwise.

6 - Dip the banana slices into the coconut mixture and then coat with the remaining rice flour, followed by the sesame seeds.

7 - Set the temperature of Ninja Air Fryer to 392 degrees F to preheat for 5 minutes.

8 - After preheating, line the Air Fryer Basket with a greased and floured piece of foil.

9 - Arrange the banana slices into the prepared Air Fryer Basket in a single layer.

10 - Slide the basket into Air Fryer and set the time for 15 minutes.

11 - While cooking, flip the banana slices once halfway through.

12 - When cooking time is completed, transfer the banana slices onto plates to cool slightly

13 - Serve warm.

Nutrition: Calories: 121 Fat: 3g Carbohydrates: 23.1g Fiber: 2.6g Sugar: 7.3g Protein: 2.2g

511.   Nutty Pears

Preparation Time: 10 minutes
Cooking Time: 30 minutes
Servings: 2

Ingredients:
- 1 ripe pear, halved and cored
- 1/8 teaspoon ground cinnamon
- 6 semisweet chocolate chips
- 2 tablespoons pecans, chopped
- 1 teaspoon pure maple syrup

Directions:

1 - Set the temperature of Air Fryer to 350 degrees F to preheat for 5 minutes.

2 - After preheating, arrange the pear halves into the greased Air Fryer Basket, cut sides up and sprinkle with cinnamon.

3 - Top each half with chocolate chips and pecans and drizzle with maple syrup.

4 - Slide the basket into Air Fryer and set the time for 30 minutes.

5 - When cooking time is completed, transfer the pear halves onto a platter.

6 - Serve warm.

Nutrition: Calories: 136 Fat: 7.5g Carbohydrates: 18.5g Fiber: 3.4g Sugar: 12.5g Protein: 1.1g

512.   Stuffed Apples

Preparation Time: 10 minutes
Cooking Time: 20 minutes
Servings: 2

Ingredients:

*   2 tablespoons raisins
*   2 tablespoons walnuts, chopped
*   1 teaspoon coconut oil, melted
*   ¼ teaspoon ground nutmeg
*   ¼ teaspoon ground cinnamon
*   1 medium apple
*   ¼ cup water

Directions:

1 - In a bowl, mix together the raisins, walnut, coconut oil, cinnamon and nutmeg.

2 - Cut the apple in half around the middle and with a scooper, scoop out some flesh.

3 - Stuff each apple half with raisin mixture.

4 - Set the temperature of Air Fryer to 350 degrees F to preheat for 5 minutes.

5 - After preheating, arrange the apple halves into the Air Fryer pan.

6 - Carefully place the water into the Air Fryer Pan.

7 - Slide the pan into Air Fryer and set the time for 20 minutes.

8 - When cooking time is completed, transfer the apple halves onto a platter.

9 - Serve warm.

Nutrition: Calories: 155 Fat: 7.2g Carbohydrates: 23.7g Fiber: 3.8g Sugar: 17.1g Protein: 2.5g

513.   Black and White Brownies

Preparation Time: 10 minutes
Cooking Time: 20 minutes
Servings: 8

Ingredients:

*   1 flax egg
*   ¼ cup brown sugar
*   2 tablespoons white sugar
*   2 tablespoons safflower oil
*   1 teaspoon vanilla
*   ¼ cup cocoa powder
*   1/3 cup all-purpose flour
*   ¼ cup white chocolate chips
*   Non-stick baking spray with flour

Directions:

1 - In a medium bowl, beat the flax egg with brown sugar and white sugar. Beat in the oil and vanilla.

2 - Add the cocoa powder and flour, and stir just until combined. Fold in the white chocolate chips.

3 - Spray a 6-by-6-by-2-inch baking pan with non-stick spray. Spoon the brownie batter into the pan.

4 - Air Frying. Bake for 20 minutes or until the brownies are set when lightly touched with a finger. Let cool for 30 minutes before slicing to serve.

Nutrition: Calories: 81 Fat: 4 g Protein: 1 g Fiber 1 g

514.   Baked Apple

Preparation Time: 5 minutes
Cooking Time: 20 minutes
Servings: 4

Ingredients:

*   ¼ cup water
*   ¼ teaspoon nutmeg
*   ¼ teaspoon cinnamon
*   1-½ teaspoons melted ghee
*   2 tablespoons raisins
*   2 tablespoons chopped walnuts
*   1 medium apple

Directions:

1 - Preheat your Air Fryer to 350°Fahrenheit.

2 - Slice an apple in half and discard some of the flesh from the center.

3 - Place into the frying pan.

4 - Mix remaining ingredients together except water. Spoon mixture to the middle of apple halves.

5 - Pour water overfilled apples.

6 - Air Frying. Place pan with apple halves into the Kalorik Maxx Air Fryer, bake 20 minutes.

Nutrition: Calories: 199 Fat: 9 g Protein: 1 g Sugar 3 g

515.   Cinnamon Fried Bananas

Preparation Time: 5 minutes

Cooking Time: 10 minutes
Servings: 2-3
Ingredients:
- 1 cup panko breadcrumbs
- 3 tablespoon cinnamon
- ½ cup almond flour
- 3 flax eggs
- 8 ripe bananas
- 3 tablespoon vegan coconut oil

Directions:
1 - Heat coconut oil and add breadcrumbs. Mix around 2-3 minutes until golden. Pour into a bowl.
2 - Peel and cut bananas in half. Roll half of each banana into flour, eggs, and crumb mixture.
3 - Air Frying. Place into the Kalorik Maxx Air Fryer. Cook 10 minutes at 280°Fahrenheit.
4 - A great addition to a healthy banana split!
Nutrition: Calories: 219 Fat: 10 g Protein: 3 g Sugar 5 g

516. Awesome Chinese Doughnuts

Preparation Time: 10 minutes
Cooking Time: 8 minutes
Servings: 8
Ingredients:
- 1 tablespoon baking powder
- 1 tablespoon coconut oil
- ¾ cup coconut milk
- 6 teaspoons sugar
- 2 cup all-purpose flour
- ½ teaspoon sea salt

Directions:
1 - Preheat the Air Fryer to 350°Fahrenheit.
2 - Mix baking powder, flour, sugar, and salt in a bowl.
3 - Add coconut oil and mix well. Add coconut milk and mix until well combined.
4 - Knead the dough for 3-4 minutes.
5 - Roll dough half-inch thick and using a cookie cutter cut doughnuts.
6 - Place doughnuts in a cake pan and brush with oil. Place cake pan in Air Fryer basket and air fry doughnuts for 5 minutes. Turn doughnuts to the other side and air fry for 3 minutes more.
7 - Serve and enjoy.
Nutrition: Calories: 259 Fat: 15.9 g Carbohydrates: 27 g Protein: 3.8 g

517. Crispy Bananas

Preparation Time: 10 minutes

Cooking Time: 10 minutes
Servings: 4
Ingredients:
- 4 sliced ripe bananas
- 1 flax egg
- ½ cup breadcrumbs
- 1-½ tablespoons cinnamon sugar
- 1 tablespoon almond meal
- 1-½ tablespoons coconut oil
- 1 tablespoon crushed cashew
- ¼ cup cornflour

Directions:
1 - Set the pan on fire to heat the coconut oil over medium heat and add breadcrumbs in the pan and stir for 3-4 minutes.
2 - Remove pan from heat and transfer breadcrumbs to a bowl.
3 - Add almond meal and crush cashew in breadcrumbs and mix well.
4 - Dip banana half in cornflour then in flax egg and finally coat with breadcrumbs.
5 - Place coated banana in Air Fryer basket. Sprinkle with cinnamon sugar.
6 - Air fry at 350°Fahrenheit/176°Celsius for 10 minutes.
7 - Serve and enjoy.
Nutrition: Calories: 282 Fat: 9 g Carbohydrates: 46 g Protein: 5 g

518. Air Fried Banana and Walnuts Muffins

Preparation Time: 10 minutes
Cooking Time: 10 minutes
Servings: 2
Ingredients:
- ¼ cup flour
- ½ teaspoon baking powder
- ¼ cup mashed banana
- ¼ cup butter
- 1 tablespoon chopped walnuts
- ¼ cup oats

Directions:
1 - Spray four muffin molds with cooking spray and set them aside.
2 - In a bowl, mix together mashed bananas, walnuts, sugar, and butter.
3 - In another bowl, mix oat flour, and baking powder.
4 - Combine the flour mixture with the banana mixture.
5 - Pour batter into the muffin mold.

6 - Place in Air Fryer basket and cook at 320°Fahrenheit/160°Celsius for 10 minutes.

7 - Remove muffins from the Air Fryer and allow them to cool completely.

8 - Serve and enjoy.

Nutrition: Calories: 192 Fat: 12.3 g Carbohydrates: 19.4 g Protein: 1.9 g

519. Nutty Mix

Preparation Time: 5 minutes
Cooking Time: 4 minutes
Servings: 6
Ingredients:

- 2 cup mix nuts
- 1 teaspoon ground cumin
- 1 teaspoon chili powder
- 1 tablespoon melted butter
- 1 teaspoon salt
- 1 teaspoon pepper

Directions:

1 - Set all ingredients in a large bowl and toss until well coated.

2 - Preheat the Air Fryer at 350°Fahrenheit for 5 minutes.

3 - Add mix nuts in the Air Fryer basket and air fry for 4 minutes. Shake basket halfway through.

4 - Serve and enjoy.

Nutrition: Calories: 316 Fat: 29 g Carbohydrates: 11.3 g Protein: 7.6 g

520. Chocolate Cup Cakes

Preparation Time: 5 minutes
Cooking Time: 12 minutes
Servings: 6
Ingredients:

- 3 eggs
- ¼ cup caster sugar
- ¼ cup cocoa powder
- 1 teaspoon baking powder
- 1 cup coconut milk
- ¼ teaspoon vanilla essence
- 2 cup all-purpose flour
- 4 tablespoons butter

Directions:

1 - Preheat your Air Fryer to a temperature of 400°Fahrenheit (200°Celsius).

2 - Beat eggs with sugar in a bowl until creamy.

3 - Add butter and beat again for 1-2 minutes.

4 - Now add flour, cocoa powder, milk, baking powder, and vanilla essence, mix with a spatula.

5 - Fill ¾ of muffin tins with the mixture and place them into the Air Fryer basket.

6 - Let cook for 12 minutes.

Nutrition: Calories: 289 Fat: 11.5 g Carbohydrates: 38.94 g Protein: 8.72 g

521. Air Baked Cheesecake

Preparation Time: 20 minutes
Cooking Time: 20 minutes
Servings: 8-12
Ingredients:
Crust:

- ½ cup dates, chopped, soaked in water for at least 15 min., soaking liquid reserved
- ½ cup walnuts
- 1 cup quick oats

Filling:

- ½ cup vanilla almond milk
- ¼ cup coconut palm sugar
- ½ cup coconut flour
- 1 cup cashews, soaked in water for at least 2 hours
- 1 teaspoon vanilla extract
- 2 tablespoons lemon juice
- 1 to 2 teaspoons grated lemon zest
- ½ cup fresh berries or 6 figs, sliced
- 1 tablespoon arrowroot powder

Directions:

1 - Make the crust: in a food processor, process together with all the crust ingredients until smooth and press the mixture into the bottom of a springform pan.

2 - Make the filling: add cashews along with soaking liquid to a blender and process until very smooth; add milk, palm sugar, coconut flour, lemon juice, lemon zest, and vanilla and blend until well combined; add arrowroot and continue blending until mixed and pour into the crust. Smooth the top and cover the springform pan with foil.

3 - Place the pan in your air fry toaster oven and bake at 375°Fahrenheit for 20 minutes.

4 - Carefully remove the pan from the fryer and remove the foil; let the cake cool completely and top with fruit to serve.

Nutrition: Calories: 423 Fat: 3.1 g Carbohydrates: 33.5 g Protein: 1.2 g

522. Air Roasted Nuts

Preparation Time: 10 minutes
Cooking Time: 20 minutes
Servings: 8

Ingredients:
* 1 cup raw peanuts
* ½ teaspoon cayenne pepper
* 3 teaspoons seafood seasoning
* 2 tablespoons olive oil
* Salt to taste

Directions:
1 - Preheat your Air Fryer toast oven to 320ºFahrenheit.
2 - In a bowl, whisk together cayenne pepper, olive oil, and seafood seasoning; stir in peanuts until well coated.
3 - Transfer to the fryer basket and air roast for 10 minutes; toss well and then cook for another 10 minutes.
4 - Transfer the peanuts to a dish and season with salt. Let cool before serving.
Nutrition: Calories: 193 Fat: 17.4 g Carbohydrates: 4.9 g Protein: 7.4 g

523. Air Fried White Corn

Preparation Time: 10 minutes
Cooking Time: 40 minutes
Servings: 8

Ingredients:
* 2 cups giant white corn
* 3 tablespoons olive oil
* 1-½ teaspoons sea salt

Directions:
1 - Soak the corn in a bowl of water for at least 8 hours or overnight; drain and spread in a single layer on a baking tray; pat dry with paper towels.
2 - Preheat your Air Fryer toast oven to 400°Fahrenheit.
3 - In a bowl, mix corn, olive oil, and salt and toss to coat well.
4 - Air fry corn in batches in the preheated Air Fryer toast oven for 20 minutes, shaking the basket halfway through cooking.
5 - Let the corn cool for at least 20 minutes or until crisp.
Nutrition: Calories: 225 Fat: 7.4 g Carbohydrates: 35.8 g Protein: 5.9 g

524. Fruit Cake

Preparation Time: 5 minutes
Cooking Time: 45 minutes

Servings: 4-6

Ingredients:
Dry Ingredients:
* 1 teaspoon sea salt
* ½ teaspoon baking powder
* ½ teaspoon baking soda
* ½ teaspoon ground cardamom
* 1-¼ cups whole wheat flour

Wet Ingredients:
* 2 tablespoons coconut oil
* ½ cup unsweetened nondairy milk
* 2 tablespoons ground flax seeds
* ¼ cup agave
* 1-½ cups water

Mix-Ingredients:
* ½ cup chopped cranberries
* 1 cup chopped pear

Directions:
1 - Grease a Bundt pan; set aside.
2 - In a mixing, mix all dry ingredients together. In another bowl, combine together the wet ingredients; whisk the wet ingredients into the dry until smooth.
3 - Fold in the add-ins and spread the mixture into the pan; cover with foil.
4 - Place pan in your Air Fryer toast oven and add water in the bottom and bake at 370°Fahrenheit for 35 minutes.
5 - When done, use a toothpick to check for doneness. If it comes out clean, then the cake is ready, if not, bake for 5-10 more minutes, checking frequently to avoid burning.
6 - Remove the cake and let stand for 10 minutes before transferring from the pan.
Nutrition: Calories: 309 Fat: 27 g Carbohydrates: 14.7 g Protein: 22.6 g

525. Banana Walnut Bread

Preparation Time: 5 Minutes
Cooking Time: 50 Minutes
Servings: 1

Ingredients:
* 1/2 cups whole wheat flour
* ¾ teaspoon baking soda
* 1 very ripe banana, mashed
* ½ cup maple syrup
* ¼ cup unsweetened applesauce

- 2 tablespoons aquafaba (the liquid from a can of chickpeas)
- 1 teaspoon vanilla extract
- 1 teaspoon pink Himalayan salt
- ¾ cup chopped walnuts

Directions:
1. Preheat the oven to 180 C or 350 F.
2. Line the pan using parchment paper or a silicone liner.
3. In a mixing bowl, sift the flour and baking soda together.
4. In a separate container, combine the mashed bananas, maple syrup, applesauce, aquafaba, vanilla, and salt. Mix well. Stir in the flour mixture and mix well. Gently stir the walnuts.
5. Transfer the combination into the arranged pan. Bake it for 40 to 50 minutes, until brown on the top and edges. Enjoy right after it cools or store it in a reusable container at room temperature for up to 5 days.

Nutrition: Calories: 541 Fats: 17g Carbs: 96g Proteins: 12g Fibers: 11g

526. Cashew Chickpea Bars

Preparation Time: 5 Minutes
Cooking Time: 15 Minutes
Servings: 1
Ingredients:
- 1 Medjool dates, pitted
- 1/4 cup cashews
- 1/4 cup cooked chickpeas (drained and rinsed, if canned)
- 1 tablespoon sunflower seed
- 1 tablespoon pumpkin seed
- 1 teaspoon vanilla extract
- 8 ounces (227 g) vegan dark mini chocolate chips

Directions:
1. Line a baking sheet with parchment paper or a silicone liner.
2. In a food processor, combine the dates, cashews, chickpeas, sunflower seeds, pumpkin seeds, and vanilla. Blend, but leave the mixture a little chunky.
3. Shape the mixture into bars and place them on the prepared baking sheet. Bake for 15 minutes, or until the edges become lightly browned.

Remove from the oven and let cool for 10 minutes.
4. In a small saucepan over low heat, stir the chocolate chips until melted. Coat the top of the bars with the melted chocolate and let cool to room temperature.

Nutrition: Calories: 299 Fats: 15g Carbs: 42g Proteins: 5g Fibers: 5g

527. Chocolate Avocado Pudding

Preparation Time: 5 Minutes
Cooking Time: 0 Minutes
Servings: 1
Ingredients:
- 2 ripe avocados, pitted and peeled
- ¼ cup unsweetened plant-based milk
- 1/3 cup coconut sugar
- 1/3 cup cocoa powder
- 1 teaspoon vanilla extract

Directions:
1. In a food processor, combine all the ingredients and blend until you achieve a smooth pudding consistency. Serve immediately.

Nutrition: Calories: 457 Fats: 29g Carbs: 56g Proteins: 6g Fibers: 17g

528. Cranberry and Almond Muffins

Preparation Time: 10 Minutes
Cooking Time: 20 Minutes
Servings: 1
Ingredients:
- 1/2 cups whole wheat flour (or gluten-free flour)
- 1 teaspoon baking soda
- 1 teaspoon baking powder
- ½ teaspoon pink Himalayan salt
- 1/4 cup unsweetened plant-based milk
- 1/8 cup dried cranberries, soaked in water for 1 hour to soften
- 1/8 cup maple syrup
- 1/8 cup chopped almonds
- 1/8 cup unsweetened applesauce
- 1 tablespoon freshly squeezed lemon juice
- 1 tablespoons aquafaba (the liquid from a can of chickpeas)
- ½ teaspoon vanilla extract

Directions:

1. Preheat the oven to 375°F (190°C). Insert silicone muffin cups into a muffin pan.
2. In a bowl, combine the flour, baking soda, baking powder, and salt and mix well.
3. In a separate bowl, combine the milk, cranberries, maple syrup, almonds, applesauce, lemon juice, aquafaba, and vanilla and mix well.
4. Combine the wet and dry ingredients and mix well.
5. Fill each muffin cup a little more than half full with batter. Bake for 20 minutes, or until lightly browned and a toothpick inserted into the center of a muffin comes out clean. Enjoy as soon as they cool or store in a reusable container at room temperature.

Nutrition: Calories: 143 Fats: 2g Carbs: 31g Proteins: 3g Fibers: 3g

529. Chocolate Chip Cashew Bites

Preparation Time: 10 Minutes
Cooking Time: 0 Minutes
Servings: 1
Ingredients:
- ¼ cup rolled oats
- ½ cup cashews
- 3 tablespoons whole wheat flour (or gluten-free flour)
- ½ teaspoon ground flaxseed
- ¼ teaspoon Himalayan pink salt
- 2 tablespoons maple syrup
- 1 teaspoon vanilla extract
- 2 tablespoons vegan dark chocolate chips

Directions:
1. In a food processor, combine the oats, cashews, flour, flaxseed, and salt. When the dry ingredients are fully mixed, add the maple syrup and vanilla and continue to mix in the processor.
2. Add the chocolate chips and mix them in with a spoon. Using your hands, shape the mixture into 1-inch balls. Enjoy immediately or store in a reusable container in the refrigerator for up to 5 days.

Nutrition: Calories: 81 Fats: 4g Carbs: 10g Proteins: 2g Fibers: 1g

530. Banana Orange Nice Cream

Preparation Time: 5 Minutes
Cooking Time: 0 Minutes
Servings: 1
Ingredients:
- 1 orange, peeled, separated into segments, and frozen
- 2 bananas, peeled, sliced, and frozen
- ½ teaspoon vanilla extract
- ¼ teaspoon hemp seeds

Directions:
1. In a food processor or blender, combine all the ingredients and blend until smooth and creamy. Enjoy immediately or store in a reusable container in the freezer for up to 1 month.

Nutrition: Calories: 283 Fats: 1g Carbs: 70g Proteins: 4g Fibers: 9g

531. Pineapple Coconut Macaroons

Preparation Time: 5 Minutes
Cooking Time: 20 Minutes
Servings: 1
Ingredients:
- 1/3 cups unsweetened coconut shreds
- ½ cup chopped pineapple
- ½ cup coconut sugar
- ½ banana
- 3 tablespoons wheat flour (or gluten-free flour)

Directions:
1. Preheat the oven to 350°F (180°C). Line a baking sheet with parchment paper or a silicone liner.
2. In a food processor, combine all the ingredients and process until almost smooth.
3. Use a tablespoon to make 10 heaping macaroons. Space them evenly on the prepared baking sheet.
4. Bake for 20 minutes, or until the tops and bottoms are light browns.
5. Let cool on a wire rack for 10 minutes before serving. Store in a reusable container in the refrigerator for up to 5 days.

Nutrition: Calories: 90 Fats: 4g Carbs: 15g Proteins: 1g Fibers: 1g

532. Hydrated Apples

Preparation Time: 5 minutes
Cooking Time: 15 minutes
Servings: 6
Ingredients:

- 6 Apples, cored
- 1 teaspoon cinnamon powder
- ½ cup sugar
- 1 cup red wine
- ¼ cup raisins

Directions:

1 - Add apples to your Air Fryer toast oven's pan and then add wine, cinnamon powder, sugar and raisins.

2 - Hydrate for 20 minutes and remove from air fry toaster oven.

3 - Serve the apples in small serving bowls drizzled with lots of cooking juices.

Nutrition: Calories: 229 Fat: 0.4 g Carbohydrates: 53.3 g Protein: 0.8 g

533.   Banana and Walnut Bread

Preparation Time: 5 minutes

Cooking Time: 1 hour and 10 minutes

Servings: 6-8

Ingredients:

- 1-½ cups unbleached flour
- ½ cup sugar or sugar substitute
- 2 teaspoons baking powder
- ½ teaspoon baking soda
- ½ teaspoon vanilla extract
- ½ teaspoon sea salt
- 1 cup ripe bananas, mashed
- 1 cup softened butter
- ¼ cup almond milk
- 1 flax egg
- ¼ cup walnuts chopped

Directions:

1 - Combine the flour, sugar, baking powder, baking soda, and salt in a large mixing bowl; whisk until the ingredients are well mixed.

2 - Fold in the bananas, butter, milk, egg, and vanilla extract. Use an electric mixer to mix until the batter has a uniform thick consistency.

3 - Fold in chopped walnuts.

4 - Grease the bottom of the Air Fryer oven pan with non-stick cooking spray.

5 - Pour batter into Air Fryer oven pan and cook for 1 hour. Transfer to plate and let cool for one hour before serving.

Nutrition: Calories: 255 Fat: 11 g Carbohydrates: 36.1 g Protein: 4.6 g Sodium 211 mg Fiber 1.4 g

534.   Choco-Peanut Mug Cake

Preparation Time: 5 minutes

Cooking Time: 20 minutes

Servings: 1

Ingredients:

- 1 teaspoon softened butter
- 1 falx egg
- 1 teaspoon butter
- 1 teaspoon vanilla extract
- 2 tablespoons erythritol
- 2 tablespoons unsweetened cocoa powder
- ¼ teaspoon baking powder
- 1 tablespoon heavy cream

Directions:

1 - Preheat the Air Fryer for 5 minutes.

2 - Combine all ingredients in a mixing bowl.

3 - Pour into a greased mug.

4 - Set in the Air Fryer basket and cook for 20 minutes at 400°Fahrenheit.

Nutrition: Calories: 293 Fat: 23.3 g Carbohydrates: 8.5 g Protein: 12.4 g

535.   Raspberry-Coco Desert

Preparation Time: 5 minutes

Cooking Time: 20 minutes

Servings: 12

Ingredients:

- 1 teaspoon vanilla bean
- 1 cup pulsed raspberries
- 1 cup coconut milk
- 3 cups desiccated coconut
- ¼ cup coconut oil
- 1 cup erythritol powder

Directions:

1 - Preheat the Air Fryer for 5 minutes.

2 - Combine all ingredients in a mixing bowl.

3 - Pour into a greased baking dish.

4 - Bake in the Air Fryer for 20 minutes at 375°Fahrenheit.

Nutrition: Calories: 132 Fat: 9.7 g Carbohydrates: 9.7 g Protein: 1.5 g

536.   Almond Cherry Bars

Preparation Time: 5 minutes

Cooking Time: 35 minutes

Servings: 12

Ingredients:

- 1 tablespoon xanthan gum
- 1-½ cups almond flour

- ½ teaspoon salt
- 1 cup pitted fresh cherries
- ½ cup softened butter
- 2 eggs
- ¼ cup water
- ½ teaspoon vanilla
- 1 cup erythritol

Directions:

1 - Combine almond flour, softened butter, salt, vanilla, eggs, and erythritol in a large bowl until you form a dough.

2 - Press the dough in a baking dish that will fit in the Air Fryer.

3 - Set in the Air Fryer and bake for 10 minutes at 375°Fahrenheit.

4 - Meanwhile, mix the cherries, water, and xanthan gum in a bowl.

5 - Take the dough out and pour over the cherry mixture.

6 - Cook again for 25 minutes more at 375°Fahrenheit in the Air Fryer.

Nutrition: Calories: 99 Fat: 9.3 g Carbohydrates: 2.1 g Protein: 1.8 g

537. Coffee Flavored Doughnuts

Preparation Time: 5 minutes
Cooking Time: 6 minutes
Servings: 6
Ingredients:

- 1 teaspoon baking powder
- ½ teaspoon salt
- 1 tablespoon sunflower oil
- ¼ cup coffee
- ¼ cup coconut sugar
- 1 cup white all-purpose flour
- 2 tablespoons aquafaba

Directions:

1 - Combine sugar, flour, baking powder, salt in a mixing bowl.

2 - In another bowl, combine the aquafaba, sunflower oil, and coffee.

3 - Mix to form a dough.

4 - Let the dough rest inside the fridge.

5 - Preheat the Air Fryer to 400°Fahrenheit.

6 - Knead the dough and create doughnuts.

7 - Arrange inside the Air Fryer in a single layer and cook for 6 minutes.

8 - Do not shake so that the donut maintains its shape.

Nutrition: Calories: 113 Fat: 2.54 g Carbohydrates: 20.45 g Protein: 21.6 g

538. Simple Strawberry Cobbler

Preparation Time: 10 minutes
Cooking Time: 25 minutes
Servings: 4
Ingredients:

- ¼ cup heavy whipping cream
- 1-½ teaspoons cornstarch
- 1-½ teaspoons white sugar
- ½ cup water
- ¼ teaspoon salt
- 2 teaspoons butter
- 1-½ cups hulled strawberries
- 1-½ teaspoons white sugar
- 1 tablespoon diced butter
- 1 tablespoon butter
- ½ cup all-purpose flour
- ¾ teaspoon baking powder

Directions:

1 - Lightly grease baking pan of Air Fryer with cooking spray. Add water, cornstarch, and sugar. Cook for 10 minutes 390°Fahrenheit or until hot and thick. Add strawberries and mix well. Dot tops with 1 tablespoon butter.

2 - In a bowl, mix well salt, baking powder, sugar, and flour. Cut in 2 teaspoons butter. Mix in cream. Spoon on top of berries.

3 - Cook for 15 minutes at 390°Fahrenheit, until tops, are lightly browned.

Nutrition: Calories: 255 Fat: 13 g Carbohydrates: 32 g Protein: 2.4 g

539. Easy Pumpkin Pie

Preparation Time: 5 minutes
Cooking Time: 35 minutes
Servings: 8
Ingredients:

- 3 flax eggs
- ½ teaspoon ground ginger
- ½ teaspoon fine salt
- 1 teaspoon Chinese 5-spice powder
- 19-inch unbaked pie crust
- ¼ teaspoon freshly grated nutmeg
- 14 ounces almond milk
- 15 ounces pumpkin puree
- 1 teaspoon ground cinnamon

Directions:

1 - Lightly grease baking pan of Air Fryer with cooking spray. Press pie crust on the bottom of the pan, stretching up to the sides of the pan. Pierce all over with a fork.

2 - In a blender, blend well flax eggs, and pumpkin puree. Add Chinese 5-spice powder, nutmeg, salt, ginger, cinnamon, and milk. Pour on top of pie crust.

3 - Cover pan with foil.

4 - For 15 minutes, cook on preheated 390°Fahrenheit Air Fryer.

5 - Cook for 20 more minutes at 330°Fahrenheit without the foil until the middle is set.

6 - Allow cooling in the Air Fryer completely.

Nutrition: Calories: 326 Fat: 14.2 g Carbohydrates: 41.9 g Protein: 7.6 g

540. Simple Cheesecake

Preparation Time: 10 minutes
Cooking Time: 19 minutes
Servings: 5

Ingredients:

- 1 cup crumbled graham crackers
- ½ teaspoon vanilla extract
- 4 tablespoons sugar
- 2 tablespoons butter
- 1 pound cream cheese
- 2 eggs

Directions:

1 - Mix crackers with the butter in a bowl.

2 - Press crackers mixture on the bottom of a lined cake pan.

3 - Transfer to the Air Fryer to cook at 350°Fahrenheit for 4 minutes.

4 - Meanwhile, in a bowl, mix eggs, cream cheese, sugar and vanilla, then whisk well.

5 - Spread filling over crackers crust and cook in the Air Fryer at 310°Fahrenheit for 15 minutes.

6 - Cool and keep in the refrigerator for 3 hours.

7 - Slice and serve.

Nutrition: Calories: 245 Fat: 12 g Carbohydrates: 20 g Protein: 3 g

541. Strawberry Donuts

Preparation Time: 10 minutes
Cooking Time: 15 minutes
Servings: 4

Ingredients:

- 4 ounces whole coconut milk
- 1 flax egg
- 1 teaspoon baking powder
- 1 tablespoon brown sugar
- 1 tablespoon white sugar
- 8 ounces flour
- ½ tablespoons butter

For the strawberry icing:

- 1 tablespoon whipped cream
- ½ teaspoon pink coloring
- 2 tablespoons butter
- ¼ cup chopped strawberries

Directions:

1 - In a bowl, mix flour, 1 tablespoon white sugar, 1 tablespoon brown sugar and butter, and stir.

2 - Stir together the flax egg with almond milk, and 1-½ tablespoon butter in another bowl.

3 - Combine the 2 mixtures, stir, then shape donuts from this mix.

4 - Cook the doughnuts in the Air Fryer at 360°Fahrenheit for 15 minutes.

5 - Mix strawberry puree, whipped cream, food coloring, icing sugar, and 1 tablespoon butter, and whisk well.

6 - Arrange donuts on a platter and serve with strawberry icing on top.

Nutrition: Calories: 250 Fat: 12 g Carbohydrates: 32 g Protein: 4 g

542. Apricot Blackberry Crumble

Preparation Time: 10 minutes
Cooking Time: 20 minutes
Servings: 8

Ingredients:

- 1 cup flour
- 2 tablespoons lemon juice
- 2 ounces cubed and deseeded fresh apricots
- ½ cup sugar
- 2 tablespoons cold butter
- 5-½ ounces fresh blackberries
- Salt to taste

Directions:

1 - Put the apricots and blackberries in a bowl. Add lemon juice and 2 tablespoons of sugar. Mix until combined. Transfer the mixture to a baking dish.

2 - Mix flour, the rest of the sugar, and a pinch of salt in a bowl.

3 - Add a tablespoon of cold butter. Combine the mixture until it becomes crumbly. Put this on top of the fruit mixture and press it down lightly.

4 - Move the baking dish to the cooking basket. Cook for 20 minutes at 390°Fahrenheit.

5 - Allow cooling before slicing and serving.

Nutrition: Calories: 217 Fat: 7.44 g Carbohydrates: 36.2 g Protein: 2.3 g

543.   Chocolate Coconut Cookies

Preparation Time: 15 minutes
Cooking Time: 12 minutes
Servings: 8
Ingredients:
- 1 tablespoon ground flaxseed
- 3 tablespoons water
- 2¼ ounces caster sugar
- 3½ ounces coconut oil
- 1 teaspoon vanilla extract
- 5 ounces self-rising flour
- 1¼ ounces vegan chocolate, chopped
- 3 tablespoons desiccated coconut

Directions:
1 - In a small bowl, add flaxseed and water and mix well. Set aside for about 5 minutes.

2 - In a large bowl, add the sugar and coconut oil and beat until fluffy and light

3 - Add the flaxseed mixture and vanilla extract and beat until well combined

4 - Now, add the flour and chocolate and mix well.

5 - In a shallow bowl, place the coconut.

6 - With your hands, make small balls from the mixture.

7 - Roll each dough ball into the coconut evenly.

8 - Press each ball slightly.

9 - Set the temperature of Air Fryer to 355 degrees F to preheat for 5 minutes.

10 - After preheating, place the cookies into the Air Fryer Basket.

11 - Slide the basket into Air Fryer and set the time for 8 minutes.

12 - When cooking time is completed, remove the basket from Air fryer and place onto a wire rack to cool for about 5 minutes.

13 - Now, invert the cookies onto the wire rack to cool completely before serving.

Nutrition: Calories: 238 Fat: 14.8g Carbohydrates: 24.7g Fiber: 1g Sugar: 10.5g Protein: 2.4g

544.   Shortbread Fingers

Preparation Time: 15 minutes
Cooking Time: 12 minutes
Servings: 10
Ingredients:
- 1 2/3 cups all-purpose flour
- 1/3 cup caster sugar
- ¾ cup coconut oil

Directions:
1 - In a large bowl, mix together the sugar and flour.

2 - Add the coconut oil and mix until a smooth dough forms.

3 - Cut the dough into 10 equal-sized fingers.

4 - With a fork, lightly prick the fingers.

5 - Arrange fingers onto the greased baking sheet in a single layer.

6 - Set the temperature of Air Fryer to 350 degrees F to preheat for 5 minutes.

7 - After preheating, arrange the baking sheet into the Air Fryer Basket.

8 - Slide the basket into Air Fryer and set the time for 12 minutes.

9 - Remove the baking sheet from Air Fryer and place onto a wire rack to cool for about 5-10 minutes.

10 - Now, invert the shortbread fingers onto the wire rack to completely cool before serving.

Nutrition: Calories: 242 Fat: 16.6g Carbohydrates: 22.6g Fiber: 0.6g Sugar: 6.7g Protein: 2.2g

545.   Cinnamon Rolls

Preparation Time: 15 minutes
Cooking Time: 7 minutes
Servings: 8
Ingredients:
For Cinnamon Rolls:
- ¼ cup coconut oil, softened
- 6 tablespoons brown sugar
- 1 tablespoon ground cinnamon
- 1 frozen vegan puff pastry sheet, thawed
For Icing:
- ½ cup powdered white sugar
- 1 tablespoon unsweetened almond milk
- 2 teaspoons fresh lemon juice

Directions:
1 - In a small bowl, add the coconut oil, sugar and cinnamon and mix well.

2 - Place the puff pastry onto a smooth surface and gently roll it.

3 - Place the cinnamon mixture over the pastry in a thin layer.

4 - Starting from the shorter end, roll the pastry gently and loosely.

5 - With a serrated knife, cut the pastry into 1-inch pieces.

6 - Set the temperature of Air Fryer to 400 degrees F to preheat for 5 minutes.

7 - After preheating, arrange the roll pieces into the greased Air Fryer Basket.

8 - Slide the basket into Air Fryer and set the time for 7 minutes.

9 - When cooking time is completed, remove the roll pieces and place onto a platter to cool slightly before icing.

10 - For icing: in a bowl, add all the ingredients and beat until well combined.

11 - Drizzle the rolls with icing and serve warm.

Nutrition: Calories: 285 Fat: 18.5g Carbohydrates: 28.6g Fiber: 0.9g Sugar: 14.2g Protein: 2.3g

546.   Fudge Brownies

Preparation Time: 10 minutes
Cooking Time: 15 minutes
Servings: 4

Ingredients:

- ½ cup all-purpose flour
- ¾ cup white sugar
- 6 tablespoons unsweetened cocoa powder
- ¼ teaspoon baking powder
- ¼ teaspoon salt
- ½ cup unsweetened applesauce
- ¼ cup coconut oil, melted
- 1 tablespoon vegetable oil
- ½ teaspoon vanilla extract

Directions:

1 - In a large bowl, mix together the flour, sugar, cocoa powder, baking powder and salt.

2 - Add the remaining ingredients and mix until well combined.

3 - Place the mixture into a generously greased 7-inch baking pan evenly.

4 - Set the temperature of Air Fryer to 330 degrees F to preheat for 5 minutes.

5 - After preheating, arrange the baking pan into the Air Fryer Basket.

6 - Slide the basket into Air Fryer and set the time for 15 minutes.

7 - When cooking time is completed, remove the baking pan and place onto a wire rack to cool completely.

8 - Cut into desired sized squares and serve.

Nutrition: Calories: 379/ Fat: 18.3g/ Carbohydrates: 57.5g/ Fiber: 3.5g / Sugar: 40.8g/ Protein: 3.3g

Chapter 25. Sauces and Condiments

547. Mild Harissa Sauce

Preparation time: 5 minutes
Cooking time: 20 minutes
Servings: 3 to 4 cups

Ingredients:

- 1 large red bell pepper, deseeded, cored, and cut into chunks
- 4 garlic cloves, peeled
- 1 yellow onion, cut into thick rings
- 1 cup no-sodium vegetable broth or water
- 2 tbsp tomato paste
- 4 garlic cloves, peeled
- 1 tbsp low-sodium soy sauce or tamari
- 1 tsp ground cumin

Directions:

1 - Preheat the oven to 450°F (235°C). Line a baking sheet with aluminum foil or parchment paper.
2 - Put the bell pepper, flesh-side up, on the baking sheet and spread the garlic and onion around the bell pepper.
3 - Roasted in the preheated oven for 20 minutes until the pepper is lightly charred.
4 - Remove from the heat and let it cool for a few minutes.
5 - Place the bell pepper in a blender, along with the remaining ingredients, and process until smoothly puréed.
6 - Serve immediately or store in a sealed container in the refrigerator for up to 2 weeks or in the freezer for up to 6 months.

Nutrition: Calories: 16 Fat: 0.9 g Carbohydrates: 3.1 g Protein: 1.1 g Fiber: 1.3 g

548. Satay Sauce

Preparation time: 5 minutes
Cooking time: 8 minutes
Servings: 2 cups

Ingredients:

- 1/2 yellow onion, diced
- 3 garlic cloves, minced
- 1 fresh red chili, thinly sliced (optional)
- 1-inch (2.5-cm) piece fresh ginger, peeled and minced
- 1/4 cup smooth peanut butter
- 2 tbsp coconut amino
- 1 (13 1/2 oz. / 383-g) can unsweetened coconut milk
- 1/4 tsp freshly ground black pepper
- 1/4 tsp salt (optional)

Directions:

1 - Heat a large nonstick skillet over medium-high heat until hot.
2 - Add the onion, garlic cloves, chili (if desired), and ginger to the skillet, and sauté for 2 minutes.
3 - Pour in the peanut butter and coconut amino and stir well. Add the coconut milk, black pepper, and salt (if desired) and continue whisking, or until the sauce is just beginning to bubble and thicken.
4 - Remove the sauce from the heat to a bowl. Taste and adjust the seasoning if necessary.

Nutrition: (1/2 cup): Calories: 322 Fat: 28.8 g Carbohydrates: 9.4 g Protein: 6.3 g Fiber: 1.8 g

549. Edamame Hummus

Preparation time: 15 minutes
Cooking time: 11 minutes
Servings: 5

Ingredients:

- 10 oz. frozen edamame pods
- 1 ripe avocado, peeled, pitted, and chopped roughly
- 1/2 cup fresh cilantro, chopped
- 1/4 cup scallion, chopped
- 1 jalapeno pepper
- 1 garlic clove, peeled
- 2 to 3 tbsp fresh lime juice
- Salt and ground black pepper to taste
- 1/4 cup avocado oil
- 2 tbsp fresh basil leaves
- Water to taste

Directions:

1 - In a small pot of boiling water, cook the edamame pods for 6 to 8 minutes.
2 - Drain the edamame pods and let them cool completely.
3 - Remove soybeans from the pods.
4 - In a food processor, add edamame and the remaining ingredients (except for oil) and pulse until mostly pureed.

5 - While the motor is running, add the reserved oil and pulse until light and smooth.

6 - Transfer the hummus into a bowl and serve with the garnishing of the remaining basil leaves.

Nutrition: Calories: 339 Fat: 33.8 g Saturated fat: 4.3 g Cholesterol: 0 mg Sodium: 27 mg

550. Beans Mayonnaise

Preparation time: 10 minutes
Cooking time: 2 minutes
Servings: 4
Ingredients:

- 1 (15 oz.) can of white beans, drained and rinsed
- 2 tbsp apple cider vinegar
- 1 tbsp fresh lemon juice
- 2 tbsp yellow mustard
- 3/4 tsp salt
- 2 garlic cloves, peeled
- 2 tbsp aquafaba (liquid from the can of beans)
- 1 tbsp Olive oil

Directions:

1 - In a food processor, add all ingredients (except for oil) and pulse until mostly pureed.

2 - While the motor is running, add the reserved oil and pulse until light and smooth.

3 - Transfer the mayonnaise into a container and refrigerate to chill before serving.

Nutrition: Calories: 8 Fat: 1.1 g Saturated fat: 0.1 g Cholesterol: 0 mg Sodium: 559 mg

551. Cashew Cream

Preparation time: 10 minutes
Cooking time: 0 minutes
Servings: 5
Ingredients:

- 1 cup raw, unsalted cashews, soaked for 12 hours and drained
- 1/2 cup water
- 1 tbsp nutritional yeast
- 1 tsp fresh lemon juice
- 1/8 tsp salt

Directions:

1 - In a food processor, add all ingredients and pulse at high speed until creamy and smooth.

2 - Serve immediately.

Nutrition: Calories: 165 Fat: 12.8 g Saturated fat: 2.5 g Cholesterol: 0 mg Sodium: 65 mg Carbohydrates: 9.9 g

552. Lemon Tahini

Preparation time: 15 minutes
Cooking time: 0 minutes
Servings: 4
Ingredients:

- 1/4 cup fresh lemon juice
- 4 medium garlic cloves, pressed
- 1/2 cup tahini
- 1/2 tsp fine sea salt
- A pinch of ground cumin
- 6 tbsp ice water

Directions:

1 - In a medium bowl, combine the lemon juice and garlic and set aside for 10 minutes.

2 - Through a fine-mesh sieve, strain the mixture into another medium bowl, pressing the garlic solids.

3 - Discard the garlic solids.

4 - In the bowl of lemon juice, add the tahini, salt, and cumin, and whisk until well blended.

5 - Slowly, add water, 2 tbsp at a time, whisking well after each addition.

Nutrition: Calories: 187 Fat: 16.3 g Saturated fat: 2.4 g Cholesterol: 0 mg Sodium: 273 mg

553. Pecan Butter

Preparation Time: 10 minutes
Cooking Time: 10 minutes
Servings: 8
Ingredients:

- 3 cups pecans, soaked well for at least 3 hours, rinsed, strained and dried

Directions:

1 - Add the pecans to a food processor and blend until a smooth and creamy consistency is achieved. Scrape down the sides of the bowl when necessary.

2 - Transfer to a Mason jar and store in the refrigerator. Can be stored in the refrigerator for several months. Makes a great spread on toast and sandwiches and a great fruit and veggie dip.

Nutrition: Fat: 25 g Cholesterol 0 mg Sodium 0 mg Carbohydrates: 5 g

554. Keto Vegan Ranch Dressing

Preparation Time: 5 minutes
Cooking Time: 10 minutes
Servings: 3
Ingredients:
- 1 cup vegan mayonnaise
- 1-½ cups coconut milk
- 2 scallions
- 2 garlic cloves, peeled
- 1 cup fresh dill
- 1 teaspoon garlic powder
- Salt and pepper to taste

Directions:
1 - Add scallion, fresh dill, and garlic cloves to a food processor and pulse until finely chopped.
2 - Add the rest of the ingredients and blend until a smooth, creamy consistency is achieved. Makes a great creamy salad dressing.
3 - Store in the refrigerator.
Nutrition: Fat: 11.9 g Cholesterol 0 mg Sodium 50 mg Fiber 4 g

555. Cauliflower Hummus
Preparation Time: 10 minutes
Cooking Time: 20 minutes
Servings: 7
Ingredients:
- 1 large head cauliflower
- 1 tablespoon almond butter
- 1 garlic clove, finely chopped
- 1 tablespoon lemon juice
- 2 teaspoons olive oil
- ¼ teaspoon cumin
- Salt and pepper to taste

Directions:
1 - Cut cauliflower into florets and place in a large microwave-safe bowl. Microwave for 10 minutes on high heat or until completely cooked through.
2 - Transfer cauliflower florets to a food processor. Add the rest of the ingredients
3 - Blend until a smooth, creamy consistency is reached. Can be stored in the refrigerator in an airtight container for up to 5 days. Makes a great dip for fruits and veggies.
Nutrition: Fat: 2.7 g Cholesterol 0 mg Sodium 12 mg Carbohydrates: 2.7 g

556. Healthier Guacamole
Preparation Time: 10 minutes

Cooking Time: 10 minutes
Servings: 4
Ingredients:
- ¾ cup crumbled tofu
- 2 avocados, peeled and pitted, divided
- 1 teaspoon salt
- 1 teaspoon minced garlic
- A pinch cayenne pepper (optional)

Directions:
1 - Prepare a food processor then put one avocado and tofu in it then blend well until it becomes smooth. Combine salt, lime juice, and the left avocado in a bowl.
2 - Add in the garlic, tomatoes, cilantro, onion, and tofu-avocado mixture. Put in cayenne pepper.
3 - Let it chill in the refrigerator for 1 hour to enhance the flavor or you can serve it right away.
Nutrition: Calories: 534 Fat: 5 g Carbohydrates: 23 g Protein: 11 g

557. Chocolate Coconut Butter
Preparation Time: 10 minutes
Cooking Time: 20 minutes
Servings: 20
Ingredients:
- ½ pound unsweetened shredded coconut
- 3 tablespoons cocoa butter
- 1 teaspoon salt

Directions:
1 - Preheat your oven to 350°Fahrenheit.
2 - Place shredded coconut on a greased baking sheet. Spread out into a thin, even layer.
3 - Bake for up to 15 minutes or until the coconut flakes are golden brown. Stir the coconut shreds every 3 minutes and watch them closely because they burn very easily and quickly.
4 - Allow the coconut flakes to cool for 15 minutes.
5 - Add coconut flakes to a food processor and blend until smooth and creamy.
6 - Adding cocoa butter and salt and blend to mix well.
7 - Pour into an airtight jar and seal the lid. The consistency will thicken up as the butter cools. The oil may separate and float to the top of the container as the butter cools.
8 - Simply reheat a portion in the microwave just before using. Can be stored for up to a whole year at room temperature!

Nutrition: Fat: 17.4 g Cholesterol 0 mg Sodium 17 mg Carbohydrates: 0.9 g Fiber 0.6 g Protein: 0.3 g

558. Orange Dill Butter

Preparation Time: 10 minutes
Cooking Time: 15 minutes
Servings: 12
Ingredients:
- ½ cup vegan butter
- 2 tablespoons fresh dill, finely chopped
- 2 tablespoons orange zest
- 1 teaspoon salt

Directions:
1 - Add 4 cups of water to a small pot and bring to a boil over high heat. Reduce heat to low and allow water to simmer.
2 - Add vegan butter to a glass Mason jar and screw on the lid loosely.
3 - Place Mason jar in the boiling water. Ensure the jar does not get submerged or over-turn.
4 - Allow the butter to melt and add the remaining ingredients.
5 - Remove the Mason jar from the pot and allow it to cool until the mixture becomes partially solidified.
6 - Can be used alongside your favorite veggies to infuse them with flavor and fat. Can be stored in the refrigerator for up to 2 weeks.
Nutrition: Fat: 1.5 g Cholesterol 0 mg Sodium 199 mg Carbohydrates: 1 g Fiber 0.3 g Protein: 0.1 g

559. Spiced Almond Butter

Preparation Time: 10 minutes
Cooking Time: 5 minutes
Servings: 10
Ingredients:
- 2 cups raw almond
- 1 teaspoon allspice
- 1 teaspoon cinnamon
- 1 teaspoon cardamom
- 1 teaspoon ground ginger
- 1 teaspoon ground cloves
- ½ teaspoon salt

Directions:
1 - Place all ingredients in a food processor and blend until a smooth consistency is achieved. Makes a delicious fruit and veggie dip and can be added to smoothies, on toast, on pancakes and waffles.

Nutrition: Fat: 9.5 g Cholesterol 0 mg Sodium 117 mg Carbohydrates: 4.1 g Fiber 2.4 g Protein: 4 g

560. Keto Strawberry Jam

Preparation Time: 25 minutes
Cooking Time: 5 minutes
Servings: 18
Ingredients:
- 1 cup fresh strawberries, chopped
- 1 tablespoon lemon juice
- 4 teaspoons xylitol
- 1 tablespoon water

Directions:
1 - Add all ingredients to a small saucepan and place over medium heat. Stir to combine and cook for about 15 minutes. Stir occasionally.
2 - After 15 minutes are up, mash up strawberries with a potato masher or fork.
3 - Pour into a heat-safe container such as a mason jar.
4 - Allow cooling then cover with a lid and refrigerate. Can be stored in the refrigerator for up to 3 days. Goes great with toast and sweet sandwiches.
Nutrition: Fat: 0 g Cholesterol 0 mg Sodium 0 mg Carbohydrates: 1 g Fiber 0.2 g Protein: 0.1 g

561. Spicy Avocado Mayonnaise

Preparation Time: 10 minutes
Cooking Time: 10 minutes
Servings: 8
Ingredients:
- 2 ripe avocados, pitted and peeled
- ¼ jalapeno pepper, minced
- 2 tablespoons lemon juice
- ½ teaspoon onion powder
- 2 tablespoons fresh cilantro, chopped
- Salt to taste

Directions:
1 - Add all ingredients to a food processor and blender until a smooth creamy consistency is achieved.
2 - The jalapeno peppers can be foregone if you prefer a cooler mayo. Can be enjoyed in sandwiches, on toast, as a topping, in veggie wraps and salads.
Nutrition: Fat: 9.8 g Cholesterol 0 mg Sodium 23 mg Carbohydrates: 4.6 g Fiber 3.4 g Protein: 1 g

562. Green Coconut Butter

Preparation Time: 10 minutes
Cooking Time: 10 minutes

Servings: 8

Ingredients:
- 2 cups unsweetened shredded coconut
- 2 teaspoons matcha powder
- 1 tablespoon coconut oil

Directions:

1 - Add shredded coconut to a food processor and blend for 5 minutes or until a smooth but runny consistency is achieved.

2 - Add matcha powder and olive oil. Blend for 1 more minute.

3 - Can be stored in an airtight container at room temperature for up to 2 weeks. Makes a delicious fruit dip and can be added to smoothies, on pancakes and toast.

Nutrition: Fat: 5.2 g Cholesterol 0 mg Sodium 3 mg Carbohydrates: 1.7 g Fiber 1.2 g Protein: 0.7 g

563. Chimichurri

Preparation Time: 10 minutes
Cooking Time: 5 minutes
Servings: 8

Ingredients:
- ½ yellow bell pepper, deseeded and finely chopped
- 1 green chili pepper, deseeded and finely chopped
- 1 lemon juice and zest
- 1 cup olive oil
- ½ cup parsley, chopped
- 2 garlic cloves, grated
- Salt and pepper to taste

Directions:

1 - Add all ingredients to a large mixing bowl. Can be mixed by hand or with an immersion blender. Mix until desired consistency is achieved.

2 - Can be served over burgers, sandwiches, salads, and more. Can be stored in the refrigerator for up to 5 days or for longer in the freezer.

Nutrition: Fat: 25.3 g Sodium 3 mg Fiber 2 g

564. Keto Vegan Raw Cashew Cheese Sauce

Preparation Time: 5 minutes
Cooking Time: 5 minutes
Servings: 6

Ingredients:
- 1 cup raw cashews, soaked in water for at least 3 hours before making the recipe

- 2 tablespoons olive oil
- 2 tablespoon nutritional yeast
- ¼ teaspoon garlic powder
- 2 tablespoons fresh lemon juice
- ½ cup water
- Salt to taste

Directions:

1 - To prepare cashews before making the sauce, boil 2 cups of water turn off the heat and add cashews. This can be allowed to soak overnight. Rinse and strained cashews. Discard water.

2 - Add all ingredients to a food processor and blend until a smooth consistency is achieved. Can be used to make pizzas, over roasted veggies, in lasagna, as a dip and more.

Nutrition: Fat: 15.5 g Sodium 34 mg Carbohydrates: 9.23 g Protein: 5.1 g

565. Homemade Hummus

Preparation Time: 15 minutes
Cooking Time: 0 minutes
Servings: 8

Ingredients:
- 30 ounces (2 cans) garbanzo beans
- 1 cup chickpea liquid
- ½ cup tahini
- ¼ cup olive oil
- 2 lemons, juiced
- 2 teaspoons garlic, minced
- ½ teaspoon salt

Directions:

1 - Add all ingredients to a blender.

2 - Blend until smooth for about 30 seconds.

3 - Transfer to an airtight container and sprinkle with additional seasonings or olive oil if desired.

Nutrition: Calories: 330 Fat: 17 g Protein: 12 g Carbohydrates: 35 g

566. Spinach and Artichoke Dip

Preparation Time: 20 minutes
Cooking Time: 10 minutes
Servings: 10

Ingredients:
- 1 tablespoon olive oil
- 2 teaspoons garlic, minced
- 12 ounces marinated artichoke hearts
- 4 cups baby spinach, roughly chopped
- ¼ cup vegan mayonnaise

- 8 ounces vegan cream cheese
- ½ teaspoon onion powder
- ½ teaspoon salt

Directions:

1 - Preheat the oven to 400°Fahrenheit. Add olive oil, garlic, artichoke hearts, and spinach to the skillet. Sauté for about 3 minutes to soften the vegetables.

2 - Add cream cheese, mayo, and spices. Mix until well incorporated. Add the mixture to an oven-safe baking dish. Broil for 5 minutes.

3 - Remove from the oven and serve warm with crackers or chips. This recipe is great to bring to social events.

Nutrition: Calories: 75 Fat: 6 g Protein: 3 g Carbohydrates: 5 g

567. Pineapple Mint Salsa

Preparation Time: 10 minutes
Cooking Time: 0 minutes
Servings: 3

Ingredients:

- 1 pound (454 g) fresh pineapple, finely diced and juices reserved
- 1 bunch mint, leaves only, chopped
- 1 minced jalapeno, (optional)
- 1 white or red onion, finely diced
- Salt, to taste (optional)

Directions:

1 - In a medium bowl, mix the pineapple with its juice, mint, jalapeno (if desired), and onion, and whisk well. Season with salt to taste, if desired.

2 - Refrigerate in an airtight container for at least 2 hours to better mix the flavors.

Nutrition: Calories: 58 Fat: 0.1 g Carbohydrates: 13.7 g Protein: 0.5 g Fiber 1.0 g

568. Healthy Grandma's Applesauce

Preparation time: 10 minutes
Cooking time: 25 minutes
Servings: 4

Ingredients:

- 3 lb. cooking apples
- 1/2 cup water
- 8 fresh dates, pitted
- 2 tbsp lemon juice
- A pinch of salt
- A pinch of grated nutmeg
- 1/4 tsp ground cloves

- 1/2 tsp ground cinnamon

Directions:

1 - Prepare apples by peeling, removing their core, and cutting them into dice.

2 - Add the apples and water to a heavy-bottomed pot and cook for about 20 minutes.

3 - Meanwhile, mix your dates and 1/2 cup water using a high-speed blender. Process until completely smooth.

4 - Then, mash the cooked apples with a potato masher; stir the pureed dates into the mashed apples and stir to combine well.

5 - Continue to simmer until the applesauce has thickened to your desired consistency. Add in the lemon juice and spices and stir until everything is well incorporated.

Nutrition: Calories: 73 Fat: 0.2 g Carbohydrates: 19.3 g Protein: 0.4 g

569. Homemade Chocolate Sauce

Preparation time: 10 minutes
Cooking time: 10 minutes
Servings: 4

Ingredients:

- 5 tbsp coconut oil, melted
- 3 tbsp agave syrup
- 3 tbsp cacao powder
- A pinch of grated nutmeg
- A pinch of kosher salt
- 1/2 tsp cinnamon powder
- 1/2 tsp vanilla paste

Directions:

1 - Thoroughly combine all the ingredients using a wire whisk.

2 - Store the chocolate sauce in your refrigerator.

3 - To soften the sauce, heat it over low heat just before serving.

Nutrition: Calories: 95 Fat: 7.6 g Carbohydrates: 7.5 g Protein: 0.2 g

570. French Mignonette Sauce

Preparation time: 5 minutes
Cooking time: 15 minutes
Servings: 4

Ingredients:

- 3/4 cup red wine vinegar
- 2 tsp mixed peppercorns, freshly cracked

- 1 small eschalot, finely chopped
- Sea salt, to taste

Directions:

1 - Combine the vinegar, peppercorns, and eschalot in a mixing bowl—season with salt.

2 - Leave it for at least 15 minutes. Serve with grilled oyster mushrooms.

Nutrition: Calories: 14 Fat: 0 g Carbohydrates: 1.9 g Protein: 0.2 g

571. Easy Homemade Pear Sauce

Preparation time: 10 minutes
Cooking time: 25 minutes
Servings: 4

Ingredients:

- 2 lb. pears, peeled, cored, and diced
- 1/4 cup water
- 1/4 cup brown sugar
- 1/2 tsp fresh ginger, minced
- 1/2 tsp ground cloves
- 1 tsp ground cinnamon
- 1 tsp fresh lime juice
- 1 tsp cider vinegar
- 1 tsp vanilla paste

Directions:

1 - Add the pears, water, and sugar to a heavy-bottomed pot and cook for about 20 minutes.

2 - Then, mash the cooked pear with a potato masher.

3 - Finally, add in the remaining ingredients.

4 - Continue to simmer until the pear sauce has thickened to your desired consistency.

Nutrition: Calories: 76 Fat: 0.3 g Carbohydrates: 19.2 g Protein: 0.6 g

572. Cinnamon Vanilla Sunflower Butter

Preparation time: 10 minutes
Cooking time: 10 minutes
Servings: 1

Ingredients:

- 2 cups roasted sunflower seeds, hulled
- 1/2 cup maple syrup
- 1 tsp vanilla extract
- 1 tsp cinnamon powder
- A pinch of grated nutmeg
- A pinch of sea salt

Directions:

1 - Blitz the sunflower seeds in your food processor until butter forms.

2 - Add in the remaining ingredients and continue to blend until creamy, smooth, and uniform.

3 - Taste and adjust the flavor as needed. Bon appétit!

Nutrition: Calories: 129 Fat: 9 g Carbohydrates: 10.1 g Protein: 3.6 g

573. Garlic Cilantro Dressing

Preparation time: 10 minutes
Cooking time: 10 minutes
Servings: 5

Ingredients:

- 1/2 cup almonds
- 1/2 cup water
- 1 bunch cilantro
- 1 red chili pepper, chopped
- 2 garlic cloves, crushed
- 2 tbsp fresh lime juice
- 1 tsp lime zest
- Sea salt and ground black pepper to taste
- 5 tbsp extra-virgin olive oil

Directions:

1 - Add almonds and water to your blender. Mix until creamy and smooth.

2 - Add in the cilantro, chili pepper, garlic, lime juice, lime zest, salt, and black pepper; blitz until everything is well combined.

3 - Slowly add olive oil and mix until smooth. Store in your refrigerator for up to 5 days.

Nutrition: Calories: 181 Fat: 18.2 g Carbohydrates: 4.8 g Protein: 3 g

574. Lime Coconut Sauce

Preparation time: 10 minutes
Cooking time: 15 minutes
Servings: 4

Ingredients:

- 1 tsp coconut oil
- 1 large garlic clove, minced
- 1 tsp fresh ginger, minced
- 1 cup coconut milk
- 1 lime, freshly squeezed and zested
- A pinch of Himalayan rock salt

Directions:

1. In a saucepan, warm the coconut oil over medium heat.
2. Once hot, cook the garlic and ginger for about 1 minute or until aromatic.
3. Lower heat and simmer, then add in the coconut milk, lime juice, lime zest, and salt.
4. Let it simmer for more minutes or until heated through.

Nutrition: Calories: 87 Fat: 8.8 g Carbohydrates: 2.6 g Protein: 0.8 g

575. Creamy Mustard Sauce

Preparation time: 10 minutes
Cooking time: 30 minutes
Servings: 4

Ingredients:
- 1/2 plain hummus
- 1 tsp fresh garlic, minced
- 1 tbsp deli mustard
- 1 tbsp extra-virgin olive oil
- 1 tbsp fresh lime juice
- 1 tsp red pepper flakes
- 1/2 tsp sea salt
- 1/4 tsp ground black pepper

Directions:
1 - Prepare and mix well all the ingredients in a mixing bowl.
2 - Keep it in the refrigerator for about 30 minutes before serving.

Nutrition: Calories: 73 Fat: 4.2 g Carbohydrates: 7.1 g Protein: 1.7 g

576. Traditional Balkan-Style Ajar

Preparation time: 10 minutes
Cooking time: 30 minutes
Servings: 4

Ingredients:
- 4 red bell peppers
- 1 small eggplant
- 1 garlic clove, smashed
- 2 tbsp olive oil
- 1 tsp white vinegar
- 1/2 tbsp Kosher salt
- Ground black pepper, to taste

Directions:

1 - Grill the peppers and eggplant until they are soft and charred.
2 - Arrange peppers in a plastic bag and let them steam for about 15 minutes.
3 - Remove the skin, seeds, and core of the peppers and eggplant.
4 - Then, transfer them to the bowl of your food processor.
5 - Add in the garlic, olive oil, vinegar, salt, and black pepper and continue to blend until well combined.

Nutrition: Calories: 93 Fat: 4.9 g Carbohydrates: 11.1 g Protein: 1.8 g

577. Authentic French Remoulade

Preparation time: 10 minutes
Cooking time: 10 minutes
Servings: 4

Ingredients:
- 1 cup plant-based mayonnaise
- 1 tbsp Dijon mustard
- 1 scallion, finely chopped
- 1 tsp garlic, minced
- 2 tbsp capers, coarsely chopped
- 1 tbsp hot sauce
- 1 tbsp fresh lemon juice
- 1 tbsp flat-leaf parsley, chopped

Directions:
1 - Thoroughly combine all the ingredients in your food processor or blender.
2 - Blend until uniform and creamy. Bon appétit!

Nutrition: Calories: 121 Fat: 10.4 g Carbohydrates: 1.3 g Protein: 6.2 g

578. Mexican-Style Chili Sauce

Preparation time: 5 minutes
Cooking time: 5 minutes
Servings: 5

Ingredients:
- 10 oz. canned tomato sauce
- 2 tbsp apple cider vinegar
- 2 tbsp brown sugar
- 1 Mexican chili pepper, minced
- 1/2 tsp dried Mexican oregano
- 1/4 tsp ground allspices
- Ground black pepper, to taste
- Sea salt, to taste

Directions:

1 - Prepare a medium mixing bowl, set, and combine well all the ingredients.

2 - Store in a glass jar in your refrigerator. Bon appétit!

Nutrition: Calories: 35 Fat: 0.2 g Carbohydrates: 7.1 g Protein: 0.8 g

579. Sunflower Seed Pasta Sauce

Preparation time: 10 minutes

Cooking time: 10 minutes

Servings: 3

Ingredients:

- 1/2 cup sunflower seeds, soaked overnight
- 1/2 cup almond milk, unsweetened
- 2 tbsp lemon juice
- 1 tsp granulated garlic
- 1/4 tsp dried oregano
- 1/2 tsp dried basil
- 1 tsp dried dill
- Ground black pepper, to taste
- Sea salt to taste

Directions:

1 - Set all the ingredients in the bowl of your food processor or a high-speed blender.

2 - Puree until the sauce is uniform and smooth.

3 - Serve the sauce over the cooked pasta or vegetable noodles. Bon appétit!

Nutrition: Calories: 164 Fat: 13.1 g Carbohydrates: 7.6 g Protein: 6.2 g

580. Keto Salsa Verde

Preparation Time: 10 minutes

Cooking Time: 5 minutes

Servings: 5

Ingredients:

- 4 tablespoons fresh cilantro, finely chopped
- ¼ cup fresh parsley, finely chopped
- 2 garlic cloves, grated
- 2 teaspoons lemon juice
- ¾ cup olive oil
- 2 tablespoons small capers
- 1 teaspoon salt
- ½ teaspoon black pepper

Directions:

1 - Add all ingredients to a large mixing bowl. Can be mixed by hand or with an immersion blender. Mix until desired consistency is achieved.

2 - Can be served over burgers, sandwiches, salads and more. Can be stored in the refrigerator for up to 5 days or for longer in the freezer.

Nutrition: Fat: 25.3 g Cholesterol 0 mg Sodium 475 mg Protein: 0.2 g

581. Cilantro Coconut Pesto

Preparation Time: 5 minutes

Cooking Time: 0 minutes

Servings: 2

Ingredients:

- 1 (13-½ ounces/383 g) can unsweetened coconut milk
- 2 jalapenos, seeds and ribs removed
- 1 bunch cilantro, leaves only
- 1 tablespoon white miso
- 1-inch (2-½ cm) piece ginger, peeled and minced
- Water, as needed

Directions:

1 - Pulse all the ingredients in a blender until creamy and smooth.

2 - Thin with a little extra water as needed to reach your preferred consistency.

3 - Store in an airtight container in the fridge for up to 2 days or in the freezer for up to 6 months.

Nutrition: Calories: 141 Fat: 13.7 g Carbohydrates: 2.8 g Protein: 1.6 g Fiber 0.3 g

582. Fresh Mango Salsa

Preparation Time: 10 minutes

Cooking Time: 0 minutes

Servings: 6

Ingredients:

- 2 small mangoes, diced
- 1 red bell pepper, finely diced
- ½ red onion, finely diced
- ½ lime juice, or more to taste
- 2 tablespoons low-sodium vegetable broth
- Handful cilantro, chopped
- Freshly ground black pepper, to taste
- Salt, to taste (optional)

Directions:

1 - Stir together all the ingredients in a large bowl until well mixed.

2 - Taste and add more lime juice or salt, if needed.

3 - Store in an airtight container in the fridge for up to 5 days.

Nutrition: Calories: 86 Fat: 1.9 g Carbohydrates: 13.3 g Protein: 1.2 g Fiber 0.9 g

583. Spicy and Tangy Black Bean Salsa

Preparation Time: 15 minutes
Cooking Time: 0 minutes
Servings: 3

Ingredients:
- 1 (15 ounces/425 g) can cooked black beans, drained and rinsed
- 1 cup chopped tomatoes
- 1 cup corn kernels, thawed if frozen
- ½ cup cilantro or parsley, chopped
- ¼ cup finely chopped red onion
- 1 tablespoon lemon juice
- 1 tablespoon lime juice
- 1 teaspoon chili powder
- ½ teaspoon ground cumin
- ½ teaspoon regular or smoked paprika
- 1 medium garlic clove, finely chopped

Directions:
1 - Put all the ingredients in a large bowl and stir with a fork until well mixed.
2 - Serve immediately, or chill for 2 hours in the refrigerator to let the flavors blend.
Nutrition: Calories: 83 Fat: 0.5 g Carbohydrates: 15.4 g Protein: 4.3 g Fiber 4.6 g

584. Homemade Chimichurri

Preparation Time: 5 minutes
Cooking Time: 0 minutes
Servings: 1

Ingredients:
- 1 cup finely chopped flat-leaf parsley leaves
- 2 lemons zest and juice
- ¼ cup low-sodium vegetable broth
- 4 garlic cloves
- 1 teaspoon dried oregano

Directions:
1 - Place all the ingredients into a food processor, and pulse until it reaches the consistency you like.
2 - Refrigerate the chimichurri in an airtight container for up to 5 days. It's best served within 1 day.
Nutrition: Calories: 19 Fat: 0.2 g Carbohydrates: 3.7 g Protein: 0.7 g Fiber 0.7 g

585. Beer Cheese Dip

Preparation Time: 10 minutes
Cooking Time: 7 minutes
Servings: 3

Ingredients:
- ¾ cup water
- ¾ cup brown ale
- ½ cup raw walnuts, soaked in hot water for at least 15 minutes, then drained
- ½ cup raw cashews, soaked in hot water for at least 15 minutes, then drained
- 2 tablespoons tomato paste
- 2 tablespoons fresh lemon juice
- 1 tablespoon apple cider vinegar
- ½ cup nutritional yeast
- ½ teaspoon sweet or smoked paprika
- 1 tablespoon arrowroot powder
- 1 tablespoon red miso

Directions:
1 - Place the water, brown ale, walnuts, cashews, tomato paste, lemon juice, apple cider vinegar into a high-speed blender, and puree until thoroughly mixed and smooth.
2 - Transfer the mixture to a saucepan over medium heat. Add the nutritional yeast, paprika, and arrowroot powder, and whisk well. Bring to a simmer for about 7 minutes, stirring frequently, or until the mixture begins to thicken and bubble.
3 - Remove from the heat and whisk in the red miso. Let the dip cool for 10 minutes and refrigerate in an airtight container for up to 5 days.
Nutrition: Calories: 113 Fat: 5.1 g Carbohydrates: 10.4 g Protein: 6.3 g Fiber 3.8 g

586. Creamy Black Bean Dip

Preparation Time: 10 minutes
Cooking Time: 0 minutes
Servings: 3

Ingredients:
- 4 cups cooked black beans, rinsed and drained
- 2 tablespoons Italian seasoning
- 2 tablespoons minced garlic
- 2 tablespoon low-sodium vegetable broth
- 2 tablespoons onion powder
- 1 tablespoon lemon juice, or more to taste
- ¼ teaspoon salt (optional)

Directions:

1 - In a large bowl, mash the black beans with a potato masher or the back of a fork until mostly smooth.

2 - Add the remaining ingredients to the bowl and whisk to combine.

3 - Taste and add more lemon juice or salt, if needed.

4 - Serve immediately, or refrigerate for at least 30 minutes to better incorporate the flavors.

Nutrition: Calories: 387 Fat: 6.5 g Carbohydrates: 63.0 g Protein: 21.2 g Fiber 16.0 g

587.   Avocado-Chickpea Dip

Preparation Time: 15 minutes
Cooking Time: 0 minutes
Servings: 2

Ingredients:

- 1 (15 ounces/425 g) can cooked chickpeas, drained and rinsed
- 2 large, ripe avocados, chopped
- ¼ cup red onion, finely chopped
- 1 tablespoon Dijon mustard
- 1 to 2 tablespoons lemon juice
- 2 teaspoons chopped fresh oregano
- ½ teaspoon garlic clove, finely chopped

Directions:

1 - In a medium bowl, mash the cooked chickpeas with a potato masher or the back of a fork, or until the chickpeas pop open (a food processor works best for this).

2 - Stir in the remaining ingredients and continue to mash until completely smooth.

3 - Place in the refrigerator to chill until ready to serve.

Nutrition: Calories: 101 Fat: 1.9 g Carbohydrates: 16.2 g Protein: 4.7 g Fiber 4.6 g

588.   Slow-Cooker Applesauce

Preparation time: 10 minutes
Cooking time: 4 to 5 hours
Servings: 4 cups

Ingredients:

- 6 large apples, peeled, cored, and chopped into 1- to 2-inch pieces
- 1/2 cup water
- 1 tbsp freshly squeezed lemon juice
- 2 (3-inch) cinnamon sticks
- 1/4 tsp salt (optional)

Directions:

1 - Add the apple pieces, water, lemon juice, cinnamon sticks, and salt (if desired) to a slow cooker and stir to combine.

2 - Cover and cook on High for about 4 to 5 hours, stirring twice during cooking, or until the apples are very softened.

3 - If you prefer smooth applesauce, you can puree the applesauce with an immersion blender until the desired consistency is reached.

4 - Allow the applesauce to cool for 5 minutes and serve hot.

Nutrition: Calories: 173 Fat: 0.4 g Carbohydrates: 41.6 g Protein: 0.8 g Fiber: 4.2 g

589.   Creamy Alfredo Pasta Sauce

Preparation time: 5 minutes
Cooking time: 6 minutes
Servings: 4 cups

Ingredients:

- 2 tbsp olive oil (optional)
- 6 garlic cloves, minced
- 3 cups unsweetened almond milk
- 1 head cauliflower, cut into florets, about 1 pound (454 g) total
- 1 tsp salt (optional)
- 1/4 tsp freshly ground black pepper
- 4 tbsp nutritional yeast
- Juice of 1 lemon

Directions:

1 - In a medium saucepan over medium-high heat, heat the olive oil, if desired. Add the garlic to the pan and sauté for 1 minute, or until fragrant. Stir in the almond milk and bring to a boil.

2 - Gently fold in the cauliflower florets. Stir in the salt (if desired) and pepper and return to a boil. Cook over medium-high heat for an additional 5 minutes, or until the cauliflower is tender, stirring constantly.

3 - Carefully transfer the cauliflower along with the cooking liquid to a blender. Add the nutritional yeast and lemon and blend for 1 to 2 minutes, or until smooth and creamy.

4 - Store in an airtight container and refrigerate for up to 5 days.

Nutrition: Calories: 108 Fat: 7.1 g Carbohydrates: 6.9 g Protein: 4.2 g Fiber: 3.1 g

590.   Creamy Mushroom Sauce

Preparation time: 10 minutes
Cooking time: 22 minutes
Servings: 2 cups
Ingredients:
- 1/4 lb. (113 g) mushrooms, sliced
- 1 leek, rinsed and sliced
- 2 cups water, divided
- 1 tbsp soy sauce
- 1 tsp parsley flake
- 1/4 tsp dried oregano
- 1/4 tsp dried sage
- 1/8 tsp paprika
- Freshly ground white pepper, to taste
- 2 tbsp cornstarch

Directions:
1 - In a medium saucepan over medium-high heat, heat 1/2 cup of water. Add the mushrooms and leek to the pan and sauté for 5 minutes.
2 - Pour in 1 cup of the water and stir in all the seasonings. Reduce to low heat and continue to cook for 15 minutes.
3 - In a small bowl, mix the cornstarch in the remaining 1/2 cup of water. Slowly add to the sauce while stirring. Cook for 2 more minutes, or until thickened and clear, stirring constantly.
4 - Serve immediately.
Nutrition: Calories: 35 Fat: 0.6 g Carbohydrates: 6.5 g Protein: 0.8 g Fiber: 0.9 g

591. Enchilada Sauce
Preparation time: 10 minutes
Cooking time: 25 minutes
Servings: 2 1/2 cups
Ingredients:
- 1 (8 oz. / 227-g) can tomato sauce
- 1 1/2 cups water
- 2 garlic cloves, minced
- 1 large onion, chopped
- 1 tbsp chili powder
- 1/2 tsp dried oregano
- 1/2 tsp ground cumin
- 2 tbsp cornstarch, mixed with 1/4 cup cold water
Directions:
1 - Combine all the ingredients except the cornstarch mixture in a small saucepan and bring to a boil over medium-high heat.

2 - Reduce the heat to low, cover, and allow to simmer for 20 minutes, whisking occasionally.
3 - Stir in the cornstarch mixture and cook for about 5 minutes until the sauce thickens, whisking constantly.
4 - Remove from the heat and allow the sauce to cool to room temperature. Serve warm.
Nutrition: Calories: 21 Fat: 0.2 g Carbohydrates: 4.3 g Protein: 0.5 g Fiber: 1.0 g

592. Garlic Mushroom Sauce
Preparation time: 10 minutes
Cooking time: 6 minutes
Servings: 2 cups
Ingredients:
- 1 3/4 cups water, divided
- 1 cup sliced mushrooms
- 2 tbsp low-sodium soy sauce
- 1 garlic clove, crushed
- 1 tsp grated fresh ginger
- 2 1/2 tbsp cornstarch, dissolved in 1/4 cup water
- A dash sesame oil (optional)
- Freshly ground pepper, to taste
Directions:
1 - Combine 1/4 cup of water and mushrooms in a saucepan. Stir in the soy sauce, garlic, and ginger and sauté for about 4 minutes, or until the mushrooms are slightly softened.
2 - Whisk in the remaining 1 1/2 cups of water and cornstarch mixture and continue stirring until the sauce begins to thicken and bubble.
3 - Drizzle with the sesame oil, if desired. Season with the pepper to taste before serving.
Nutrition: Calories: 25.6 Fat: 1.2 g Carbohydrates: 3.4 g Protein: 0.3 g Fiber: 0.1 g

593. Homemade Tomato Sauce
Preparation time: 20 minutes
Cooking time: 40 minutes
Servings: 6 cups
Ingredients:
- 4 lb. (1.8 kg) tomatoes, coarsely chopped
- 2 to 3 garlic cloves, minced
- 1 large onion, chopped
- 1 tbsp chopped fresh thyme
- 1 tbsp chopped fresh oregano

- 1 bay leaf
- 1/4 tsp crushed red pepper flakes
- 1/4 cup chopped fresh basil
- Freshly ground pepper, to taste

Directions:

1 - Combine all the ingredients except the basil and pepper in a large saucepan and bring to a boil over medium-high heat.

2 - When it starts to boil, reduce the heat, and simmer uncovered for about 30 minutes, stirring occasionally.

3 - Discard the bay leaf and stir in the basil and pepper. Serve warm.

Nutrition: Calories: 35.1 Fat: 0.3 g Carbohydrates: 6.2 g Protein: 1.9 g Fiber: 1.6 g

594. Homemade Tzatziki Sauce

Preparation time: 20 minutes
Cooking time: 0 minutes
Servings: 1 cup

Ingredients:

- 2 oz. (57 g) raw, unsalted cashews (about 1/2 cup)
- 2 tbsp lemon juice
- 1/3 cup water
- 1 small clove garlic
- 1 cup chopped cucumber, peeled
- 2 tbsp fresh dill

Directions:

1 - In a blender, add the cashews, lemon juice, water, and garlic. Keep it aside for at least 15 minutes to soften the cashews.

2 - Blend the ingredients until smooth. Stir in the chopped cucumber and dill, and continue to blend until it reaches your desired consistency. It doesn't need to be totally smooth. Feel free to add more water if you like a thinner consistency.

3 - Transfer to an airtight container and chill for at least 30 minutes for the best flavors.

4 - Bring the sauce to room temperature and shake well before serving.

Nutrition: Calories: 208 Fat: 13.5 g Carbohydrates: 15.0 g Protein: 6.7 g Fiber: 2.8 g

595. Hot Buffalo Sauce

Preparation time: 5 minutes
Cooking time: 15 minutes
Servings: 2 cups

Ingredients:

- 1/4 cup olive oil (optional)
- 1 small red onion, roughly chopped
- 4 garlic cloves, roughly chopped
- 6 cayenne chiles, roughly chopped
- 1 cup water
- 1/2 cup apple cider vinegar
- 1/2 tsp salt (optional)
- 1/2 tsp freshly ground black pepper

Directions:

1 - In a large sauté pan over medium high heat, heat the olive oil, if desired. Add the onion, garlic, and chiles to the pan and sauté for 5 minutes, or until the onion is tender.

2 - Pour in the water and bring to a boil. Cook for about 10 minutes, or until the water has nearly evaporated.

3 - Transfer the cooked onion and chili mixture to a blender and blend briefly to combine.

4 - Add the apple cider vinegar, salt (if desired), and pepper to the blender. Blend again for 30 seconds.

5 - Using a mesh sieve, strain the sauce into a bowl. Use a spoon to scrape and press all the liquid from the pulp.

6 - Serve immediately or refrigerate in an airtight container for up to 2 weeks.

Nutrition: Calories: 76 Fat: 7.1 g Carbohydrates: 2.9 g Protein: 1.1 g Fiber: 1.2 g

596. Avocado-Dill Dressing

Preparation time: 20 minutes
Cooking time: 0 minutes
Serving: 1 cup

Ingredients:

- 2 ounces (57 g) raw, unsalted cashews (about ½ cup)
- ½ cup water
- 3 tablespoons lemon juice
- ½ medium, ripe avocado, chopped
- 1 medium clove garlic
- 2 tablespoons chopped fresh dill
- 2 green onions, white and green parts, chopped

Directions:

1 - Put the cashews, water, lemon juice, avocado, and garlic into a blender. Keep it aside for at least 15 minutes to soften the cashews.

2 - Blend until everything is fully mixed. Fold in the dill and green onions, and blend briefly to retain some texture.

3 - Store in an airtight container in the fridge for up to 3 days and stir well before serving.

Nutrition: Calories: 312 | fat: 21.1g | carbs: 22.6g | protein: 8.0g | fiber: 7.1g

597. Cilantro-Chili Dressing

Preparation time: 5 minutes
Cooking time: 0 minutes
Serving: ¾ cups
Ingredients:

* 1 (4-ounce / 113-g) can chopped green chilies
* 1 to 2 cloves garlic
* ¼ cup fresh lime juice
* ¼ cup water
* ¼ cup chopped fresh cilantro
* 2 teaspoons maple syrup (optional)
* Freshly ground pepper, to taste

Directions:
1 - Combine all the ingredients in a food processor and pulse until creamy and smooth.

Nutrition: Calories: 50 | fat: 2.1g | carbs: 5.5g | protein: 2.3g | fiber: 0.3g

598. Citrus Tahini Dressing

Preparation time: 5 minutes
Cooking time: 0 minutes
Serving: 1 cup
Ingredients:

* ½ cup orange juice
* ¼ cup tahini
* ¼ cup lemon juice
* 1 small clove garlic
* 1 teaspoon grated or finely chopped fresh ginger

Directions:
1 - Put all the ingredients in a blender and pulse until smooth.

2 - Chill for an hour in the refrigerator to thicken and blend the flavors.

3 - Refrigerate in an airtight container for up to 5 days.

Nutrition: Calories: 57.6 | fat: 4.0g | carbs: 4.0g | protein: 1.4g | fiber: 0.8g

599. Creamy Avocado Cilantro Lime Dressing

Preparation time: 5 minutes
Cooking time: 0 minutes
Serving: 2 cups
Ingredients:

* 1 avocado, diced
* ½ cup water
* ¼ cup cilantro leaves
* ¼ cup fresh lime or lemon juice (about 2 limes or lemons)
* ½ teaspoon ground cumin
* ¼ teaspoon salt (optional)

Directions:
1 - Put all the ingredients in a blender, and pulse until well combined. Taste and adjust the seasoning as needed. It is best served within 1 day.

Nutrition: Calories: 94 | fat: 7.4g | carbs: 5.7g | protein: 1.1g | fiber: 3.5g

600. Creamy Spinach and Avocado Dressing

Preparation time: 10 minutes
Cooking time: 0 minutes
Serving: 1 cup
Ingredients:

* 2 ounces (57 g) spinach leaves (about 1 cup chopped and packed)
* ¼ medium, ripe avocados
* ¼ cup water, plus more as needed
* 1 small clove garlic
* 1 tablespoon Dijon mustard
* 1 green onion, white and green parts, sliced

Directions:
1 - Blitz all the ingredients in a blender until thoroughly mixed. Add a little more water if a thinner consistency is desired.

2 - Refrigerate in an airtight container for 3 days and shake before using.

Nutrition: Calories: 14.6 | fat: 1.0g | carbs: 1.0g | protein: 0.4g | fiber: 0.7g

601. Easy Lemon Tahini Dressing

Preparation time: 5 minutes
Cooking time: 0 minutes
Serving: 1¼ cups

Ingredients:
- ½ cup tahini
- ¼ cup fresh lemon juice (about 2 lemons)
- 1 teaspoon maple syrup
- 1 small garlic clove, chopped
- 1/8 Teaspoon black pepper
- ¼ teaspoon salt (optional)
- ¼ to ½ cup water

Directions:

1 - Process the tahini, lemon juice, maple syrup, garlic, black pepper, and salt (if desired) in a blender (high-speed blenders work best for this). Gradually add the water until the mixture is completely smooth.

2 - Store in an airtight container in the fridge for up to 5 days.

Nutrition: Calories: 128 | fat: 9.6g | carbs: 6.8g | protein: 3.6g | fiber: 1.9g

602. Maple Dijon Dressing

Preparation time: 5 minutes
Cooking time: 0 minutes
Serving: ½ cups

Ingredients:
- ¼ cup apple cider vinegar
- 2 teaspoons Dijon mustard
- 2 tablespoons maple syrup
- 2 tablespoons low-sodium vegetable broth
- ¼ teaspoon black pepper
- Salt, to taste (optional)

Directions:

1 - Mix together the apple cider vinegar, Dijon mustard, maple syrup, vegetable broth, and black pepper in a resealable container until well incorporated. Season with salt, if desired.

2 - The dressing can be refrigerated for up to 5 days.

Nutrition: Calories: 82 | fat: 0.3g | carbs: 19.3g | protein: 0.6g | fiber: 0.7g

603. Orange-Mango Dressing

Preparation time: 5 minutes
Cooking time: 0 minutes
Serving: ¾ cup

Ingredients:
- 1 medium mango, peeled and cut into chunks
- 1 clove garlic, crushed
- ½ cup orange juice

- 1 teaspoon soy sauce
- ¼ teaspoon curry powder

Directions:

1 - Place all the ingredients in a blender and blend until creamy and smooth.

Nutrition: Calories: 51 | fat: 0.5g | carbs: 11.3g | protein: 0.7g | fiber: 1.0g

604. Sweet Mango and Orange Dressing

Preparation time: 5 minutes
Cooking time: 0 minutes
Serving: 1½ cups

Ingredients:
- 1 cup (165 g) diced mango, thawed if frozen
- ½ cup orange juice
- 2 tablespoons rice vinegar
- 2 tablespoons fresh lime juice
- ¼ teaspoon salt (optional)
- 1 teaspoon date sugar (optional)
- 2 tablespoons chopped cilantro

Directions:

1 - Pulse all the ingredients except for the cilantro in a food processor until it reaches the consistency you like. Add the cilantro and whisk well.

2 - Store in an airtight container in the fridge for up to 2 days.

Nutrition: Calories: 32 | fat: 0.1g | carbs: 7.4g | protein: 0.3g | fiber: 0.5g

605. Vinegary Maple Syrup dressing

Preparation time: 5 minutes
Cooking time: 0 minutes
Serving: 2/3 cups

Ingredients:
- ¼ cup rice vinegar
- ¼ cup balsamic vinegar
- 2½ tablespoons maple syrup (optional)
- 1½ tablespoons Dijon mustard
- Freshly ground pepper, to taste

Directions:

1 - Combine all the ingredients in a jar. Cover and shake until well blended.

Nutrition: Calories: 49 | fat: 0.2g | carbs: 11.5g | protein: 0.3g | fiber: 0.2g

Conclusion

The topic of plant-based eating is a complicated one. As a result, there is not only confusion with regards to how to cook and eat it, but also concern about the healthiness of it as well. Here are some basic facts that you'll need once you're ready to take the step into a plant-based diet.

Plant-based eating refers to a diet that focuses mainly on veggies, fruits and grains. It's also known as vegetarian or vegan. There are variations of this diet, which typically includes aspects of veganism and also takes into account the consumption of plant foods (as opposed to animal foods) in general. This style of eating is not just limited to a restricted food list, but it also involves strict avoidance of specific ingredients. It's important to note that in many parts of the world plant-based eating can be considered the norm since it encompasses various cultural customs such as the Mediterranean Diet and others.

Although plant-based eating has been around for a long time, it's only recently that the health benefits of this diet have been widely acknowledged. One of the most talked about health benefits is the associated lowered risk of obesity, which is attributed to decreased intake of animal fats and cholesterol. In addition to this, plant-based diets overall provide higher levels of fiber and nutrients and lower levels of saturated fat compared to other diets. Plant-based diets are also great if you are trying to lower your intake of simple sugars since they typically contain greater amounts of complex carbohydrates than animal products do.

Plant-based diets also have other potential health benefits, such as prevention and/or treatment of heart diseases and certain cancers. They may also prevent, slow or reverse the process of osteoporosis. Plant-based diets are typically much lower in sodium than the typical western diet is. This is great since high sodium intake has been linked to increased risk of cardiovascular disease, hypertension and stomach cancer.

Low fat plant-based eating is associated with decreased risk of colon cancer (and all other types of cancer), as well as lowered blood cholesterol levels. The vitamins from plant-based sources are thought to be major contributors to these improved health outcomes.

Although there are many benefits associated with plant-based eating, it's important to note that not everyone can be on a plant-based diet. In fact, there are some people who should never turn to a plant-based diet. If you have certain medical conditions or have had major surgery in the past year, then your doctor may advise against this type of eating. When eating a well-balanced diet, vegans who eat dairy and eggs have similar health outcomes to non-vegetarians. They would have to stay away from their eggs and dairy products to achieve the same results as those on a fully plant-based diet. However, vegans can only get their essential amino acids from animal products, so they need to be careful about their intake and must consult a physician before deciding on this type of diet.

As previously stated, there are many studies that have been conducted on the potential health benefits of plant-based eating. The American Dietetic Association has published a comprehensive guide with suggestions for how to incorporate plant-based foods into a healthy diet. Another good resource is The China Study, which was first published in 2006 and is the product of decades of research by nutritionist T. Colin Campbell and his son, Dr. Thomas M., who were colleagues in nutritional epidemiology at Cornell University.

A food pyramid for a plant-based diet is similar to the typical "food pyramid" you see depicted in restaurants, schools and grocery stores. The plant-based food pyramid emphasizes the importance of legumes, whole grains and what it calls "unrefined carbs" at its base as opposed to meat and dairy products. In addition to this, it also advocates for a much higher intake of fruits and vegetables than the traditional food pyramid does. Although this diet may seem restrictive at first, there are plenty of delicious dishes that you can prepare with various veggies. There is no need for you to miss out on your favorite meals since the Chinese cuisine is full of vegan-friendly dishes that are just as tasty as their meat-based counterparts.

Printed in Great Britain
by Amazon

83660445R00147